Springer
Tokyo
Berlin
Heidelberg
New York
Barcelona
Budapest
Hong Kong
London
Milan
Paris
Singapore

M. Ando, C. Uyama (Eds.)

Medical Applications of Synchrotron Radiation

With 116 Figures, Including 3 in Color

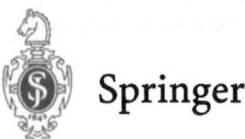 Springer

Masami Ando
Professor, Photon Factory, KEK
1-1 Oho, Tsukuba, Ibaraki,
305-0801 Japan

Chikao Uyama
Director, Department of Investigative Radiology
Research Institute, National Cardiovascular Center
5-7-1 Fujishiro-dai, Suita, Osaka,
565-8565 Japan

ISBN-13: 978-4-431-68487-9   e-ISBN-13: 978-4-431-68485-5
DOI: 10.1007/978-4-431-68485-5

Printed on acid-free paper

© Springer-Verlag Tokyo 1998
Softcover reprint of the hardcover 1st edition 1998

Typesetting: Camera-ready by authors

SPIN: 10676853

Looking Toward the Future

Immediately after their discovery by Roentgen in 1895, X-rays became a powerful tool for medical diagnosis. Since then, most X-ray clinical imaging has been by absorption. X-ray computed tomography (CT) was a substantial innovation because of its capacity for three-dimensional imaging of internal organs. Other CT techniques that were devised later, such as magnetic resonance imaging, single photon emission CT, and positron emission CT, have shared with X-ray imaging in medical diagnosis.

Synchrotron radiation (SR), which is characterized by its photon energy tunability and small divergence, will certainly be a very powerful X-ray source for further innovation in clinical imaging. Energy-subtraction intravenous coronary angiography (CA) using SR has been proposed by Professor Edward Rubenstein. Many facilities are currently gathering clinical data on outpatients for CA using SR. Those who have been engaged in development of this method are watching with great interest to see how the clinical community will assess current and future CA programs, and what their decision will be on whether or not they will implement their own clinical SR sources at their hospitals.

Other potential applications of SR such as mammography and bronchography are in the intensive clinical trial stage. Additional new imaging tools based on phase, refraction, or scattering have been introduced quite recently. These, too, are powerful candidates for clinical use because they are capable of revealing lesions that otherwise are difficult to visualize. The history of medical imaging studies, from fundamental research to a clinical application, could be likened to a marathon race. A current leading runner is CA, while newcomers such as phase-contrast CT and phase-shift imaging are moving through the field to join the leading group of competitors. Because there is still a long distance left to go in this "diagnosis race," all of the competitors are still potential winners. In addition to diagnosis, an ambitious program of SR therapy is at the planning stage.

It was fortunate that the International Workshop on Medical Applications of Synchrotron Radiation (HAGA '97) could be held August 8—11th, 1997, when everyone joined in sharing their knowledge and experience in the field for three days at a small hot-spring spa in the sparsely populated forestry town of Haga, in Hyogo Prefecture. We tried to invite as many medical doctors as possible, and we were gratified that eighteen could join us. Twenty-five talks and eight posters were presented from among the 53 participants, 16 of whom were from overseas. The discussions that took place were quite open, thus achieving one of the most important purposes of the workshop. We are working both in competition and in harmony, because although we are competing to develop each system to its fullest potential, we still need this type of rewarding exchange of knowledge and experience.

To convey to readers the atmosphere of the discussions, transcripts of the question-and-answer sessions were included with papers when possible, depending on the clarity of the recording made at the time. Minor modifications, such as filling in correct numbers, were made by the Editorial Board. Additional summaries made by the chairpersons were included in the Workshop program. All manuscripts were reviewed for publication. Presentation of R. Tatchyn's paper on X-ray optics was welcomed by the Program Committee although he could not be present himself at HAGA '97 because of a scheduling conflict. Also, a paper was submitted by A.M. Charver and his group after the Workshop

although they had been unable to participate. The paper went through the review process and is included here. In 1992, we held a similar meeting, DAIGO '92, The International Workshop on Medical Applications of Synchrotron Radiation, in the town of Daigo in Ibaraki Prefecture. We have included here some of the papers presented at DAIGO '92 which had not published previously. Thus a total of 28 papers have been selected for publication in this volume.

As described above, the invention and development of new techniques and devices for medical imaging are expected to proceed very rapidly, and a substantially better quality of imaging in diagnosis will be in strong demand. For these reasons, we hope that this book will be of great help not only for those who are engaged in medical imaging but also for others who want to bring about innovations in medical synchrotron applications. We also hope that everyone, including those who are new to this field, will join us in looking toward a new horizon with the advent of the 21st century.

May 1998
Masami Ando and Chikao Uyama
Chairpersons, Editorial Board

Contents

*papers submitted at DAIGO'92

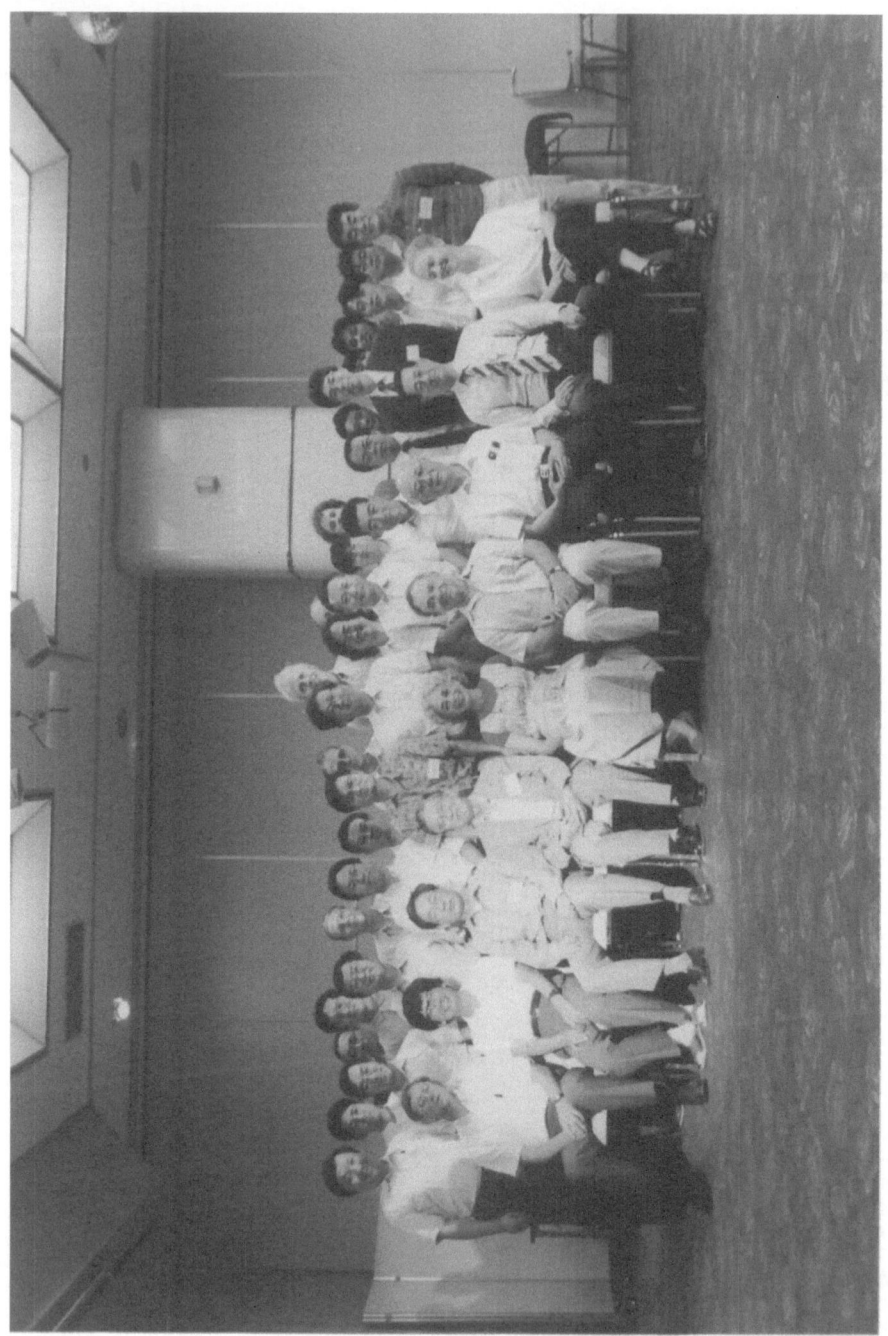

HAGA '97

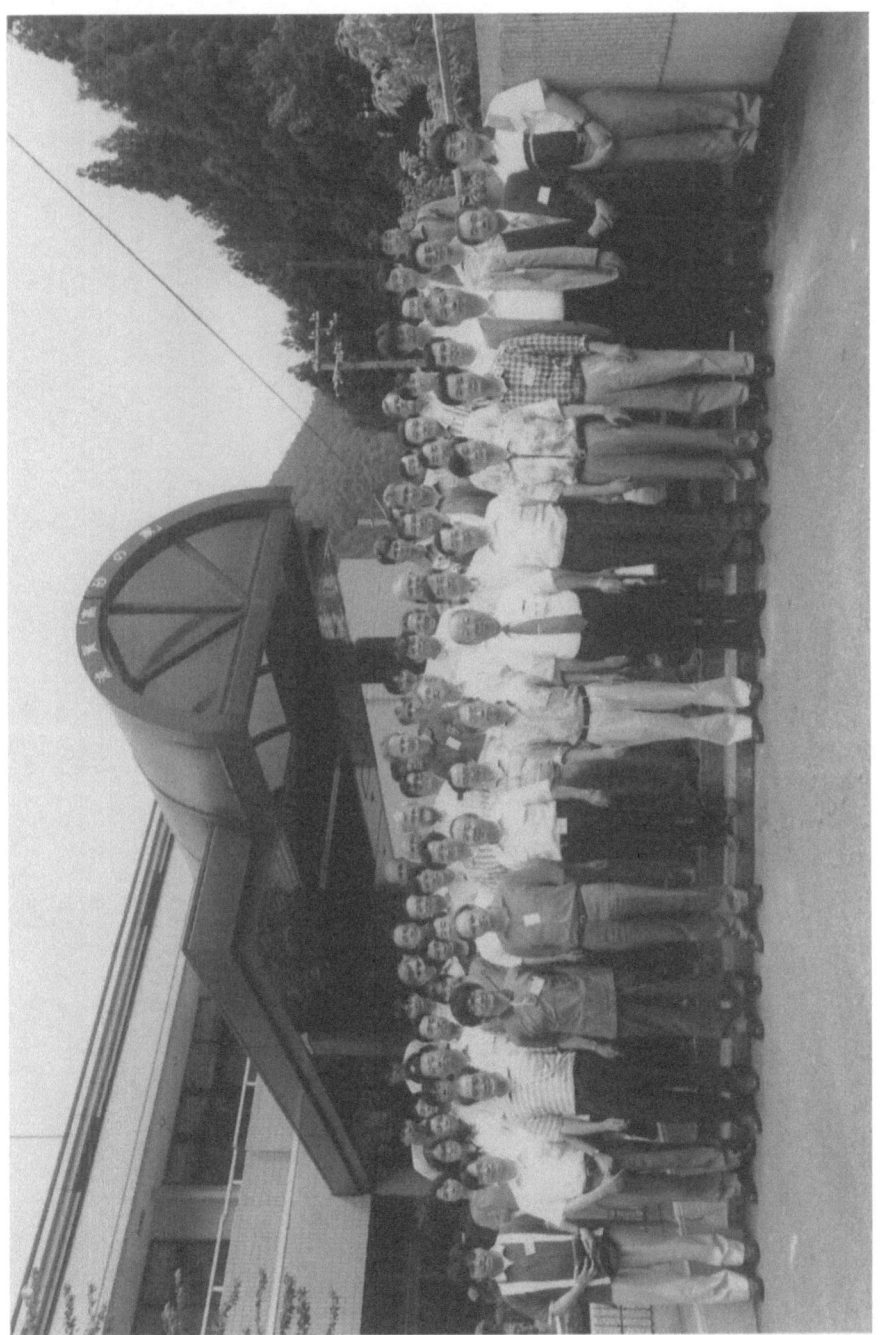

DAIGO '92

Opening Remark

Michio Kono, M.D.
Professor and Chairman
Department of Radiology,
Kobe University School of Medicine
Kusuniki-machi7-5-1, Tyuouku, Kobe-shi, 650-0017, JAPAN

Currently, synchrotron radiation has become an important topics in clinical medicine, contributing to such applications as coronary angiography, mammography, bronchograhy, and monochromatic X-ray computed tomography (CT), etc. It was fortunate, therefore, that the International Workshop on Medical Applications of Synchrotron Radiation could be held in the town of Haga, Hyogo Prefecture, Japan, August 8-11, 1997.

More than 50 excellent physicists and medical doctors who are interested in SR came from all over the world to participate in the workshop and to present excellent papers. As a radiologist, I believe that medical doctors and physicists must engage much more they now do in exchanges of opinions and ideas about the medical use of SR.

At present, if SR can be used for diagnostic imaging, the results should be far superior to those of high resolution CT, magnetic resonance imaging, and digital subtraction angiography because it will enable imaging vessels down to 200 micrometers in diameter. Among clinical practitioners there are high expectations for synchrotron radiation in diagnostic imaging, for instance, pathologic diagnosis without biopsies or resected specimens.

Imaging techniques that make possible clinical views on a very small clinical scale with use of SR should be developed much further. For this reason, medical doctors should communicate their clinical requirements to physicists.

Physicists should thoroughly discuss these needs with medical doctors and provise them with the necessary technological skills and concepts. At present, there still is a conceptual gap between medical doctors and physicists with regard to the clinical use of SR, and we must make a continuous effort to solve this problem. I believe that the 197 Workshop in Haga will provide valuable contributions in the filed of clinical medicine. I hope that the Workshop will grow year by year.

I will express my sincere gratitude to all participants for their contributions.

Synchrotron Radiation Applications in Medical Research

W. Thomlinson

National Synchrotron Light Source, Brookhaven National Laboratory, Upton, NY 11973

SUMMARY. Over the past two decades there has been a phenomenal growth in the number of dedicated synchrotron radiation facilities and a corresponding growth in the number of applications in both basic and applied sciences. The high flux and brightness, tunable beams, time structure and polarization of synchrotron radiation provide an ideal x-ray source for many applications in the medical sciences. There is a dual aspect to the field of medical applications of synchrotron radiation. First there are the important in-vitro programs such as structural biology, x-ray microscopy, and radiation cell biology. Second there are the programs that are ultimately targeted at in-vivo applications. The present status of synchrotron coronary angiography, bronchography, multiple energy computed tomography, mammography and radiation therapy programs at laboratories around the world is reviewed.

KEY WORDS: synchrotron, medical applications, angiography, mammography, radiation therapy

INTRODUCTION

In order to understand the role of the synchrotron in medicine it is necessary to be aware of competing technologies that are presently utilized as well as their potential. The medical community already utilizes many advanced imaging and therapy modalities, and the technologies are always advancing in areas such as digital mammography and angiography, nuclear medicine, ultrasound, MRI and radiotherapy. These are the modalities with which synchrotron based applications must successfully compete. The discussions in this paper will be limited to those areas where the fields of medicine and synchrotron radiation science have joined to create new tools for medical research, diagnosis, and treatment.

Figure 1 is a representation of the many fields of medicine presently being studied. The accompanying Table I is a summary of the status of each program, indicating where they have progressed to the human and animal research stages. The sections below will concentrate on those applications which involve in-vivo research or which are directly associated with such programs. Details of in-vivo and in-vitro biomedical research at synchrotron facilities have been presented elsewhere [1,2].

2

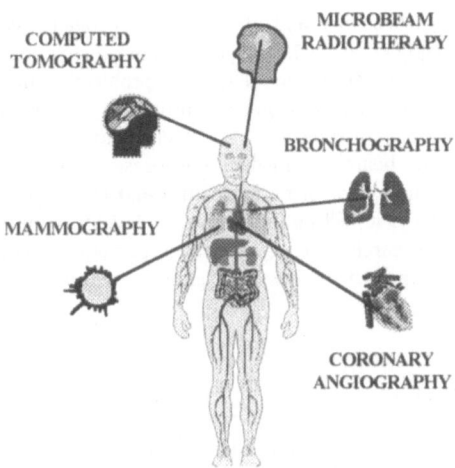

Fig. 1. The medical research areas presently active at synchrotron facilities

Table 1. Synchrotron based medical research programs

	TYPE OF IMAGE OR THERAPY	**PRIMARY ANATOMY**	**RESEARCH STATUS**
Angiography	Projection Image	Coronary Arteries	Human Studies
Bronchography	Projection Image	Lungs	Human Studies
Computed Tomography	CT Image	Head and Neck	Animal Models
Mammography	Projection Image	Breast Tumors	In-Vitro Tissues
Radiotherapy	Microbeam Therapy	Brain Tumors	Animal Models

UNIQUE PROPERTIES OF SYNCHROTRON RADIATION

The properties of synchrotron beams which make them applicable to medical research are their extremely high intensity and broad-band energy spectrum. Several orders of magnitude more flux and the smooth, continuous spectrum of the synchrotron as compared to the sharply peaked characteristic emission peaks from a tube. Basically, the high intensity and tunability allow monochromatic beams to be generated at virtually any energy. The standard problem of beam hardening in both medical imaging and therapy is eliminated by the monochromatic beams since the energy spectrum does not change with passage through tissue, only the intensity changes. The tunable spectrum allows enhancement of images and therapeutic dose by selection of the most effective energy for a given procedure. Benefits to the patients come from more effective dose delivery in therapeutic modalities and less dose with greater image quality in imaging procedures.

The advantages of the synchrotrons and their powerful beams come with some distinct disadvantages for medical applications. The planar beam is a distinct disadvantage when one tries to create a large two-dimensional image. The real problem comes when considering the application of synchrotrons to clinical diagnostic programs for humans or even large scale research programs involving human subjects. At present, and in the foreseeable future, there is little access to the synchrotron beams for medical purposes, due both to lack of development of such programs and the very high cost of both facilities and research beamlines. Assuming that technical matters can be solved, it will be imperative to develop compact sources which will be cost effective for hospitals, research centers, or medical centers. Without such development, the medical applications will be limited to a few well defined research programs and will not greatly influence the clinical technologies.

SYNCHROTRON SOURCES

Each synchrotron source has unique characteristics so it is necessary to make decisions regarding the medical programs which can be effectively pursued. The most important parameter is usually the flux available in the energy range required by the application. A careful analysis of the source and programmatic needs must be made. Not all storage rings or magnetic devices provide the necessary beam for all applications. Experience has shown that new advanced medical technologies can only be developed in a timely fashion if the experimental facility is dedicated to the program and sufficient beam time is available. Although a dedicated clinical facility called SMERF was constructed at NSLS [3], it shares beam time with many other medical and non-medical programs. Due partly to the long development time necessitated by lack of beam time, the angiography project is now on hold with no new studies planned at this time. It is fortunate that at both the ESRF [4] and ELETTRA [5] dedicated beamlines have been built for medical research. At HASYLAB, the angiography beamline has been dedicated for an extended period of time to carry out a large trial of the technology [6]. When medical programs are started at new or existing facilities, it is imperative that the need for dedicated operations be considered.

MULTIPLE-ENERGY COMPUTED TOMOGRAPHY

Monochromatic synchrotron x-rays have two distinct advantages over the radiation obtained from x-ray tubes for radiology in general and for computed tomography (CT) in particular. The monochromatic x-rays do not beam harden. Beam hardening is particularly troublesome for image reconstruction of CT images. Second, the tunability of the spectrum allows both dual-photon absorptiometry (DPA) and K-edge subtraction (KES) imaging. Multiple Energy Computed Tomography was first developed at Brookhaven National Laboratory to utilize synchrotron radiation beams for DPA and KES [7]. That program has advanced to the stage of imaging small mammals, but its long range goal is to image the human head and neck. Another long term goal is to do high resolution in-situ imaging for patient orientation and positioning for subsequent radiotherapy treatment. A new human studies CT program is just starting experimentation at the ESRF [4]. In addition, developments in Japan are focusing on the fundamental technology of synchrotron computed tomography; for example, phase-contrast x-ray computed tomography [8].

The synchrotron geometry is ideal for doing CT of the brain, since beams are naturally collimated in the vertical direction and are fan shaped in the horizontal plane. In addition, the highly collimated beams allow the detector to be placed far behind the patient, thus reducing the problem of subject to detector scatter. The CT configuration is that of a fixed, horizontal fan beam and a subject seated in a rotating chair. The KES studies will image the brain, large blood vessels of the head and neck, and arteriovenous malformations. DPA will obtain images that map the low Z and intermediate Z elements. Progress to human studies will eventually occur at NSLS and ESRF.

MAMMOGRAPHY

It has been suggested that the use of the synchrotron source for mammography with its monochromatic, highly collimated, tunable radiation could increase the signal to noise and increase the contrast resolution in the images, possibly at lower dose to the patient. Burattini, et al [9], recently reported their work using synchrotron radiation and conclude that the monochromatic images have higher contrast, better resolution, and similar or less radiation dose. A dedicated mammography beamline is being constructed at the ELETTRA facility in Trieste, Italy [5].

Experiments have been done at the NSLS by Dr. R. Eugene Johnston from the University of North Carolina and his collaborators using monoenergetic x-rays to explore the potential of monoenergetic photons for mammographic imaging [10]. The experiments done on the X27 beamline have shown that superior image contrast can be obtained relative to the conventional film-screen techniques. Images of various mammographic phantoms and real tissue have been carried out in the energy range 16 to 24 keV. In these early experiments, it was clear that improved contrast at equivalent or less dose is obtained. Scoring of the phantom images according to American College of Radiology criteria shows improvement over the conventional systems, with similar or less mean glandular dose. The early work at the NSLS has utilized available image plate and conventional mammographic film detectors. It is planned to study digital detectors and new imaging optical configurations. The elimination of scatter is expected to produce images with higher contrast than conventional imaging systems. Complimentary experiments studying diffraction and image quality are underway at Daresbury Laboratory [11]

Recently, a new radiographic imaging modality called Diffraction Enhanced Imaging (DEI) has been developed by D. Chapman and co-workers at the NSLS [12,13]. This new modality uses an x-ray analyzer crystal (Bragg or Laue geometry) as a scatter rejection optic that diffracts the beam which is transmitted through the object being imaged. Experiments performed with this scatter rejection optic revealed that the system is sensitive to refractive index effects within the object in addition to the x-ray absorption and small angle scattering by the object. A simple algorithm has been developed to separate refractive index effects from absorption effects. The measured absorption is really an apparent absorption since it is the combination of absorption and extinction processes. Extinction is the loss of intensity due to diffraction occurring as the beam traverses the object In some phantom details, enhancement in the apparent absorption of an object has been as much as a factor of 17 when compared with a conventional synchrotron radiograph. Direct comparisons between the synchrotron DEI system and conventional systems are being made using mammography phantoms and tissue samples obtained from patient specimens containing different types of cancers (masses, calcifications, and architectural distortions). In the long term, it may be possible to advance the program to human studies in the medical research facility at the NSLS.

CORONARY ANGIOGRAPHY

Certainly the most advanced of the applied medical research programs at synchrotron facilities are those doing human coronary angiography. The field traces its origins back to the proposal that the intensity of the synchrotron x-ray beams would be high enough to allow imaging of the coronary arteries following venous injection of an iodine containing contrast agent [14]. Differences in x-ray optics and types of detectors appear among the experimental groups depending upon the needs of the technology. The pioneering work in angiography in Russia at the Institute of Nuclear Physics [15] and the programs at the NSLS [16] and HASYLAB [17], as well as the planned work at the ESRF [4], move the patient through a stationary one-dimensional fan beam. The programs in Japan at the Photon Factory are taking very rapid, two-dimensional exposures [18,19]. They use a single energy above the K-edge of iodine with transvenous injection. Thus far, four patients have been imaged.

The concept of synchrotron based coronary angiography was first developed at Stanford University and the early human studies were done at the Stanford Synchrotron Radiation Laboratory [20]. The NSLS program has been a collaboration between Stanford University, North Shore University Hospital and SUNY Stony Brook. Thus far a total of 28 patients have been imaged, 7 at SSRL and 21 at the NSLS [21].

In Germany at HASYLAB the researchers have developed a system similar to the Stanford/NSLS system. Two of the major goals of the transvenous imaging have been to advance to where the contrast agent can be injected into a peripheral vein and the images can be gated on the ECG signal. The German group headed by Dr. W.-R. Dix has made major advances in each of these areas of the technology having imaged over 150 patients [22,23]. Excellent images of the right coronary artery and of the left anterior descending coronary artery have been obtained at the NSLS and HASYLAB, but the circumflex artery has been more difficult to image, although the HASYLAB group is making significant progress. The technology is now at a point where definitive medical research can begin. In order to evaluate the true clinical potential of synchrotron coronary angiography, the HASYLAB team is carrying out a major study involving over 400 patients [6]. The outcome of that study will certainly influence the continuation or commencement of projects around the world.

BRONCHOGRAPHY

Recently, Rubenstein et al have described a medical imaging procedure using xenon as a contrast agent for K-edge dichromography of the respiratory air passages [24]. The process could provide the opportunity to image anatomic structures and pathologic processes that cannot be visualized by conventional x-ray based imaging methods. For example, detection of lung cancer, the leading cause of cancer related deaths in the US, is an important application. At present, standard x-ray procedures cannot detect tumors less than 1 cm in diameter. It has been calculated that synchrotron imaging with xenon could detect significantly smaller, earlier tumors leading to enhanced five-year survival For the synchrotron bronchography, the airway structures are imaged after inhalation of a gas mixture containing stable xenon. The amount of inhaled gas is limited to the anatomic dead space volume of the upper and lower air passages. The subjects hold their breath for several seconds while the images are recorded using the dual-energy imaging system developed at SSRL and the NSLS for coronary angiography. Initial studies on human volunteers have been carried out at the NSLS in recent experiments [25]. For these studies, the X17 beamline was aligned to bracket the xenon K-edge at 34.56 keV. The procedure was identical to the angiography imaging except that the contrast agent was inhaled instead of being injected. In these preliminary experiments the trachea and bronchi to the tertiary level could be seen.

MICROBEAM RADIATION THERAPY

The application of synchrotron radiation to radiotherapy was first suggested by Larsson [26]. The inherent collimation of the synchrotron beams allows the creation of beams which optimize dose delivery to the tumor site but also effectively spare intervening normal tissue. The synchrotron geometry is ideal for stereotactic radiosurgery and the monochromatic beams will not beam harden. Hence, the radiation dose to the patient will be efficiently delivered. Microbeam Radiation Therapy (MRT) is a concept developed at Brookhaven National Laboratory by which a lesion is irradiated in a stereotactic fashion using synchrotron radiation collimated into microscopically thin parallel arrays of planar beams[27]. The energy range required is 50-150 keV. The microbeams are planes several millimeters high and 25-50 μm wide. The beams in each bundle are separated by 75-200 μm on center. The central phenomenon is that endothelium and other kinds of dividing cells that are destroyed by absorbed doses in the direct paths of microbeams regenerate from similar cells in the minimally irradiated contiguous segments between the microbeams. Tissue necrosis is thus avoided except in the crossfired zone.

Experiments have been carried out at the NSLS in which it has been shown that MRT is effective in increasing the survival of rats with imminently lethal brain tumors [28]. The present efforts at the NSLS and in Grenoble at the ESRF [4,29] are continuing both experimentally and by carrying out simulations in order to determine the optimal beam parameters for MRT.

DISCUSSION

The projects discussed in this paper are, for the most part, still in their infancies. There is a lot of competition from advances in conventional imaging with the development of digital angiography, advanced mammography systems, magnetic resonance imaging and fast computed tomography. The synchrotron programs will have to provide significant advantages over these modalities in order to be accepted by the medical profession. The development of compact sources will be required in order to move the synchrotron developed imaging technologies into the clinical world. In any event, it can be expected that the images produced by the synchrotron technologies will establish "gold standards" to be targeted by conventional modalities. A lot more work needs to be done in order to bring synchrotron radiation therapy and surgery to the level of human studies and, subsequently, to clinical applications.

8

ACKNOWLEDGMENT

This work was supported by the US Department of Energy under contract #DE-AC02-76CH00016.

REFERENCES

1. Thomlinson W (1992) Medical Applications of Synchrotron Radiation. Nucl. Instr. and Meth. A319: 295-304.
2. Thomlinson W (1995) Synchrotron Radiation Applications in Medical Research. Proceedings of the International Conference on Industrial Applications of Synchrotron Radiation, Hyogo Prefecture, Japan, pp 98-126.
3. Thomlinson W, Gmür N, Chapman D, Garrett R, Lazarz N, Moulin H, Thompson AC, Zeman HD, Brown GS, Morrison J, Reiser P, Padmanabhan V, Ong L, Green S, Giacomini J, Gordon H, Rubenstein E (1992) First Operation of the Synchrotron MedicalResearch Facility for Coronary Angiography. Rev. Sci. Instrum. 63: 625-628.
4. Charvet AM, LeBas JF, Elleaume H, Schulze C, Suortti P, Spanne P (1995) Medical Applications of Synchrotron Radiation at the ESRF. Proceedings of the International School E. Fermi - CXXVIII Course - Biomedical Applications of Synchrotron Radiation, eds. E. Burattini and A. Balerna. IOS Press, Amsterdam, pp 355-377.
5   Arfelli F, Barbiellini G, Bernstorff S, Bravin A, Cantatore G, Castelli E, Dalla Palma L, Di Michiel M, Longo R, Poropat P, Rosei R, Sessa M, Tromba G, Vacchi A (1995) Digital Mammography with Synchrotron Radiation. Rev. Sci. Instrum. 66: 1325-1328.
6. Dix W-R. Private Communication.
7. Dilmanian FA, Wu XY, Kress J, Ren B, Button TM, Chapman D, Coderre JA, Giron F, Greenberg D, Krus DJ, Liang Z, Marcovici S, Parsons E, Petersen MJ, Roque CT, Shleifer M, Slatkin DN, Thomlinson WC, Yamamoto K, Zhong Z (1997) Single and Dual-Energy CT with Monochromatic Synchrotron X-Rays. Phys. Med. Biol. 42:371-387.
8. Momose, T. Takeda, Y. Itai (1995) Rev. Sci. Instrum. 66: 1434.
9. Burattini E, Cossu E, Di Maggio C, Gambaccini M, Indovina P, Maryiani M, Porek M, Simeoni S, Simonetti G (1994) Mammography with Synchrotron Radiation. Radiology 125: 239-244
10. Johnston RE, Washburn D, Pisano E, Thomlinson WC, Chapman LD, Arfelli F, Gmür NF, Zhong Z, Sayers D (1996) Preliminary Experience with Monoenergetic Photon Mammography. Medical Imaging 1995: Physics of Medical Imaging, SPIE 1995: 2432; pp 434-441
11. Rogers K, Towns-Andrews E, Boggis C, Lewis RA, Hufton A (1997) Initial studies of breast tissue microcalcification structure using synchrotron radiation. Abstract submitted to Radiology 1997, 19-21 May 1997, Birmingham, UK.
12. Chapman D, Thomlinson W, Arfelli F, Gmür N, Zhong Z, Menk R, Johnston RE, Washburn D, Pisano E, Sayers D (1996) Mammography Imaging Studies Using a Laue Crystal Analyzer. Rev. Sci. Instrum. 67: Published on CD ROM.
13. Chapman D, Thomlinson W, Johnston RE, Washburn D, Pisano E, Gmür N, Zhong Z, Menk R, Arfelli F, Sayers D (1997) Diffraction Enhanced Imaging. Phys. Med. Biol. (to be published).

14. Rubenstein E, Hughes EB, Campbell LE, Hofstadter R, Kirk RL, Krolicki TJ, Stone JP, Wilson S, Zeman HD, Brody WR, Macovski A, Thompson AC (1981) Synchrotron Radiation and Its Application to Digital Subtraction. SPIE 1981: 314: 42-49.

15. Dementiev EN, Dolbnya IP, Zagorodnikov EI, Kolesnikov KA, Kulipanov GN, Kurylo G, Medvedko AS, Mezentsev NA, Pindyurin VF, Cheskidov V, Sheromov MA (1989) Dedicated X-ray Scintillator Detector for Digital Subtraction Angiography Using Synchrotron Radiation. Rev. Sci. Instrum. 60: 2264-2267.

16. Thomlinson W (1995) Transvenous Coronary Angiography in Humans. Proceedings of the International School E. Fermi - CXXVIII Course - Biomedical Applications of Synchrotron Radiation, eds. E. Burattini and A. Balerna. IOS Press, Amsterdam, pp 127-153.

17. Dix W-R. Intravenous Coronary Angiography with Synchrotron Radiation. Prog. Biophys. Molec. Biol. 1995: 63; 159-191.

18. Takeda T, Itai Y, Wu J, Ohtsuka S, Hyodo K, Ando M, Nishimura K, Hasegawa S, Akatsuka T, Akisada M (1995) Two Dimensional Intravenous Coronary Arteriography Using Above-K-Edge Monochromatic Synchrotron X-ray. Acad. Radiol. 2: 602-608.

19. Ando M, Hyodo K, Nishimura K, Ohtsuka S, Takeda T, Sugishita Y, Itai Y (1997) The Medical Application Programme Using AR & PF Ring at KEK. Physica Medica (to be published)

20. Rubenstein E, Hofstadter R, Zeman HD, Thompson AC, Otis JN, Brown GS, Giacomini J, Gordon HJ, Kernoff RS, Harrison DC, Thomlinson W (1986) Transvenous Coronary Angiography in Humans Using Synchrotron Radiation. Proc. Nat. Acad. Sci. USA 83: 9724-9728.

21 Rubenstein E, Brown GS, Chapman D, Garrett RF, Giacomini JC, Gmür N, Gordon HJ, Lavender WM, Morrison J, Thomlinson W, Thompson AC, Zeman H (1994) Synchrotron Radiation Coronary Angiography in Humans. Synchrotron Radiation in the Biosciences, eds. B. Chance, et al. Oxford University Press, New York. 1994, pp 639-645.

22. Dix W-R, Besch HJ, Graeff W, Hamm CW, Illing G, Kupper W, Lohmann M, Meinertz T, Menk RH, Beime B, Rust C, Schildwaechter L, Walenta AH (1996) Intravenous Coronary Angiography with Synchrotron Radiation. Physica Scripta T61: 51-56.

23. Hamm CW, Meinertz T, Dix W.-R, Rust C, Graeff W, Illing G, Lohmann M, Menk R, Reime B, Schildwaechter L, Besch HJ, Kupper W (1996) Intravenous Coronary Angiography with Dichromography Using Synchrotron Radiation. Herz 21: 127-131.

24. Rubenstein E, Giacomini JC, Gordon HJ, Rubenstein JA, Brown G (1995) Xenon K-edge Dichromographic Bronchography: Synchrotron Radiation Based Medical Imaging. Nucl. Instr. and Meth. A364: 360-361.

25. Giacomini J, Gordon H, O'Neil R, VanKessel A, Cason B, Chapman D, Lavender W, Gmür N, Menk R, Thomlinson W, Zhong Z, Rubenstein E (1997) Bronchial Imaging Using Xenon K-Edge Dichromography. American College of Chest Physicians (to be published).

26. Larsson B (1983) Potentialities of Synchrotron Radiation in Experimental and Clinical Radiation Surgery. Acta. Radiol. Suppl. 365: 58-64.

27. Slatkin DN, Spanne P, Dilmanian FA, Sandburg M (1992) Microbeam Radiation Therapy. Med. Phys. 19: 1395-1400.

28. Slatkin DN, Spanne P, Dilmanian FA, Gebbers J-O, Laissue JA (1995) Subacute Neuropathological Effects of Microplanar Beams of X-rays from a Synchrotron Wiggler. Proc. Natl. Acad. Sci. USA 92: 8783-8787.

29. Spanne P. Microbeam Radiation Therapy. Abstract submitted to Biophysics and Synchrotron Radiation Conference, Grenoble, France, Aug. 21-25, 1995.

A perspective view of the medical applications of synchrotron radiation in Japan

Yuji Itai

Department of Radiology, Institute of Clinical Medicine, University of Tsukuba 1-1-1 Tennodai, Tsukuba 305-0006 Japan

SUMMARY: In this review article, the medical applications of synchrotron radiation in Japan are briefly described, principally on angiography and monochromatic x-ray CT, covering the past, present, and near future. † The history of our medical application began in 1983, when a diagnostic group was formed in Tsukuba. In 1985, the first video image of the cardiovascular system in a cat was successfully taken with K-edge subtraction. Based on the experiences with cats, studies on dogs and goats were carried out, and later human studies were performed in 1996. † Intravenous angiography with synchrotron radiation in Japan is characterized by the two-dimensional method. For that purpose, much attention has been given to the technical efforts of increasing the beam size and the photon flux density. Nevertheless, the image quality is still subclinical due to the lack of photon density. Coronary angiography through proximal aortic injection could be an alternative to this method and conventional coronary angiography. By using transmission monochromatic X-ray in CT, high spatial resolution CT and high contrast resolution CT have been developed. Combined transmission X-ray CT and non-transmission X-ray CT is also being developed, including fluorescent X-ray and scattering X-ray. Phase-contrast X-ray radiogram and CT have been newly developed and will be leading technologies in X-ray diagnosis in the advent of the 21st century.

KEYWORDS: Intravenous coronary angiography, Intraaortic coronary angiography, High spatial resolution CT, Simultaneous combined CTs with transmission and non-transmission X-rays, Phase-contrast X-ray CT

INTRODUCTION

Medical application of synchrotron radiation (SR) has been performed in the field of angiography in Japan, as is the case in the USA and the EU, especially Germany. The other fields include monochromatic X-ray CT, monochromatic radiogram, X-ray microscopy, in vitro fluorescent X-ray analysis of small amounts of elements such as a specific metal, and so on. In this article, angiography and monochromatic X-ray CT are mainly described.

The main target of SR angiography has been the coronary artery, especially through the intravenous approach. This is the only method which has been applied on a clinical basis to patients in the USA and Germany as well as in Japan. However, vessels of other organs are also potentially good candidates, especially for fine structures in vitro as well as in vivo. This subject has been specifically researched by Dr.Mori and his colleagues, and will be reported in another chapter.

CORONARY ANGIOGRAPHY

The history of venous SR coronary angiography is initially reviewed in brief, and this itself is a history of SR medical application in Japan. In 1983, an SR diagnostic group was formed by E.Takenaka and M.Akisada in Tsukuba. Almost all such medical work in Japan has been carried out at the National Laboratory for High Energy Physics in Tsukuba, which is known as KEK. The following year, in 1984, a two dimensional image of a rat kidney was successfully taken using

K-edge energy subtraction (1). In 1985 the cardiovascular systems including coronary arteries in a cat were taken (2), in 1987 a dog, and a goat in 1994. However, due to the lack of photon flux the images of large animals were taken at the energy above the K-edge (3). Finally, in 1996, we performed human studies, details of which will be presented by Professor Sugishita in another chapter.

Coronary angiography in Japan is characterized by two-dimensional (2D) imaging and cine mode study, in striking contrast to line scan in the USA and the EU. It is well known that there are both advantages and disadvantages in the area scan, 2D technique, and the same can be said for the line scan, 1D technique. This type of 2D imaging needs a strong light source and fast switching of X-ray energy above and below the K-edge in order to have the energy subtraction of the image. Another 2D imaging method capable of fast switching in a large view area using an iodine filter had been proposed and developed by Umetani et al (4). This method was simple and trouble-free. However, the fact that it required a 3 - 4 times higher radiation dose than the other methods was a big disadvantage if it was applied to human diagnosis.

Finally, we have stopped pursuing the energy subtraction image method and adopted the single energy radiogram above the K-edge, mainly on account of the radiation exposure and the lack of photon flux. Nevertheless, the coronary arteries are still considerably well-depicted, although the ribs are imaged in the coronary radiogram when taken at above the K-edge energy.

The advantages in intravenous SR coronary angiography of 2D cine mode include that most of the stenosis of coronary arteries can be correctly observed in dynamic study, overlap of the heart and the vessels may be evaded in some phases, and that physiological blood flow in the coronary artery and the myocardium can be evaluated. However, the quality of the images is still subclinical, even in the observation of cine mode. Obviously, the increase in photon flux with a strong light source and technical improvements in components such as the detector will improve the quality of images. Perhaps the limiting factors of this method are the low concentration of contrast agent in the coronary artery due to its venous injection, and the radiation exposure dose due to safety considerations. Non-invasive coronary angiogram has a clinical demand, especially in the follow-up care of treated patients. However, we have some potentially tough competitors in the field of non-invasive imaging of the coronary artery at the present time. These are magnetic resonance (MR) imaging and ultrafast CT. The MR imaging is capable of showing the coronary arteries quite well, especially their proximal portions, since these portions can be included in one plane and their movement is not so rapid compared with distal portions. Stenosis at the proximal left anterior descending coronary artery is nicely shown also by the MR imaging, without any contrast agent or radiation exposure. Therefore, the introduction of a higher quality SR coronary angiogram that will be achievable, for instance, by intraaortic injection (5) is needed to compete with these other technologies. Obviously, this technique may increase invasiveness, but the procedure is feasible on an outpatient basis due to the use of a thin arterial catheter. The risk factor with patients is almost the same as the intravenous method. Best of all, the quality of the image is improved to the level of a conventional coronary angiogram, or even better. The intraaortic coronary angiogram will be shown in detail by Dr.Takeda in another chapter.

However, there are several questions which need to be answered in order to decide whether or not the intraaortic coronary angiogram should substitute for the intravenous coronary angiogram: For example, (a) How much will the quality of the intravenous coronary angiogram be improved under a permissible radiation level either by the line scan method or the 2D method ? (b) How well can MR imaging and ultrafast CT depict the coronary arteries, especially their structures ?

(c) How different is the mortality rate between conventional selective coronary angiography and intraaortic coronary arteriography (perhaps the same as conventional aortography and 10 to 100 times safer than conventional selective coronary angiography) ? (d) How different is the morbidity rate among the high flow rate in VC (venous coronary) injection, insertion of a thin catheter into the aorta, and catheterization into the coronary artery ? And (e), how much difference in quality exists between conventional selective coronary angiography of cine mode and intraaortic coronary arteriogram using X-rays above the K-edge.

In order to proceed with the coronary angiography programme by any imaging method using synchrotron radiation technical difficulties have to be solved, such as in achieving X-rays above and below the K-edge in a short time, at the order of 2-4 msec, with a large view field and increased radiation dose.

MONOCHROMATIC X-RAY CT

Several kinds of SR X-ray CTs are being developed. So far only transmission X-ray has been used for CT, however, it is possible to utilize non-transmission X-ray separately or simultaneously (6-8). Thus, X-ray CTs with synchrotron radiation can be divided into two groups, transmission type and non-transmission type. The non-transmission types are further classified into scattering X-ray, fluorescent X-ray, and phase-contrast types. We have performed simultaneous operation† to obtain multiple CTs; transmission X-ray CT combined with scattering and/or fluorescent X-ray. High spatial resolution CT has been used to obtain live animal images so far, while other kinds of CTs are used in vitro, for specimen and/or phantom. In high spatial resolution CT of live animals, an image in the head of a rat was successfully obtained 4 years ago. Tooth and nostril were well depicted and the CT image correlated well with a section of a fixed rat head. Both its spatial resolution and slice thickness were 36 micrometers (6).

The high contrast CT is taken by using X-ray above the K-edge of the contrast agent, iodine or gadolinium. The purpose of high contrast CT is to obtain images with better spatial resolution than a single photon emission CT, and in good contrast resolution compared with the conventional CT that requires a much larger amount of tracer (for example 131 I-IMP). Theoretically, we expected a sensitivity of about 5 microgram iodine/ml. However, images with 50 microgram iodine/ml were hardly depicted in a previous experiment (7).

A germanium detector for fluorescent X-ray CT is located at an angle of 90 degrees, that for Compton's scattering X-ray CT at 135 degrees and that for Thomsons's scattering X-ray CT at a small angle off the direction of monochromatic X-rays (8). We have proven experimentally that a combination of simultaneous multiple CTs of Thomson's scattering X-ray, fluorescent X-ray and Compton's scattering X-ray is feasible.

Phase-contrast CT is quite a new modality which our group successfully developed two years ago (9). Its advantage over the conventional absorption imaging is noted in its high sensitivity to light elements, which are the main constituents of our body. The phase-contrast radiogram/CT is several hundreds to a thousand times more sensitive than the conventional one. Thus, since high contrast and/or high resolution images will be available even with low radiation exposure in them, the phase-contrast imaging technique could well be the shining light in the future of X-rays. For example, transplanted-liver cancer can be well-depicted without any contrast material; the viable tumour as dark areas and the necrotic portion as a white area compared with the normal liver. This subject will be presented by Dr. Momose in another chapter.

To conclude, our goals for the near future of SR CTs for different purposes are as follows: High spatial resolution -- 1 to 2 micrometer. High contrast resolution -- 5 microgram iodine/ml. Fluorescent X-ray CT -- detection of several hundred nanograms of iodine/ml. Scattering X-ray CT -- analysis of specific substances. And phase-contrast CT -- high sensitivity of weight differences in light elements of 4 mg weight difference/ml will be detected.

REFERENCES

1. Akisada M, Hyodo K, Ando M, Maruhashi A, Konishi K, Toyofuku F, Nishimura K, Hasegawa S, Suwa A, Takenaka E. (1985) K-edge subtraction using synchrotron radiation for

coronary angiography. KEK Preprint 85-18, July 1985.

2. Akisada M, Ando M, Hyodo K, Hasegawa S, Konishi K, Nishimura K, Maruhashi A, Toyofuku F, Suwa A, Kohra K (1986) An attempt at coronary angiography with a large size monochromatic SR beam. Nucl.Instrum. and Meth. A246: 713 - 718.

3. Takeda T, Itai Y, Wu J, Ohtsuka S, Hyodo K, Ando M, Nishimura K, Hasegawa S, Akatsuka T, Akisada M. (1995) Two-dimensional intravenous coronary arteriography using above K-edge monochromatic synchrotron X-ray. Acad. Radiol. 2: 602-608.

4. Umetani K, Ueda K, Takeda T, Anno I, Itai Y, Akisada M, Nakajima T. (1992) Two-dimensional real-time imaging system for subtraction angiography using an iodine filter. Rev. Sci. Instrum. 63: 629-631.

5. Takeda T, Umetani K, Doi T, Echigo J, Ueki K, Itai Y. (1997) Two-dimensional aortographic coronary arteriography with above-K-edge monochromatic synchrotron radiation. Acad. Radiol. 4: 438-445.

6 Takeda T, Itai Y, Hayashi K, Nagata Y, Yamaji H, Hyodo K. (1994) High spatial resolution CT with a synchrotron radiation system. J. Comput. Assist. Tomogr. 18: 98-101.

7. Itai Y, Takeda T, Akatsuka T, Maeda T, Hyodo K, Uchida A, Yuasa T, Kazama M, Wu J, Ando M. (1995) High contrast computed tomography with synchrotron radiation. Rev. Sci. Instrum. 66: 1385-1387.

8. Takeda T, Maeda T, Yuasa T, Akatsuka T, Ito T, Kishi K, Wu J, Kazama M, Hyodo K, Itai Y. (1995) Fluorescent scanning X-ray tomograph with synchrotron radiation. Rev. Sci. Instrum. 66: 1471-1473.

9. Momose A, Takeda T, Itai Y, Hirano K. (1996) Phase-contrast X-ray computed tomography for observing biological soft tissues. Nature Medicine 2(4): 473-475.

DISCUSSION ON OVERVIEW

C: May I say something that the situation at ESRF ? It is an European facility, and has 12 member countries and this number is going to increase in the near future. This kind of medical research is just one of the many specialized lines which is pursued. There's a policy that this medical research will be conducted at ESRF, and mostly by the researchers of the member countries. At the end the idea is the same as for the other beamlines, that the research programs will be submitted as proposals to the scientific committees, not funding agencies. The funding is there. Once a medical program is approved on the basis of scientific merit, it will get beam time. Once you get beam time, you come to Grenoble for your studies. Your travel, your hotel or guest house, your meals are paid, and so the funding is there already. So, it has scientific merit. This is like the category II (clinical research) case which was brought up. This basically belongs to that. I think that it's always in the medical application that when new techniques are developed and reach a certain maturity to be tested, they fall to the category I (routine clinical survey) soon or later. And when it comes to routine, there is need and requests for screening purposes, and it has to justify itself in another way, because it's no more new exiting research which belongs to the agenda of ESRF.

Our decision, when we suggested the programs, was that we took one program which was well advanced already, 5-7 years ago. That was angiography. There were not many patients by that time, but we were convinced it would work. We chose the approach which we knew, the line scan mode, and that's going to happen, that's going to run for some years. We have the support from the local hospital. We have the contract that if we have patients coming from other European countries they go through the hospital. That's all more or less pipeline, and it will work. The whole concept of the beamline was such that it gave possibilities for other medical research, and the computer tomography program was actually initiated by the people at Grenoble hospital. That group is actually run by them. They will use beamline. They have in the beginning exchanged their efforts, and actually put in money rather substantially, and they get free beam time over the years.

The whole concept is that we run on two tracks, one is that we want to show something which works, and things are always a mixture of scientific interest and new research, and also policy decisions, and we've got to have it relatively soon, so that we can show that it works.

So, we are building a kind of multipurpose beamline which is now being commissioned. I think we come close to your idea of this category II experiments. That has strong support and all costs are absorbed by the member countries, and we know the program will run for years without frequent requests for new funding.

Medical activities of synchrotron radiation in Japan -- Intravenous coronary cineangiography ---

Yasuro Sugishita[1], Sadanori Ohtsuka[1], Tohoru Takeda[2], Yuji Itai [2], Kazuyuki Hyodo[3], Masami Ando[3]

[1]Cardiovascular Division, Department of Internal Medicine and [2]Department of Radiology, Institute of Clinical Medicine, University of Tsukuba, 1-1-1 Ten-noudai, Tsukuba-shi, 305 Japan
[3]National Laboratory for High Energy Accelerator Research Organization, 1-1 Oho, Tsukuba-shi, 305 Japan

SUMMARY. A method of examination less invasive and more convenient than conventional coronary angiography has been sought. We have developed intravenous coronary cineangiography (cine-IVCAG) by using a two-dimensional X-ray beam from synchrotron radiation (SR). We investigated its use to visualize the coronary arteries in dogs and a goat and then used it clinically. SR, which has high intensity radiation, was reflected asymmetrically with a silicon crystal to produce an intense, wide and monochromatic (33.3 or 37 KeV) X-ray beam. The subjects received an intravenous injection of contrast agent into the central veins, then the irradiation by the two-dimensional X-ray beam was performed. Images were acquired with an image intensifier and were taken with a CCD camera for 4 msec periods at 33 msec intervals (30 images/sec), which were recorded with a digital fluorography system. The cine-IVCAG was obtained in the dogs and a goat and was shown to be able to visualize even an intentionally created coronary stenosis about 1 mm in length. Furthermore, the cine-IVCAG permitted clear visualization of the coronary arteries and enabled evaluation of coronary artery lesions in the patients with coronary artery disease. Therefore, the cine-IVCAG can be conveniently used for the evaluation of coronary arteries and may be clinically used for screening and follow-up of coronary artery disease.

KEY WORDS: Synchrotron radiation, Intravenous coronary arteriography, Coronary blood flow measurement

INTRODUCTION

Coronary artery disease, such as myocardial infarction and angina pectoris, is caused by the obstruction or stenosis of coronary arteries, and is a major cause of death in Western countries as well Japan. The diagnosis of the sites and degree of coronary stenosis needs coronary angiography (CAG). However, because CAG requires the injection of a contrast agent directly into a coronary artery, it is potentially hazardous and distressing to patients. Therefore, a method of examination less invasive and more convenient than CAG has been sought.

Intravenous CAG (IVCAG) has been developed by using synchrotron radiation (SR). Since the first report on intravenous CAG by Rubinstein et al. in 1982 [1], this procedure has been investigated at the Stanford Synchrotron Radiation Laboratory [2] and the Brookhaven National Laboratory [3,4] in the U.S.A., at DESY in Germany [5,6], and at the National Laboratory for High Energy Physics in Tsukuba (KEK), Japan [7,8]. Laboratories in the U.S.A. and Germany use two linear monochromatic X-ray beams, just above and just below the iodine K-edge, and irradiate them to a vertically moving patient to yield static K-edge subtraction images. Whereas, we have obtained a two-dimensional wide X-ray beam by reflecting asymmetrically the SR beam with a silicon crystal and have developed an intravenous coronary cineangiography (cine-IVCAG) system. Our cine-IVCAG system requires a more intense synchrotron beam, as photon density is decreased by magnification of the narrow SR to the wide X-ray beam. However, dynamic imaging may be more informative than static imaging. We have investigated its use to visualize the coronary arteries in dogs and goat and

15

16

then used it clinically.

SR BEAM AND IMAGING SYSTEM

Cine-IVCAG was performed at KEK, Japan. Details of the system have been reported previously [9]. SR is produced by a bending magnet (beamline NE5) or by an ellipsoid multipole wiggler (beamline NE1) from the accumulation ring, which was constructed as a booster ring for the high energy physics. The electron acceleration energy of the accumulation ring was 5.8 or 5.0 GeV and the average beam current was 30 mA. The SR beam was reflected asymmetrically with the (311) diffracting planes of a silicon monocrystal, and the narrow 8mm×70mm or 8mm×80mm beam was enlarged to a wide 70mm×70mm or 150mm×80mm X-ray beam, respectively. To increase the integrated photon flux by asymmetrical reflection, the silicon crystal was polished slightly with 1200 mesh silicon carbide. The wide X-ray beam obtained was parallel and monochromatic (33.3 or 37 KeV), with an energy level just above the iodine K-edge to achieve a high sensitivity to the contrast agent. The resultant intensity of the X-ray beam at the surface of an object was 2.5×10^9 photons/mm^2/sec in beamline NE5 and 2.8×10^{10} photons/mm^2/sec in beamline NE1.

X-ray imaging was acquired in animal experiments with a 9-inch image intensifier (RTP9211G, Toshiba, Tokyo, Japan) and monitored with a high signal to noise ratio charge-coupled device (CCD) camera (XC77, SONY, Tokyo, Japan). The CCD camera was adjusted to obtain an each image for 2 or 4 msec at 33-msec intervals. Thirty images per second were obtained and recorded on videotapes with a videorecorder (BVU8200, SONY). For image analysis, the recorded images were fed into a digitizer and were analyzed by a computer and image-processing equipment (VAX8250, DEC, Boston, MA, U.S.A.). Each image was digitized into a 512×480 pixel matrix that was 8 bits deep and was capable of displaying 256 shades of gray. The schema of our cine-IVCAG is shown in Fig. 1. X-ray imaging in clinical study was somewhat different and the details of the methods will be published elsewhere in the near future [10].

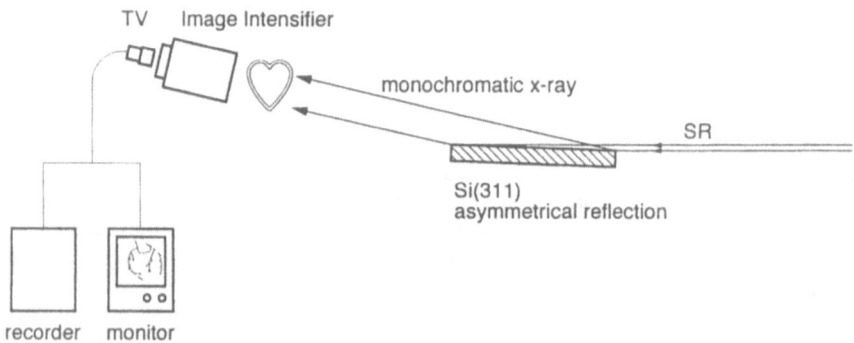

Fig. 1. Schematic diagram of imaging system [11].

ANIMAL EXPERIMENTS

Cine-IVCAG was performed in dogs and in one goat. All animal experiments were approved by the Medical Committee for the Use of Animal Subjects in Research at the University of Tsukuba.

Cine-IVCAG in dogs. Beagle dogs (9-14 Kg) were anesthetized with sodium pentobarbital (30mg/Kg, i.v.) and ventilated with a respirator. A catheter was inserted into a femoral vein and advanced to the inferior vena cava for the injection of a contrast agent (Urografin-76, Nihon Schering, Osaka, Japan). We then directed the X-ray beam from beamline NE5 at the heart in either the right or the left anterior oblique view, and determined the suitable position for CAG. After the intravenous administration of 100 μg of nitroglycerin, given to dilate the coronary arteries, 10-15 ml

(8-10 ml/sec) of the contrast agent was injected through the catheter and the X-ray beam was directed. During the intravenous CAG, the respirator was briefly interrupted.

In some dogs, a thoracotomy was performed at the fifth intercostal space in order to evaluate whether our CAG system could visualize a coronary stenosis. The proximal portion of the left anterior descending coronary artery (LAD) was dissected and was stenosed by encircling it with a thread about 1 mm in diameter. After the chest had been loosely closed with sutures with the thread in place, the X-ray beam was directed at the heart and the contrast agent was administered to obtain a cine-IVCAG.

Cine-IVCAG in a goat. Since the degree of attenuation of the X-ray beam depends on body thickness, an intense X-ray beam is required for clinical studies. Thereby, to determine whether our system is applicable to humans, we performed cine-IVCAG in a goat by using an intense X-ray beam from beamline NE1. A female goat, 40 Kg, was anesthetized with sodium pentobarbital (30 mg/Kg, i.v.) and ventilated with a respirator. The width of the animal's thorax was 28 cm in a frontal section and 40 cm in a sagittal section. A catheter was inserted into a femoral vein and advanced to the inferior vena cava for injection of the contrast agent. Following the intravenous administration of 200 μ g of nitroglycerin to dilate the coronary arteries, we directed the X-ray beam in a left anterior oblique projection and injected 25 ml (20 ml/sec) of a contrast agent (Urografin-76) for the CAG.

Visualization of coronary arteries by the cine-IVCAG
The coronary arteries were visualized immediately after the opacification of the ascending aorta by the contrast agent. Less than 10 sec was required for the contrast agent to disappear from the coronary arteries. Our IVCAG is almost real-time and is dynamic images, but it is only possible to show static images in a printed article. A representative CAG image is shown in Fig. 2. The proximal portions of the coronary arteries overlapped the left atrium, the left ventricle, and the ascending aorta; however, even those overlapped portions could be detected with somewhat less definition. Because the CAG was obtained serially in our system, the position and shape of the arteries were easily detected.

Cine-IVCAG was repeated after the LAD had been experimentally stenosed in some acutely instrumented dogs. Fig. 3 shows a representative image of a stenosed LAD. The stenosis was visible in the mid-portion of the artery and was measured about 75% in diameter. Since the length of those stenoses was equal to the diameter of the thread used to encircle the artery, our imaging system could visualize a coronary stenosis less than 1 mm in length.

Using the intense X-ray beam from beamline NE1, we also achieved a cine-IVCAG in the goat. As shown in Fig. 4, the LAD and the left circumflex coronary (LCx) arteries were clearly visualized. Accordingly, our system was shown to be capable of visualizing coronary stenosis and was suggested to be validated for human use.

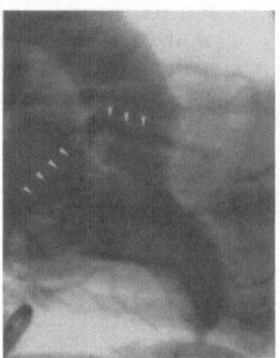

Fig. 2. Right anterior oblique projection of cine-IVCAG (intra-venous coronary angiography) in a normal dog [12]. Although the proximal portions of the coronary arteries overlap the left atrium and the ascending aorta, they were also detectable, but with less definition.

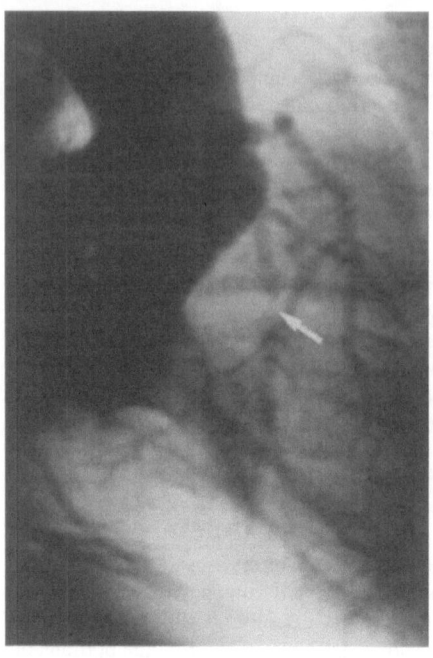

Fig. 3. Right anterior oblique projection of cine-IVCAG in a dog with an intentionally created coronary stenosis [12]. As indicated by the arrow, about 75% diameter stenosis near the mid-portion of LAD (left anterior descending coronary artery) was visualized. Since the stenosis was created by a thread 1 mm in width, a stenosis about 1 mm in length could be detected.

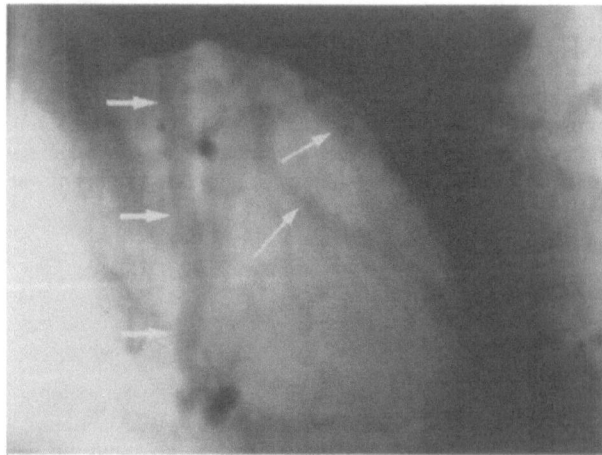

Fig. 4. Left anterior oblique projection of cine-IVCAG in a goat [12]. This IVCAG was achieved by use of the intense synchrotron radiation from beamline NE1. The LAD (indicated by the 3 thick arrows) and the left circumflex coronary artery (in-dicated by the 2 thin arrows) are visualized.

CLINICAL APPLICATION

Based on the results of animal experiments, we performed cine-IVCAG in patients with angina pectoris. This human study was approved by the Human Studies Review Committee in University of Tsukuba, by the Ministry of Education, Science and Culture, by the Ministry of Health and Welfare, and by the Institutional Review Board at KEK.

The patients underwent insertion of a catheter from the left cubital vein or the right internal jugular vein for contrast agent injection for the tip of the catheter to be placed in the central vein. Each patient was then seated in a chair and received an intravenous injection of 40 ml of a contrast agent with irradiation performed for 4 msec periods at 33 msec intervals for cine-IVCAG at 30 images/sec. Imaging was performed with a 9-inch image intensifier (RTP9211G, Toshiba, Tokyo, Japan), and the images were recorded with a digital fluorography system (DFP-2000A/C4·A4, Toshiba). The details of the instrumentations and imaging methods will be published elsewhere [11], as mentioned before.

A representative image of the cine-IVCAG is shown in Fig. 5. That is obtained in right anterior oblique projection with caudal angulation in a patient, who had undergone percutaneous transluminal coronary angioplasty (PTCA) at the proximal portion of the LAD. To minimize the silouettes of bones and soft tissues, Fig. 5 was obtained by subtracting the images between before and after the injection of the contrast agent. The large arrow indicates the site of previous PTCA and the small arrows indicate the LAD and the left circumflex coronary artery. The cine-IVCAG was shown that it enables us to visualize the coronary arteries with enough image definition and is useful for clinics with an acceptable degree of accuracy. The irradiation dose was about 25 cGy per projection.

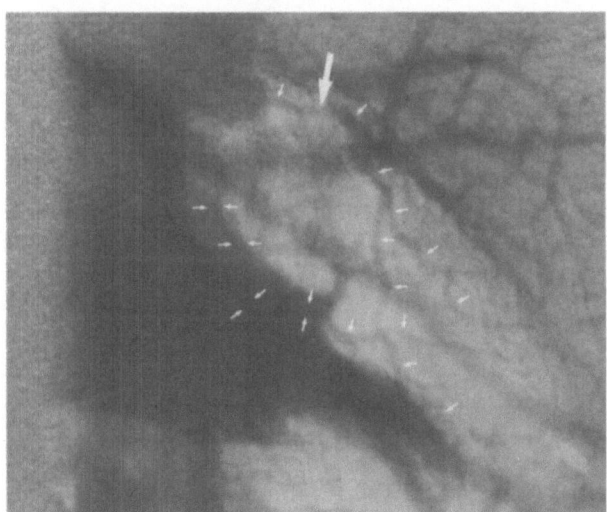

Fig. 5. Right anterior oblique projection of cine-IVCAG with caudal angulation in a patient, who had undergone PTCA (percutaneous transluminal coronary angioplasty) at the proximal portion of the LAD. The large arrow indicates the site of previous PTCA and the small arrows indicate the LAD and the left circumflex coronary artery.

DISCUSSION

IVCAG by use of SR has been developed for clinical use with two different imaging systems: one is the scanning angiographic system that uses two linear monochromatic X-ray beams, just above and just below the iodine K-edge, and radiates the two beams simultaneously by sacnning a patient to yield a few static subtracted images; the other is the cineangiographic system that uses a wide iodine-sensitive monochromatic X-ray beam and acquires dynamic images. However, because the coronary arteries move and twist as they are on the heart, the cine-IVCAG system may be suitable for such moving objects as the coronary arteries and provides much information. In general, it is easier to identify some objects when it is moving rather than when it remains static. Also, because conventional CAG has been recorded in cine-mode and cardiologists have been accustomed to evaluate coronary arteries in this mode, they believe that this mode is the best way for that. In addition, our previous study showed that cine-IVCAG enabled to estimate the coronary blood flow with a good correlation with the results measured by the electromagnetic flow meter [12]. Accordingly, cine-IVCAG seems to be expected not only anatomical diagnosis of coronary artery disease but also for functional diagnosis of coronary heart disease.

One disadvantage of the cine-IVCAG system is that SR must be more intense than that of the scanning system, because photon density is decreased by magnification of the beam size. The photon density of 33.3 KeV X-ray is decreased to about 1/1000 through a body with a thickness of 20 cm, and an intensity of more than 1×10^{10} photons/mm^2/sec is required at the surface a human subject. However, the results showed that this intense X-ray beam, such as from beamline NE1, was sufficient for cine-IVCAG even in the human. In application of our system to clinical investigations, the dose of X-rays to a patient must be minimized. We irradiated a human subject for 4 msec at 33 msec intervals with the X-ray beam from beamline NE1, by which the skin dose of radiation was 25 cGy per each injection.

Another disadvantage of our system is that we cannot produce K-edge subtraction images. The K-edge subtraction is the unique procedure allowed for synchrotron radiation due to its easy tunability for obtaining suitable X-ray energy level. However, the X-ray dose delivered must be more than doubled to perform K-edge subtraction, thereby K-edge subtraction imaging may not be allowed to our two-dimensional cineangiographic system. Alternatively, when we want to minimize the silouettes of bones and soft tissues, we can obtaine temporally subtracting images by subtracting the two-dimensional images between before and after the injection of the contrast agent.

An inevitable problem of IVCAG is to separate the overlapping portions of the coronary arteries from the left atrium, the left ventricle, and the ascending aorta. One solution is to select an optimum projection angle for the targeted coronary artery. Another solution is to increase the intensity of the SR beam. We could identify the proximal portion of the left circumflex artery as shown in Fig 2-5. Nevertheless, since the overlapped portions of the coronary arteries were more easily detected at the washout phase of the contrast medium from the left ventricle, cine-IVCAG has the advantage of reducing the imagery overlapping.

In conclusion, cine-IVCAG with a two-dimensional X-ray beam from SR permits visualization of the coronary arteries. We think it may be useful for follow-up CAG in patients who have undergone interventional coronary catheterization and for screening for coronary artery disease.

REFERENCES

1. Rubenstein E, Hughes EB, Campbell LE, Hofstadter R, Kirk RL, Krolicki TJ, Stone JP, Wilson S, Zeman HD, Brody WR, Macovski A, Thompson AC (1981) Synchrotron radiation and its application to digital subtraction angiography. SPIE Proc Conf Digital Radiogr. 314: 42-49
2. Rubenstein E, Hofstadter R, Zeman HD, Thompson AC, Otis JN, Brown GS, Giacomini JC, Gordon HJ, Kernoff RS, Harrison DC, Thomlinson W (1986) Transvenous coronary arteriography in humans using synchrotron radiation. Proc Natl Acad Sci USA 83: 9724-9728
3. Thomlinson W, Gmur N, Chapman D, Garrett R, Lazarz N, Moulin H, Thompson AC, Zeman HD, Brown G, Morrison J, Reiser P, Padmanabahn V, Ong L, Green S, Giacomini J, Gordon H, Rubenstein E (1992) First operation of the medical research facility at the NSLS for coronary angiography. Rev Sci Instrum 63: 625-628
4. Thomlinson W, Gmur N, Chapman D, Garrett R, Lazarz N, Morrison J, Reiser P, Padmanabhan V, Ong L, Green S, Thompson A, Zeman H, Hofstadter R, Brown G, Giacomini J, Gordon H, Rubenstein E (1991) Venous synchrotron coronary angiography. Lancet 337: 360 (letter)
5. Dix WR, Graeff W, Heuer J, Engelke K, Jabs H, Kupper W, Stellmaschek KH (1989) NIKOS-II-A system for noninvasive coronary angiography with synchrotron radiation. Rev Sci Instrum 60: 2238-2241
6. Dix WR, Engelke K, Graeff W, HammC, Heuer J, Kaempf W, Kupper W, Lohmann M, Reime B, Reumann R (1992) First results of patients studies with NIKOS II. Nucl Instrum and Meth A314: 307-315

7. Akisada M, Ando M, Hyodo K, Hasegawa S, Konishi K, Nishimura K, Maruhashi A, Toyofuku F, Suwa A, Kohra K (1986) An attempt at coronary angiography with a large size monochromatic SR beam. Nucl Instrum and Meth A246: 713-718

8. Sugishita Y, Kakihana M, Ohtsuka S, Takeda T, Anno I, Akisada M, Hyodo K, Ando M (1990) New trend of cardiac imaging - Intravenous coronary arteriography by synchrotron radiation. Jpn Circ J 54: 339-342

9. Hyodo K, Nishimura K, Ando M (1991) Coronary angiography project at the Photon Factory using a large monochromatic beam. In: Ebashi S, Koch M, Rubenstein E (eds) Handbook on Synchrotron Radiation vol. 4. Elsevier Science Publisher, Amsterdam, pp 55-94.

10. Hyodo K, Ando M, Oku Y, Takeda T, Itai Y, Ohtsuka S, Sugishita Y, Tada J. Development of a two-dimensional imaging system for clinical application of intravenous coronary angiography using synchrotron radiation produced by a Multipole Wiggler. *J Synchrotron Radiation* . 1998 (in press).

11. Ohtsuka S, Sugishita Y, Hyodo K (1994) Intravenous coronary arteriography using a two-dimensional imaging system. Synchrotron Radiation News 7: 21-22

12. Ohtsuka S, Sugishita Y, Takeda T, Itai Y, Hyodo K, Ando M (1997) Dynamic intravenous coronary arteriography by using synchrotron radiation and its application to measuring coronary blood flow. Jpn Circ J 61: 432-440

Intravenous Coronary Angiography with Dichromography using Synchrotron Radiation

Thorsten Dill, Rodolfo Ventura, *Wolf-Rainer Dix, *Olaf Dünger, *Meike Jung, #Michael Lohmann, *Bernd Reime, xWolfram Kupper, Christian W. Hamm.

Department of Cardiology, University Hospital Eppendorf, Hamburg; xDepartment of Cardiology II, Heart Center, Bad Bevensen; *HASYLAB, Deutsches Elektronensynchrotron (DESY), Hamburg; #Department of Physics, University Siegen, Siegen; Germany

SUMMARY: Dichromography represents a digital subtraction angiography mode based on energy substraction which allows imaging of fast moving subjects like the heart. For logarithmic subtraction two images with x-rays just below and above the iodine K-edge (33.17 keV) are simultaneously obtained in a line scan mode. Monochromatic x-rays of sufficient intensity to visualize coronary arteries of 1 mm diameter with extremely low iodine mass density (1 mg / cm2) after venous injection is only provided by synchrotron radiation. The system NIKOS at the 'Deutsche Elektronen Synchrotron' (DESY) consists of 6 components: a wiggler, a monochromator, a safety system, a scanning device, a detector and a computer system. After experimental studies in dogs patients are imaged since 1990. Results of 195 investigated patients demonstrate feasibility and safety of synchrotron radiation coronary angiography together with high diagnostic accuracy. A large scale study is underway to validate diagnostic sensitivity and specificity compared to selective coronary angiography. When compact synchrotron radiation sources become available, this technique could be used for follow-up studies and for evaluation of certain high coronary risk populations.

KEY WORDS: dichromography, synchrotron radiation, coronary angiography

Coronary angiography is the established routine imaging modality for patients with coronary artery disease. In recent years, the volume of these procedures has remarkably increased (3). Complications associated with this invasive approach are low in the range of 1,5 % and the mortality is 0,1 % (8). A further reduction of risk appears difficult to achieve because of the invasive nature of the procedure. Therefore, efforts have been made to image coronary arteries by non-invasive or minimal invasive ways.

Conventional intravenous digital subtraction angiography (DSA) uses a time subtraction mode and proved to be unsuitable for imaging of fast moving objects like the coronary arteries with diameters down to 1 mm and less. Dichromography represents a digital subtraction mode based on energy subtraction. Two images with x-rays just below and above the iodine K-edge are simultaneously obtained in a line scan mode. This requires monochromatic x-rays of sufficient intensity which today is provided only by synchrotron radiation produced in large storage rings. Accordingly, this technique can currently only be investigated at the Deutsche Elektronen Synchrotron (DESY) facilities in Hamburg (1), at the National Synchrotron Light Source (NSLS) in Brookhaven, USA (12, 13) and at the Photon Factory in Tsukuba, Japan. In the following, the technical design and the initial experience in patients at DESY is described.

Dichromography

The principle of dichromography was introduced by Jacobsen in 1953 (7). In contrast to time subtraction, the energy dependence of x-ray absorption is used to obtain two images with different contrast to the contrast agent - normally iodine - but equal contrast to other tissues like bone and soft tissue. In order to receive different contrast to iodine, the discontiniuity of the absorption at the K-edge (33.17 keV) is used (Fig. 1). Accordingly, one image is taken with monochromatic x-rays at an energy below the K-edge of iodine (mask) and the other one with an energy above the K-edge. By performing a logarithmic subtraction, the subtracted image should contain primarily the iodine image. The absorption coefficient for x-rays above the K-edge is six-fold higher than that below. For an energy separation of the two monochromatic x-ray beams of 300 eV the sensitivity for iodine is 10.000 times higher than that for soft tissue (1). This allows intravenous injection of the contrast agent, which is diluted during transit approximately by the factor 50, for imaging coronary arteries with a diameter $\geq$ 1 mm. The two images are taken simultaneously when the contrast agent fills the coronary arteries (Table 1).

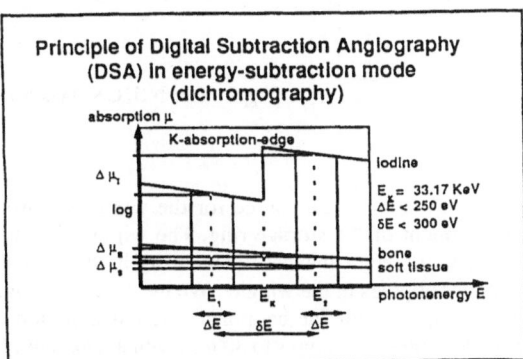

Fig. 1 Energy dependence of the absorption at the K-edge of iodine at 33.17 keV (1).

Table 1 Parameter for dichromography of the NIKOS system.

Contrast agent	370 mg/ml of iodine
Concentration of iodine in coronarty arteries	8-20 mg/ml
Mass density of iodine in coronary arteries of 1 mm diameter	0.8-2.0 mg/cm^2
K-edge of iodine	33.17 keV
Absorption length in soft tissue	2.1 cm
Bandwidth of the monochromatic beams	250 eV
Signal of a 1 mm coronary artery	3 %
Signal-to-noise ratio (SNR)	3
Statistical noise	1 %
Electronic noise	0.3 %
Dynamic range of detector	300.000:1
Exposure time per line	0.8 msec
Exposure time per image	250 msec
Speed of vertical scan	50 cm/sec
Delay for the same pixel (E1 and E2)-slow motion phase	3.2 msec
Spatial resolution	(0.4 mm) $^{-1}$
Intensity in front of the patient	3×10^{11} photons / mm^2 / s
Skin dose per subtracted image	50 mSv
Effective dose per subtracted image (male)	0.5 mSv

The NIKOS system

Dichromography requires monochromatic x-ray sources (bandwidth 250eV) of very high intensity (3x 1011 photons/mm2 / s). At present, this is only available in synchrotron laboratories. Accordingly, the system NIKOS (Non-invasive Coronary Angiography with Synchrotron Radiation) was installed in a beam line of the storage ring DORIS at DESY [1]. It consists of six main components (Fig. 2):

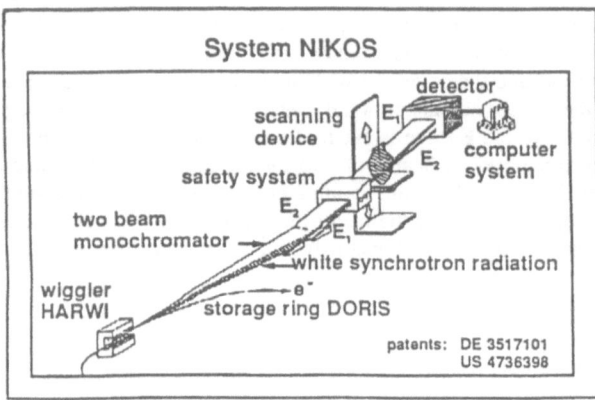

Fig.2 The NIKOS system (1).

1. The wiggler

The wiggler is a special magnetic structure which serves as a source for the white synchrotron radiation and which is installed in a straight segment of the storage ring. The wiggler forces the positrons in the storage ring into a curved path and thereby enhances the intensity in the beam. The magnitude of enhancement is related to the number of poles in the wiggler. We use a 20 pole wiggler (HARWI) (4) which has a length of 2,4 m and 0,12 m for the endpoles. After installation of a variable vacuum chamber the minimal vertical magnetic gap amounts to 30 mm with a maximum field strength of 1.26 T. The resulting critical energy is 17.0 keV and the horizontal opening angle is 6.4 mrad. At 100 mA machine current the total power in the white synchrotron radiation beam is 4 kW. During patient studies the storage ring operated at energy levels of 4.5 GeV with a current of 56 mA to 126 mA.

2. The monochromator

The two monochromatic x-ray beams are diffracted by a monchromator out of the white synchrotron radiation beam (6). For each monochromatic beam a perfect Si (111) crystal is installed in Laue geometry 31.6 m behind the wiggler. Photons of 33.17 keV are diffracted with a Bragg angle of 3.42o. To increase the photon flux to the patient the crystals are bent. They are installed in a He-filled housing and cooled by water. The bandwidth of the monochromatic beams is ∂E = 190eV to 270 eV. The flux in front of the patient was adjusted to be 2.7 x 1011 photons/mm2 / s.

Today the intensity is not limited by the system output but by the skin entry radiation dose to the patient. The upper limit is set to 50 mGy per image which results in an effective dose of 0.5 mGy (males) to 1.0 mGy (females). The effective dose is calculated on the basis of ICRP publication 60 (1990) (11). Dose adjustments are performed by reduction of the height of the white synchrotron radiation beam at the entrance of the monochromator.

3. The safety system

The critical safety issue of the present system relates to radiation. For a standard scan a skin entry dose rate of 64 Gy/s was estimated. Therefore, an immediately reacting safety system is compulsary. The safety system of NIKOS consists of three independent shutters which can switch off the monochromatic beams within less than 10 ms. Ionization chambers are used routinely for each scan to estimate the expected dose. The system can only be activated after approval of the physician based on the predicted dose.

4. The scanning device

A line scan system was developed with the aim to reduce radiation scatter and to optimize the system to the x-ray source. A chair was designed which allows vertical movements of the patient over a distance of 20 cm at a speed of 50 cm/s. Accordingly, one scan sized 12 cm x 12 cm can be performed within 250 ms. The chair is driven by a hydraulic system. During the vertical movement of the chair the readout of the detector is controlled by a precise optical scale. In addition, the chair can be rotated in the horizontal and lateral axis to allow angulated projections.

5. The detector

The detector consists of a fast low noise, two-line ionization chamber which simultaneously records the x-ray at energies above and below the K-edge. It consists of a drift cathode and 336 Cu strips per line as anodes which are directed along the monochromatic beams. The distance of the strips is 0.4 mm thus defining the horizontal pixel size of the images (10). The chamber is filled with 90% of Kr gas and 10% of CO_2 under about 13 bar pressure. The ionization current of each strip is integrated and digitized with 20 bit resolution. The dynamic range of the complete detector system is 300.000 : 1 (gain 4). Every 0.8 ms the two lines can be read in parallel. The data are transmitted to the computer via a fast glassfiber link.

6. The computer system

An Alphastation 400 4/233 is used for data acquisition, image processing and presentation. It is linked up with a VME-system for system control.

Studies

Safety and imaging potential were initially investigated experimentally in dogs. Since 1990 studies in patients are conducted. Initialy safety and feasibility was proofed. With 195 patients investigated it was demonstrated that coronary arteries can be imaged and that radiation exposure is on average half of a conventional diagnostic heart catheterization. Further technical adjustments were made constantly, e.g. improved dynamic range and noise reduction of the detector, a new monochromator and a special in different projection angles adjustable examination chair. Projection angles for different vessel regions were optimized (9). The left anterior descending coronary artery and the right coronary artery can be imaged with high diagnostic accuracy, as well as vein grafts and the internal thoracic artery (IMA). The left main stem and the circumflex artery still cause some problems for accurate imaging due to superimposed structures of the ascending aorta or the left ventricle. However, postprocedural image processing helped considerably to improve image quality (Figure 3), e.g. contrast enhancement by unsharp masking and edge preserving smoothing.
Since June 1997 a study to validate diagnostic sensitivity and specificity in a large cohort of patients compared to selective coronary angiography is underway.

System NIKOS III
(P89-2-1)

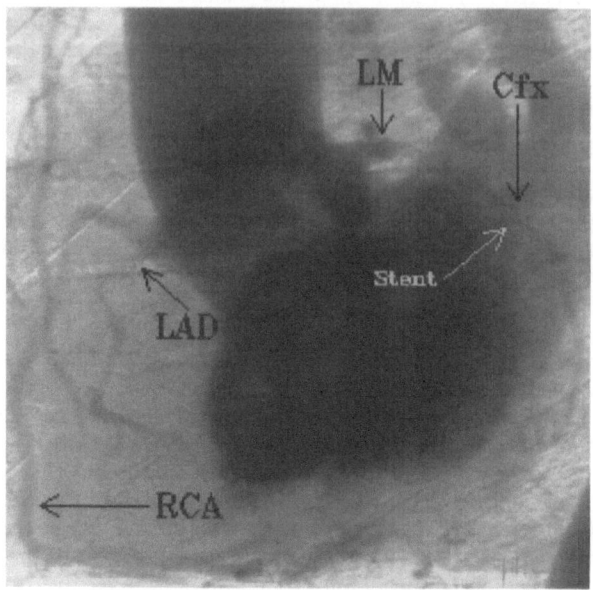

LAO60,S7F25,S

Fig 3 Intravenous synchrotron angiogram of the right coronary artery (RCA) in LAO 60° projection, also visible the circumflex (CFX) after stent implantation, the left main (LM) and the distal portion of the left anterior descending (LAD).

Conclusions

After 15 years of development, dichromography with synchrotron radiation seems to have the potential to be routinely used to image coronary arteries. The NIKOS system at HASYLAB is currently the most advanced facility available for dichromography with synchrotron radiation. It also appears at present the best minimal-invasive imaging modality for coronary arteries as compared with other approaches (2, 5, 14). Further development is necessary for wide spread use. The generation of synchrotron radiation for medical applications in compact sources is realistic and could also be cost effective. NIKOS does not aim to replace invasive coronary angiography but could find its place for follow-up of coronary interventions like percutaneous transluminal coronary angioplasty or coronary artery bypass graft operation.

27

Acknowledgments

We thank the Bundesministerium für Bildung, Forschung und Technologie (BMBF) for supporting the project (number 05350 GKA 9).

References

1. Dix W.-R.: Intravenous coronary angiography with synchrotron radiation. Prog. Biophys. Molec. Biol. 63 (1995) 159.

2. Duerinckx AJ, Urman MK.: Two-dimensional coronary MR angiography: Analysis of initial clinical results. Radiology 193 (1994) 731.

3. Gleichmann U., Mannebach H., Lichtlen P.: 11. Bericht über Struktur und Leistungszahlen der Herzkatheterlabors in der Bundesrepublik Deutschland. Z Kardiol 84 (1995) 953.

4. Graeff W., Bittner L., Brefeld W., Hahn U., Heintze G., Heuer J., Kouptsidis J., Pflüger J., Schwartz M., Weiner E.W., Wroblewski T.: HARWI-a hard x-ray wiggler beam at DORIS. Rev Sci Instrum 60 (1989) 59.

5. Hundley W.G., Clarke G.D., Landau C., Lange R.A., Willard J.E., Hillis D., Peshock R.M.: Noninvasive determination of infarct artery patency by cine magnetic resonance angiography. Circulation 91 (1995)1347.

6. Illing G., Heuer J., Reimer B., Lohmann M., Menk R.H., Schildwächter L., Dix W.-R., Graeff W.: Double beam bent Laue monochromator for coronary angiography. Rev Sci Instrum 66 (1995) 1379.

7. Jacobsen B.: Dichromatic absorption radiography. Dichromography. Acta radiol 39 (1953) 437.

8. Johnson L.W., Krone R.: Cardiac catheterization 1991: A report of the Registry of the Society of Cardiac Angiography and interventions: I. Results and complications. Cathet. Cardiovasc. Diagn. 28 (1993) 219.

9. Kupper W., Dix W.-R., Graeff W., Steiner P., Engelke K., Glüer C.C., Bleifeld W.: Projection angels for intravenous coronary angiography. Ital Phys Soc Proc 10 (1988) 165.

10. Menk R.H., Dix W.-R., Graeff W., Illing G., Reime B., Schildwächter L., Tafelmeier U., Besch H.J., Grossmann U., Langer R., Lohmann M., Schenk H.W., Wagener M., Walenta A.H., Kupper W., Hamm C., Rust C.: A dual line multicell ionization chamber for transvenous coronary angiography with synchrotron radiation. Rev Sci Instrum 66 (1995) 2327.

11. Recommendations of the international Commission on Radiological Protection. Pergamon Press, New York 1990.

12. Rubenstein E., Brown G.S., Chapman D., Garrett R.F., Giacomini J.C., Gmur N., Gordon H.J., Lavender W.M., Morrison J., Thomlinson W., Thompson A.C., Zeman H.: Synchrotron radiation coronary angiography in humans. In: Synchrotron Radiation in the Biosciences, Clarendon Press (1994) 639.

28

13. Rubenstein E., Hofstadter R., Jeman H.D., Thompson A.C., Otis J.N., Brown G.S., Giacomini J.C., Gordon J.J., Kernoff R.S., Hárrison D.C., Thomlinson W.: Transvenous coronary angiography in humans using synchrotron radiation. Proc Natl Acad Si USA 83 (1986) 9724.

14. Schmermund A., Lange S., Sehnert C., Altmaier K., Baumgart D., Görge G., Erbel R., Seibe R., Grönemeyer D.: Elektronenstrahltomographie bei koronarer Herzkrankheit. Dtsch Med Wschr 37 (1995) 1229.

Correspondence

Address all correspondence to: Dr. T. Dill, Medizinische Klinik, Abteilung Kardiologie, Universitäts-Krankenhaus Eppendorf, Martinistraße 52, 20246 Hamburg, Germany.

First tests on subtraction bronchography study at the Angiography station of the VEPP-3 storage ring

V.I. Kondratyev, G.N. Kulipanov, M.V. Kuzin* , N.A. Mezentsev, S.I. Nesterov, V.F. Pinduyrin

Budker Institute of Nuclear Physics, 630090 Novosibirsk, Russia

SUMMARY. The method of digital subtraction angiography at the K-absorption edge of Xe was applied to acquire first subtraction images of xenon distribution over a test sample. The experiments were performed at the 'Angiography' station of the VEPP-3 storage ring (Novosibirsk, Russia). The station is equipped with the dedicated X-ray monochromator providing two linear monochromatic beams with the energies above and below the K-absorption edge of iodine or xenon, and the double one-coordinate X-ray detector. Total X-ray images are obtained with the use of the line-by-line scanning of the object across the linear monochromatic beams. First results demonstrate that a thickness of Xe as small as 0.5 mm in the test sample is detected at the station.

KEYWORDS: Dichromography, Bronchography, Xenon, Synchrotron Radiation.

INTRODUCTION

The existing Angiography station at the Budker Institute of Nuclear Physics (Novosibirsk) was originally intended for experiments on dichromography imaging at the K-absorption edge of iodine (33.2 keV) [1]. The station is equipped with the special double-beam X-ray monochromator and the double one-coordinate X-ray detector, and the line-by-line scanning of the object is used for acquiring the X-ray images. The station uses synchrotron radiation (SR) from the 2 T wiggler installed in the straight section of the VEPP-3 storage ring. Earlier, the station was already used for testing the possibilities on visualization of lymphatic system of alive rats at the K-edge of iodine [2].

It was shown in Ref. [3] that there is a real necessity to improve bronchography examination, and that the technique of Digital Subtraction Angiography with SR can be employed for this purpose when is used at the K-absorption edge of xenon (34.5 keV). To investigate the VEPP-3 Angiography station capabilities for bronchography studies, the preliminary experiments on visualization of xenon distribution over the test sample (phantom) have been performed, and the obtained results are presented below.

THE ANGIOGRAPHY STATION FEATURES

The main components of the station are the double-beam X-ray monochromator, the object scanner and the double one-coordinate X-ray detector (Fig. 1). The monochromator forms two linear (about 10 cm width at the object place) monochromatic beams with the energies just above and below the K-absorption edge of xenon (34.5 keV). The monochromatic beams intersect at the object location, then they diverge and are registered simultaneously by the double one-coordinate X-ray detector. The complete images at two X-ray photon energies are taking by scanning the object vertically with a line-by-line registration of the linear beams passed through the object.

---

* Contact author: Dr. KUZIN M.V., Budker Institute of Nuclear Physics,
Ac. Lavrentyev ave., 11, 630090, Novosibirsk, Russia
Tel.: +7 (3832) 35-91-67 office   Fax: +7(3832) 35-21-63
E-mail: M.V.Kuzin@inp.nsk.su

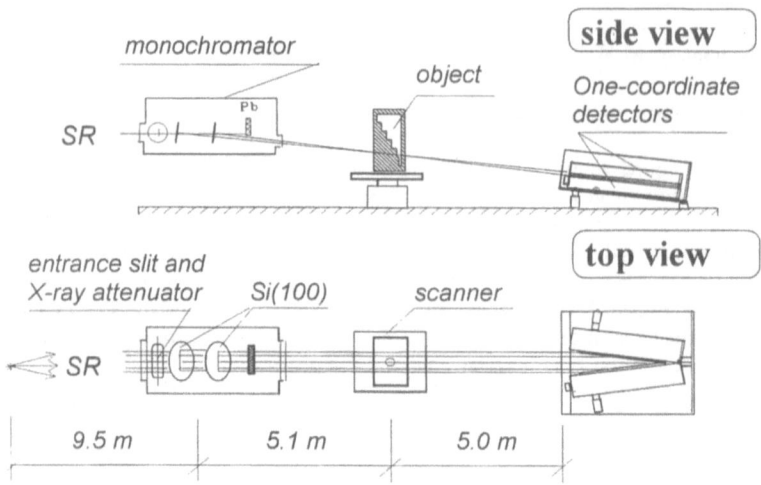

Fig. 1. Schematic layout of the VEPP-3 Angiography station.

The monochromator comprises two Si(100) crystals of a 100 mm diameter, the entrance slit and the attenuator of the white SR beam[4]. Laue diffraction on the (111) crystal plane is used for extraction the monochromatic beams. The relative energy separation of the monochromatic beams can be set in the range of $(6 \div 10) \cdot 10^{-3}$ by changing the distance between the crystals in the interval $30 \div 50$ mm. The relative energy spread of each beam can be in the range from 10^{-3} to $8 \cdot 10^{-3}$, depending on the entrance slit size. The photon flux at the object location is about 10^8 photons/s/mm² at a typical 100 mA current in the VEPP-3.

The double one-coordinate X-ray detector consists of two identical one-coordinate X-ray detectors[2,5,6]. Each one-coordinate detector has 128 separate scintillation counters with YAlO₃(Ce) scintillators. The spatial resolution δ of the detector can be set in the range from 0.2 mm to 2 mm, and total width of the X-ray sensitive area of the detector is equal to $128 \times \delta$ ($25.6 \div 256$ mm). The maximum counting rate of the each detector channel is about 6-7 MHz, and the registration efficiency is about 90%[6].

EXPERIMENT AND RESULTS

To test the station capability for Xe registration, the plexiglass phantom with xenon filled was employed (Fig. 2a). The phantom had internal cavity with different thickness of xenon along the X-ray beam (5, 4, 3, 2, 1 and 0.5 mm). The cavity was air evacuated and then filled in with xenon at about 1 atmosphere pressure. The monochromator was tuned on the K-absorption edge of xenon (34.5 keV), and the typical numbers of registered photons lied in the range of $(2-4) \times 10^5$ per a detector channel.

Figure 2b shows the usual X-ray images of the phantom at the energies above and below the xenon K-edge, as well as the subtraction image (on the right). The monochromatic beams, passed above the phantom body (white horizontal strips at the top of the images), and the beams, passed through the Xe-free part of the phantom body (black horizontal strips just under the white strips), can be observed on the usual pictures. Different thickness of xenon in the phantom, from 5 mm at the top down to 1 mm at the bottom, are clearly visualied in all pictures. The xenon distribution in the phantom along the vertical direction, corresponding to the subtraction image of Fig. 2b, is presented in Fig. 3.

Figures 2b and 3 demonstrate that a 1 mm thickness of xenon in the phantom is positively visualized. The comparison between the level of the noise and the signal value of a 1 mm xenon thickness (Fig. 3) allows us to expect that a 0.5 mm thickness of xenon must be detected, as well.

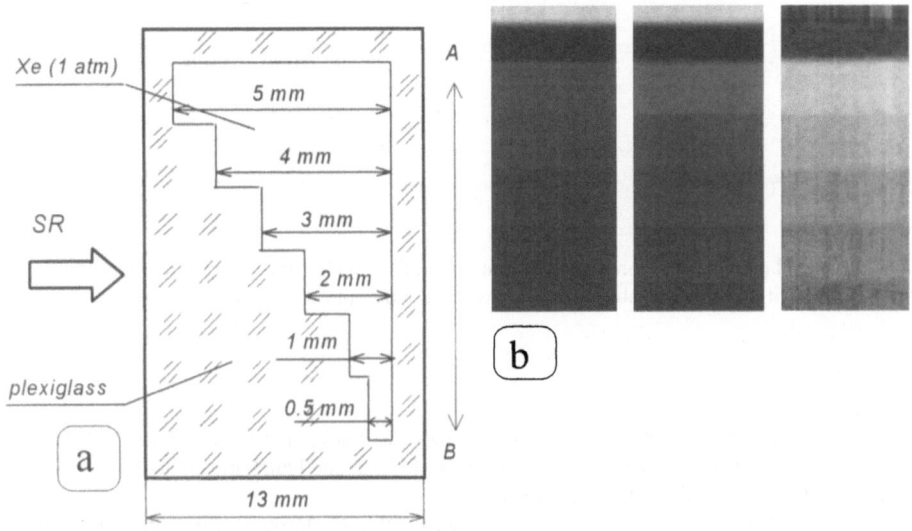

Fig. 2. Schematic drawing of the phantom (a) and its X-ray images (b): from left to right - at the energy above and below the K-edge of xenon, and the subtraction image. AB - the direction of scanning in the experiment.

A 1 mm thickness of plexiglass decreases the photon flux by 3.1%. The same values for a 1 mm thickness of xenon are 0.35% at the energy below and 1.98% at the energy above the K-absorption edge. It means that a passing from one step of the phantom to the adjoining one with the increased by a 1 mm thickness of xenon must provide a 1.63% increase in the subtraction signal. The measured value is about 1.1%. At the same time, the measured value of the X-ray absorption in the Xe-free part of the phantom body is in a good agreement with the calculated one. The most likely reason for this is that there was a mixture of xenon with air in the experiments, rather than pure xenon.

CONCLUSION

The obtained preliminary results with the phantom show that a 1 mm thickness of xenon is positively visualized and that a 0.5 mm xenon thickness must be detected, as well. It means also that the existing Angiography station of the VEPP-3, designed originally for angiography studies at the iodine K-absorption edge, can be employed for bronchography studies at the xenon K-edge.

32

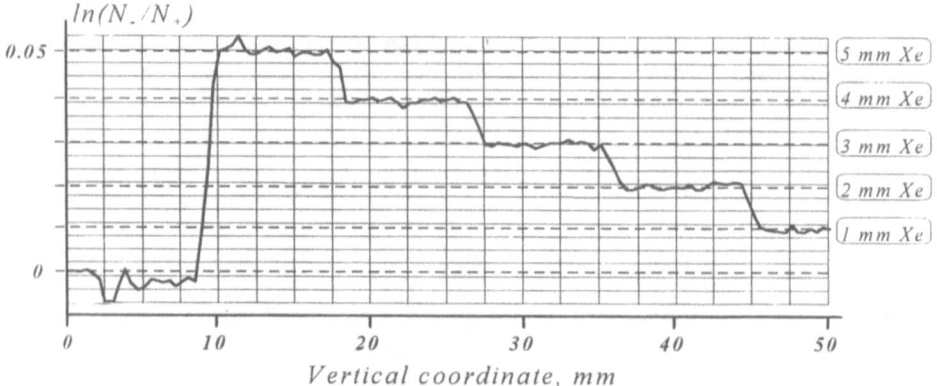

Fig. 3. The measured profile of xenon distribution in the phantom (N+ and N- are the registered numbers of photons at the energies above and below the K-absorption edge of xenon, respectively).

REFERENCES

1. Dolbnya IP, Kulipanov GN, Kurylo SG, Mezentsev NA, Pindyurin VF, Sheromov MA (1990) Application of synchrotron radiation for diagnostics of blood and lymphatic circulatory system in Novosibirsk. Physica Medica VI (3-4): 313-317
2. Kolesnikov KA, Kulipanov GN, Kuzin MV, Mezentsev NA, Nesterov SI, Pindyurin VF, Dragun GN, Zelentsov EL, Rozenberg OA (1995) Preliminary results of animal's lymphatic system study at the Angiography station of the VEPP-3 storage ring. Nucl Instr and Meth A359: 364-369
3. Rubenstein E, Giakomini JC, Gordon HJ, Rubenstein JAL, Broun G (1995) Xenon K-edge dichromographic bronchography: synchrotron radiation based medical imaging. Nucl Instr and Meth A364: 360-361
4. Barsukov VP, Dolbnya IP, Kolokolnikov YuM, Kurylo SG, Mezentsev NA, Pindyurin VF, Sheromov MA (1991) X-ray monochromator for digital subtraction angiography using synchrotron radiation. Nucl Instr and Meth A308: 419-422
5. Dementiev EN, Dolbnya IP, Zagorodnikov EI, Kolesnikov KA, Kulipanov GN, Kurylo SG, Medvedko AS, Mezentsev NA, Pindyurin VF, Cheskidov VG, Sheromov MA (1989) Dedicated X-ray scintillation detector for digital subtraction angiography using synchrotron radiation Rev. Sci. Instrum. 60 (7): 2264-2267
6. Kolesnikov KA, Kozlov RYu, Kulipanov GN, Kuzin MV, Mezentsev NA, Nesterov SI, Pindyurin VF, Dragun GN, Zelentsov EL, Rozenberg O (1996) Preliminary results of animal's lymphatic system study at the Angiography station of the VEPP-3 storage ring. In: Yoon M, Nam SH (eds) Proc 4th Intern Conf on SR Sources and 2nd Asian Forum on SR: ICSRS-AFSR'95. Kyungbuk, PAL, POSTECH, Pohang, pp 543-552

Synchrotron Radiation Coronary Angiography with Aortographic Approach

Tohoru TAKEDA, *Keiji UMETANI, Toshiki DOI, Junko ECHIGO, Syounosuke
MATSUSHITA, *Hironori UEKI, *Ken UEDA, Yuji ITAI.

Institute of Clinical Medicine, University of Tsukuba, Tsukuba-shi, Ibaraki-ken, 305 Japan
*Central Research Laboratory, Hitachi Ltd. Kokubunzi, Tokyo 185 Japan

SUMMARY. Two-dimensional synchrotron radiation (SR) coronary arteriography (CAG) with aortographic contrast injection was considered theoretically and animal experiments were performed to examine its diagnostic ability. This system consisted of a silicon monocrystal, fluorescent plate, avalanche-type pickup tube camera, and image acquisition system. The experiment was performed at synchrotron sources in the Photon Factory in Tsukuba. The x-ray energy was adjusted to just above the iodine K-edge.

Theoretical calculation described that the coronary arteries would be demonstrated with a high signal-to-noise ratio by the aortographic CAG with SR. The canine coronary arteries were demonstrated with similar clarity as the selective CAG because coronary arteries with less than a 0.2 mm diameter could be imaged. Without overlap of the left atrium and left ventricle, almost all structures of the coronary arteries could be observed. In addition, the abnormal coronary flow and the coronary arteriovenous fistula of dog were revealed clearly. SR coronary arteriography with aortographic approach provides good visualization of the coronary arteries and detailed information of coronary flow.

KEYWORDS: synchrotron radiation, coronary arteriography, aortography, above K-edge energy, coronary flow, coronary arteriovenous fistula, diagnostic radiology

INTRODUCTION

Coronary arterial disease has a high incidence and mortality rate in industrial countries. At present, selective coronary arteriography (CAG) is a gold standard to diagnose coronary arterial disease. However this procedure requires direct coronary arterial catheterization, and fatal accidents occur occasionally (0.14 % / examination). As a safer and more easily repeatable method to image the coronary arteries, Rubenstein, et. al. first suggested the use of the iodine K-edge energy subtraction CAG with synchrotron radiation (SR) [1]. Using the line scan method, human studies have been performed in the USA [2-4] and Germany [5-6].

In Japan, a two-dimensional (2D) intravenous CAG system with SR, which demonstrates the structure of coronary arteries as conventional cine angiography, has been developed [7-10]. The results of animal experiments and human studies have revealed various problems due to intravenous CAG with SR, such as the overlap of the coronary artery on cardiac chambers and other vessels, and the dilution of contrast material. 2D aortographic CAG with SR in dogs was performed to assess the diagnostic ability in visualizing coronary arteries [11-13]. In this study, we performed detailed theoretical consideration of coronary image quality above the K-edge image, and reported the results obtained by 2D aortographic CAG with SR.

THEORETICAL CONSIDERATION OF CORONARY IMAGE QUALITY

The signal-to-noise (S/N) ratio of the coronary artery was calculated corresponding to various dilutions of contrast material. The S/N ratio is defined as the ratio of the image signal to the statistical noise associated with the detection of the number of x-ray photons [14]. Without scattered radiation, the S/N ratio can be calculated as follows;

$$S/N \ ratio = (n-n')/(n+n')^{1/2}$$

where n is the transmission x-ray number near the coronary artery, and n' is the transmission x-ray number on the coronary artery.

$$n = f \, a^2 \varepsilon \, e^{-(\mu_0 b)}$$

$$n' = f \, a^2 \varepsilon \, e^{-\{\mu_0(b-d) + \mu_I^* d\}}$$

$$S/N = \frac{\left\{1 - e^{-d(\mu_I^* - \mu_0)}\right\} \sqrt{f a^2 \varepsilon e^{-b\mu_0}}}{\sqrt{1 + e^{-d(\mu_I^* - \mu_0)}}} \tag{1}$$

where f is the photon number before object to obtain one image (3 x 10^8 photon /mm^2/frame), **a** is the detector size of each pixel, ε is the efficiency of the detector (50%), μ_0 is the x-ray linear attenuation coefficient of soft tissue (0.33 cm^{-1}), μ_I^* is the x-ray linear attenuation coefficient of iodine at just above the K-edge (33.17 keV) corrected by dilution of the contrast material (35.9 x density x dilution ratio), **b** is body thickness (15, 20, 25 cm) and **d** is the diameter of the coronary artery (1 mm and 0.2 mm). To obtain 1-mm and 0.2-mm diameter coronary arteries, detector size of the pixel was set to half of the coronary arteries (a; 0.5 mm and 0.1 mm).

The relationship between the S/N ratio and contrast dilution was calculated as shown in Fig.1a and Fig.1b. In the aortographic CAG with SR (dilution ratio of 1/4), an excellent S/N ratio (more than 10) was obtained to detect a 1-mm diameter coronary artery even at a body thickness of 25 cm. When detecting a coronary artery with a 0.2-mm diameter, an image with a S/N ratio of 3 could be obtained except for the 25 cm body thickness.

The required photon flux was calculated to obtain clear images for 1-mm diameter coronary arteries with the following formula;

$$f = \frac{\{1 + e^{-d(\mu_I^* - \mu_0)}\}(S/N)^2}{\{1 - e^{-d(\mu_I^* - \mu_0)}\}^2 \{a^2 \varepsilon e^{-b\mu_0}\}} \tag{2}$$

With the aortographic approach using an x-ray dose of 3x10^8, images with a S/N ratio of 10 could be obtained even at 25 cm body thickness (Fig.2). The graph suggests that the x-ray dose can be significantly reduced with a thin object. With a thick object, the x-ray energy of 33.17 keV appears to be inadequate because x-ray exposure of the object is required in large amounts. Then, the required photon flux was also calculated by changing the x-ray energy from 33.2 keV to 50 keV (Fig.3). Here, we assumed that the ε had not changed with the x-ray energy. In the aortographic approach (dilution ratio of 1/4), the object thickness was changed to 15 cm, 20 cm and 25 cm. The adequate x-ray energy was changed to 38 keV, 41 keV and 43 keV and the x-ray exposure was reduced about 13 %, 35 % and 55 % respectively, compared to 33.17 keV (Fig.3a). If the contrast material was significantly diluted, adequate x-ray energy tended to lower the energy, and large amounts of x-ray flux would be needed (Fig.3b).

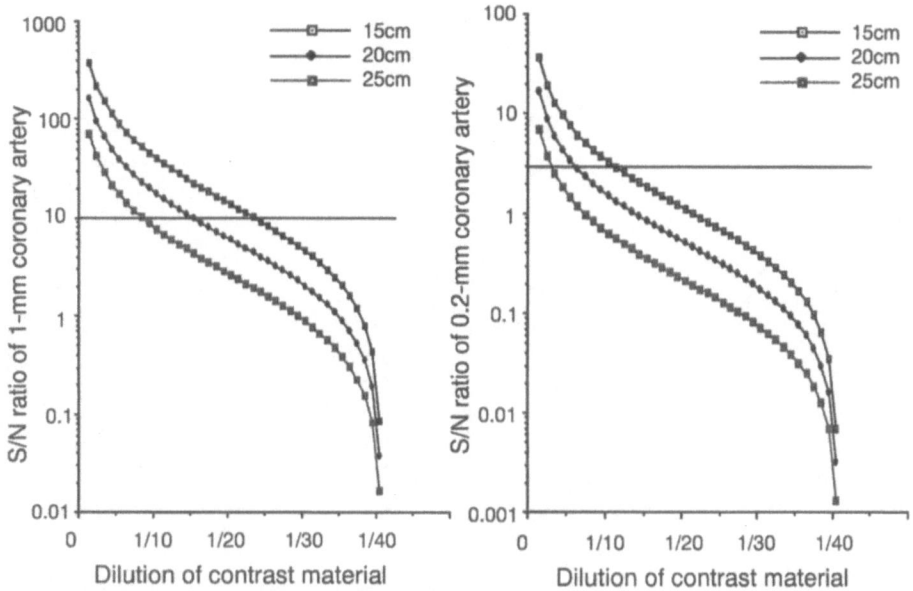

Fig.1 Relationship between the S/N ratio and the dilution of contrast material

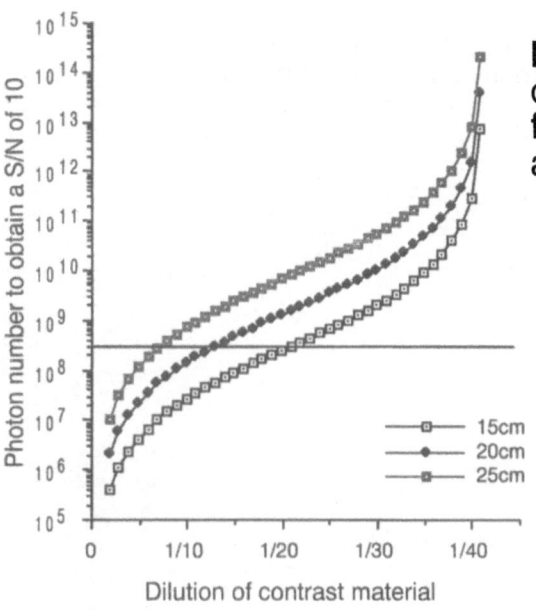

Fig.2 Photon number to obtain a S/N ratio of 10 for a 1-mm coronary artery.

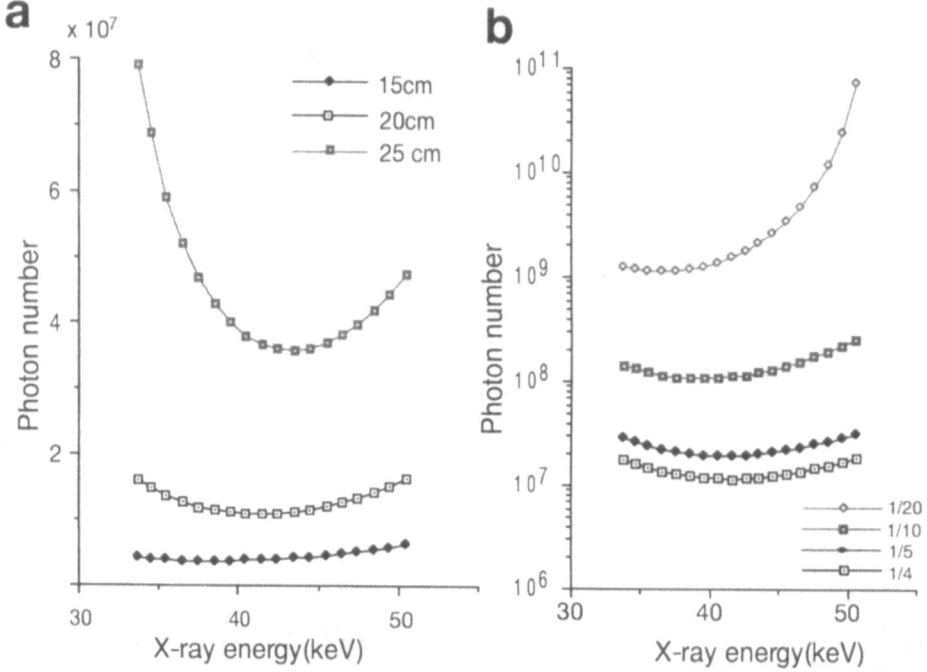

Fig.3 Relationship between x-ray energy and photon flux (photon/mm2/frame) to obtain a clear coronary image of 1-mm in diameter with a S/N ratio of 10.
a: changing the body thickness (contrast dilution is 1/4).
b: changing the contrast dilution (body thickness is 20 cm).

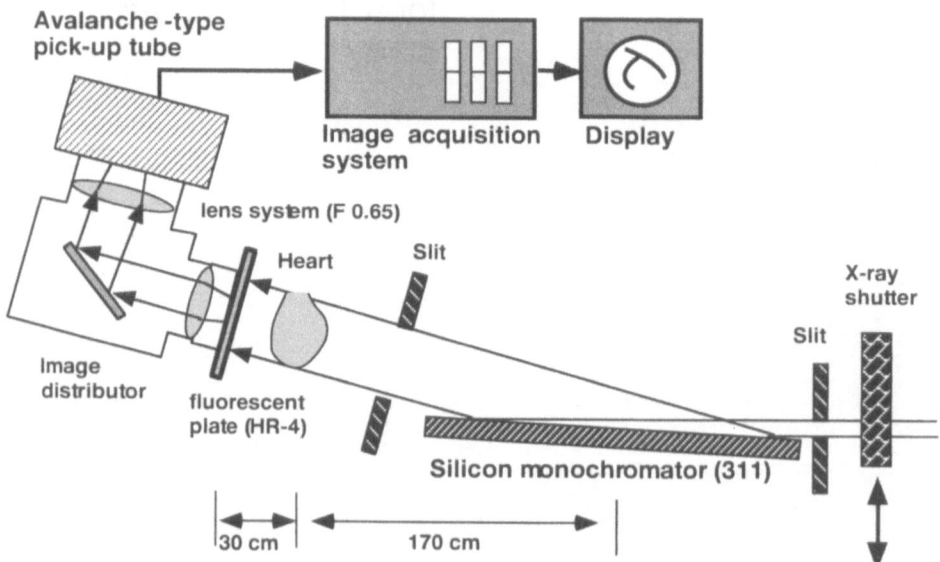

Fig.4 Schematic diagram of 2D coronary angiographic system

METHODS AND MATERIALS

The 2D-CAG system with SR was constructed at the vertical wiggler beam line of BL-14C in the Photon Factory in Tsukuba. This system consists of a silicon (311) monocrystal, fluorescent plate, avalanche-type pickup tube camera, image acquisition system and workstation (Fig.4) [11-13]. A 38 x 70 mm^2 monochromatic x-ray beam was obtained with the asymmetric reflection at the silicon planes. The beam energy was set just above the iodine K-edge with Bragg reflection on the silicon monochromator crystal (33.32 keV).

X-ray images were converted to light images with a fluorescent plate, and this light image was detected by the avalanche-type pick-up tube camera. For digital processing, x-ray TV images were digitized in a 480 x 512 pixel matrix with a 12-bit depth using a 12-bit analog-to-digital converter. A workstation (Hewlett Packard 715/33) was used for image processing and control of the image acquisition system. TV images were obtained just after the start of injection of the contrast material, and the acquisition interval of each image was set at 16.7 msec. The storage ring was operated at 2.5 GeV with a current of approximately 300 mA. A 3-pole superconducting vertical wiggler [5 tesla] was used. The incident monochromatized flux in front of the object was about 1.0 - 1.6 x 10^9 photons /mm^2 /second.

Dogs (average weight, 12 kg) were anesthetized with phenobarbital (0.9 mg/kg). A 5F catheter was inserted into the aorta via the right femoral artery. The contrast material (Iomeprol 350, 0.90 ml/kg) was injected with an injector at the rate of 10 ml/sec. Images were obtained in the lateral view. The present experiment was approved by the Medical Committee for the Use of Animals in Research of the University of Tsukuba, and it conformed to the guidelines of the American Physiological Society.

RESULTS

Typical aortographic CAG images with SR are shown in Figure 5. As the beam size in this system was limited to 38 x 70 mm^2, all canine coronary arteries were not imaged simultaneously. The coronary arteries could be imaged clearly, and the image quality was thought to be similar to selective coronary arteriography. The diameter of the main trunk of the left coronary artery was determined to be about 2.0 mm by comparison with the catheter, while the distal branches of the left anterior descending, circumferential, and right coronary arteries were about 0.2 mm in diameter. The cinematic images revealed the coronary arterial flow as clearly as selective CAG. The coronary arteriovenous fistula of dog were revealed clearly (Fig.5 a-b). In addition, the abnormal dilatation of the right coronary arterial branch and its delayed flow are shown in Fig.5b-d. The cinematic images allowed observation of the coronary flow dynamics unlike the static images. The x-ray flux in front of the sensor was estimated to be about 2.1 - 3.0 x 10^5 photons /mm^2 / frame.

DISCUSSION

Two-dimensional SR coronary arteriography

In Japan, images are acquired with a 2-dimensional TV camera system using an area shaped monochromatic x-ray, produced by asymmetric reflection on a silicon plane [7-13]. Clinically, this 2D imaging method presents many advantages compared to the line scan method used in the USA, Germany and the Nations of the former Soviet Union because the images are obtained cinematically. Therefore, the coronary arterial structures with pseudo-stereoscopic effect and coronary arterial flow can be observed sequentially.

38

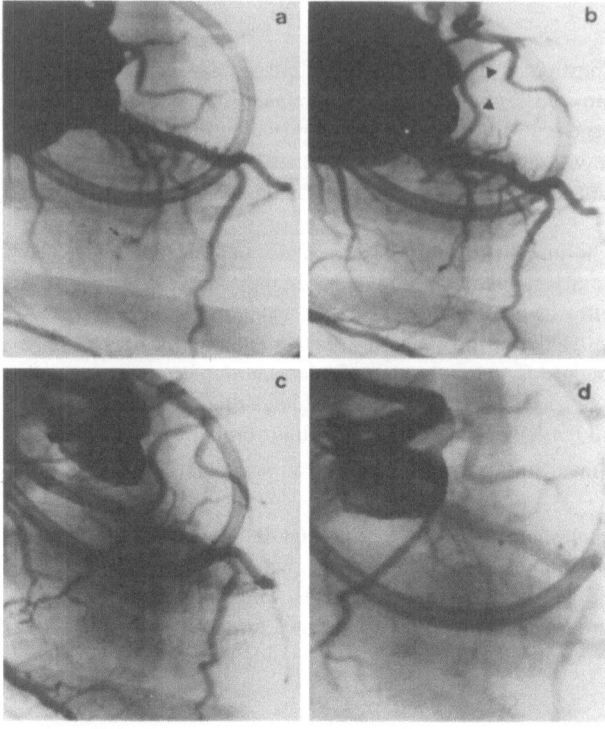

Fig.5 The cinematic images revealed the coronary arterial flow. (arrow head:AV fistula, arrow :abnormal flow & coronary dilatation)

a-b : coronary arteriovenous fistula of dog .

b-d : abnormal dilatation of right coronary arterial branch and its delayed flow.

Aortographic CAG with SR

In the 1960s, using a special loop catheter, Paulin performed aortographic CAG using the conventional x-ray system, and a considerably good coronary image was obtained [15]. However, image quality of coronary arteries is gently poor compared to selective CAG for detailed coronary diagnosis. Thus, this approach has been abandoned as a diagnostic procedure of the coronary artery, and has been applied only when the selective CAG was not technically successful. However, 2D aortographic CAG with SR provides clear images of canine coronary arteries. Even very fine coronary arteries, less than 0.2 mm in diameter, which is the detectable limitation of today's conventional selective CAG, could be revealed probably due to the high image contrast just above the iodine K-edge energy (2 fold or more) and the reduced dilution of the contrast material by the aortographic procedures (<1/4) [12].

Especially in this study, the coronary arteriovenous fistula of dog were also revealed clearly because 2D images were obtained cinematically. In addition, the abnormal dilatation of the coronary arterial branch and its delayed coronary flow were clearly shown. This phenomenon is thought to be a result of the increased resistance of coronary arteries at mico-vessel levels. Thus, cinematic images allowed superior observation of these kinds of flow abnormalities than static images. Quantitative evaluation of coronary flow using densitometry is now being planned to analyze arterial flow because the aortographic injection of contrast material is thought to be much more physiological than selective coronary arterial injection and high image contrast allows higher accuracy of data analysis.

Thus, 2D aortographic CAG with SR provides good visualization of the coronary artery and the information of detailed coronary flow.

Property of aortographic CAG with SR

The advantages and disadvantages are listed in Table.1. The fatal accidents of aortography may be reduced due to the present uses of non-ionic contrast material and improved catheterization compared to the reports of aortography in 1983 [16].

Table 1. Advantages and disadvantages of 2D aortographic CAG with SR

Advantages

    Clear coronary arterial image similar to the conventional selective CAG
       High image quality
       No overlap of coronary artery on cardiac chamber and pulmonary vessels
       No failure to visualize coronary vessels
    Imaging of coronary arterial flow
       Quantitative flow analysis at nearly physiological state
    Less invasive compared with selective CAG
       Significant reduction of fatal accidents (<1/5 compared to selective CAG)
       Simple clinical technics for clinical staff (non-selective procedure and use of small catheter)
    Reduced x-ray exposure for the patients and clinical staff
       No K-edge energy subtraction
       No hand injection of contrast material by doctor

Disadvantages

    Arterial approaches (slightly high morbidity compared to intravenous approach)

Future improvements

The image quality of 2D aortographic CAG with SR appears to resemble conventional CAG . However, from the results of the calculated S/N ratio, 0.2-mm diameter coronary arteries must be imaged more clearly. In this experiment, the significant scattered radiation from objects and the monochromator degraded the image contrast to less than 50 % because the size of the experimental hatch was very narrow. If we could employ an adequate experimental station to make the best use of the air-gap effect and a sufficient x-ray flux using a multi-pole wiggler, 2-fold improvement of image contrast would be expected by the decrement of Compton scattering (<3%) [13].

However, to obtain a good coronary image with the intravenous approach, further technical improvements will be needed in the 2D imaging method. In human studies, the ratio of contrast dilution was reported to be between 1/20 and 1/40 [4-8]. To reveal a 1-mm coronary artery at a S/N ratio of 3 without scattered radiation, the required x-ray flux ahead of the object is more than 8×10^8 photons /mm^2/frame assuming a 1/30 contrast dilution and 20-cm object thickness. A detector system with wide dynamic range (>8000:1) is indispensable. In the line scan method, the above factors are almost satisfied, and useful images of coronary artery were obtained by intravenous CAG [3-6].

X-ray exposures

In this experiment, the x-ray dose in front of the sensor to obtain one image was about 1.67 mR (3×10^5 photons/mm^2/frame). For human studies, to obtain the same quality of images as in this experiment, the entrance surface dose administered to the patient would be as 1.67 R because the x-ray absorption ratio at the body thickness of 20 cm is about 1000. The maximal allowable total entrance surface dose for a subject is 35 R for one projection [3], so the total number of frames would be limited to about 21 (4 frames/sec x 5 sec). However, due to the decrement of scatter radiation of less than 3% , the x-ray exposure could be reduced by a factor of about 1/4.

Acknowledgments
We thank Masayoshi AKISADA MD, PhD for his clinical advice. This work was performed under the approval of the Photon Factory Program Advisable Committee (Proposal No 95G238).

REFERENCES

1. Rubenstein E, Hughes EB, Campbell LE, Hofstadter R., Kirk RL., Krolicki TJ., Stone JP., Wilson S., Zeman HD., Brody WR., Macovski A., Thompson AC. (1981) Synchrotron radiation and its application to digital subtraction angiography. SPIE 314:42-48.
2. Rubenstein E., Hofstadter R., Zeman HD, Thompson AC., Otis Jn, Brown GS., Giacomini JC., Gordon HJ., Kernoff RS., Harrison DC., Thomlinson W. (1986) Transvenous coronary angiography in humans using synchrotron radiation. Proc. Natl Acad Sci USA 83:9724-9728.
3. Thomlinson W, Gmur N, Chapman D, Garrett R, Lazarz N, Moulin H, Thompson AC, Zeman HD, Brown GS., Morrison J, Reiser P, Padmanabhan V, Ong L, Green S, Giacomini JC, Gordon HJ, Rubenstein E (1992) First operation of the medical research at the NSLS for coronary angiography. Rev. Sci. Instrum. 63:625-628
4. Chapman D, Thomlinson WC, Gmur NF, Dervan JP, Stavola T, Giacomini J, Gordon H, Rubenstein E, Lavender W, Schulze C, Thompson AC. (1995) Effects of spatial resolution and spectral purity on transvenous coronary angiography images. Rev. Sci. Instrum. 66:1329-1331
5. Dix WR, Engelke K, Graeff W, Hamm C, Heuer J, Kaempf W, Kupper W, Lohmann M, Reime B, Reumann R.(1992) Coronary angiography using synchrotron radiation - Studies of human subjects with the system NIKOS II. Nucl Instr and Meth A314: 307-315
6. Dix WR. (1998) Coronary angiography at DESY. J. Synchrotron Radiation impress.
7. Akisada M, Hyodo K., Ando M., Maruhashi A., Konishi K., Toyofuku S., Nishimura K., Hasegawa S., Suwa A., Takenaka E. (1986) Synchrotron radiation at the photon factory for non-invasive coronary angiography: Experiment studies. J. Cardiography 16:527-534.
8. Hyodo K, Nishimura K, Ando M. (1991) Coronary angiography project at the photon factory using a large monochromatic beam. In: Ebashi S, Koch M, Rubenstein E ed. Handbook on Synchrotron Radiation Volume 4 North-Holland pp55-94
9. Umetani K, Ueda K, Takeda T, Itai Y, Akisada M, Nakajima T. (1993) Iodine filter imaging system for subtraction angiography using synchrotron radiation. Nucl Instr and Meth A335:569-579
10. Takeda T, Itai Y, Wu J, Ohtsuka S, Hyodo K, Ando M, Nishimura K, Hasegawa S, Akatsuka T, Akisada M.(1995) Two-dimensional intravenous coronary arteriography using above K-edge monochromatic synchrotron x-ray. Academic Radiology 2:602-608
11. Umetani K, Ueki H, Ueda K, Hirai T, Takeda T, Doi T, Wu J, Itai Y, Akisada M. (1996) High-spatial-resolution medical-imaging system using a HARPICON camera coupled with a fluorescent screen. J. Synchrotron Radiation 3: 136-144
12. Takeda T, Umetani K, Doi T, Echigo J, Ueki H, Ueda K, Itai Y. (1997) Two-dimensional aortographic coronary arteriography with above-K-edge monochromatic synchrotron radiation. Academic Radiology 4:438-445
13. Takeda T, Itai Y, Hyodo K, Ando M, Akatsuka T, Uyama C. (1998) Medical application of synchrotron radiation in Japan. J. Synchrotron Radiation impress.
14. Motz JW, Danos M.(1978) Image information content and patient exposure. Med.Phys. 5: 8-22
15. Paulin S.(1964) Coronary angiography. ACTA Radiologica Supplement 233: 5-215
16. Hessel SJ. (1983) Complications of angiography and other catheter procedures in Abrams angiography. pp 1041-1056, Little, Brown &Co., Boston

Q. Which French size do you need for the catheter?

A. I use a five French catheter a small one.

Q: I can see the advantage towards the selective coronary angiography. Once you put an arterial catheter in, it's not a big deal just to intubate the coronary selectively with a catheter, but only to stop with putting a pig tail in the aortic route, it's not a big difference for me. What is the justification for this method if you compared it as you did in the beginning with venous angiography. If you put an arterial catheter as you do, and inject contrast agent into the aortic route, it is not very much more to do to use two other catheters to inject contrast agent selectively into the left coronary artery and into the right coronary artery. That's conventional selective coronary angiography. The advantage for me is not to do it invasively with arterial puncture but to do it non-invasively with venous injection of the contrast agent.

A: I myself think that arterial punctuation is not so dangerous. Many angiographers have performed arterial punctuation, and no significant accidents have happened. Its accident rate will slightly increase compared to the intravenous method.

Q. Where did you get the complication rate for coronary injection of the contrast agent from ?

A. That number is 1.8% which corresponds to death, myocardial infarction, cerebral infarction, arrhythmia, vascular damage, contrast reaction etc. That is available from the book entitled "Cardiac catheterization and angiography 1986" by W. Grossman.

C: As a cardiologist I have the same opinion as Dr.Dill. I think there is no difference in technical problems and difficulties between intraaortic CAG and selective CAG. There are many more difficulties in arterial catheterization than in venous catheterization. I would like to emphasize mental stress and frustration on examiners and patients. As a cardiologist I would prefer the conventional selective CAG to the intraaortic CAG with SR.

C: It may be a matter of statistics. It only measured 0.025 percent. That is one in four thousand. How many patients do you have to obtain an accurate statistical calculation ? You need to study many ten thousand patients to have 0.025 as an accurate measurement, and I think that is not a case.

Q: Would you recommend this technique as a screening method ?

A: Yes, this will be a possibility for the screening of coronary artery disease.

Q: So this is for the patients with risk factors but no obvious proof of screening.

A: Yes. for patients who are suspected with coronary arterial disease. Our approach is one of the methods for screening to check coronary artery stenosis, because the fatal accident rate is very small. I think this approach might be used as one of the screening methods for all patients, all people, not only those suspected with arterial disease.

Synchrotron Radiation Micro-angiography using an Avalanche-type High-definition Video Camera

Yutaka Tanaka[1], Hidezo Mori[1], Etsuro Tanaka[1], Sumihisa Abe[1], Hiroyasu Makuuchi[1], Hiroe Nakazawa[1], Shunnosuke Handa[1], Kenkichi Tanioka**, Misao Kubota**,Seiichi Kumaoka***, Kazuyuki Hyodo[2], Masami Ando

[1]Departments of Surgery, Physiology, and Internal Medicine, Tokai
  Univ. School of Medicine, Isehara, Boseidai, Isehara, 259-11, Japan
[2]National Laboratory for High Energy Physics, Tsukuba, Japan
[3]NHK Science and Technical Research Laboratories, Tokyo
[4]SONY, Tokyo, Japan
This project was supported by a Grant-in-Aid for Scientific Research (07557060, 0967075) from the Ministry of Education, Science, and Culture, Japan, Tokai University School of Medicine Project Research (1997), and JSPS-RFTF97I00201.

SUMMARY. We improved the originally reported synchrotron radiation (SR) micro-angiographic system by applying avalanche-type high-definition (HD) video camera. The New Super Harp HDTV (NHK, Tokyo) with high contrast resolution and effective quantum ratio of 640 allowed precise assessment of configuration of small vessels (less than 100 mm after digital processing) in heart , brain, and the other organs. The originally used image-intensifier-video camera system could not delineate small vessels well. Conventional HD video system using CCD could not reveal small vessels of heart and brain in situ. This system would allow us clinical evaluation of small vessel diseases in heart , brain, and the other organs and also visualization of newly developed small vessels due to angiogenesis in malignant tumor and circulatory disorders.

KEY WORDS Synchrotron radiation, Angiography, High-definition video camera, Angiogenesis, Coronary artery

INTRODUCTION

We reported that an angiographic system using monochromatized synchrotron radiation (SR) with an energy of just above the K-absorption edge of iodine (33.3 keV) could detect a small amount of contrast material in small coronary arteries; penetrating transmural arteries and their branches, by maximizing the difference of the X-ray absorption between the contrast material (iodine) and body tissue (1, 2). However, the resolution of the detecting system (image-intensifier (II)-TV system), was not enough (approximately 200 mm) to delineate disorders of micro-circulatory system with a diameter of <100 mm. In the present study, we introduced a high-definition TV camera systems using a high-sensitive image pick-up tube camera (3,4) into SR micro-angiographic system and applied to various animal models toward clinical use in future.

METHODS

The coincidental SRs at the Beamline North-East-5 of the Accumulation Ring (ARNE5) in the National Laboratory for High Energy Physics, Tsukuba, were monochromatized at 33.3 keV (just above k-absorption edge of iodine) or and magnified 8-20 times by means of an asymmetrically cut silicon crystal in front of the objects (Bragg reflection). The parameters of the monochromatic SRs are summarized in the Table.

Table Descriptions of X-ray sources and monochromatic detecting system

synchrotron radiation source(ARNE5)		Avalanche HD video system	
light source	bending magnet	effective quantum ratio	30-640
electron energy	5.0-6.5 GeV	visual field (mm)	30 x 20
ring current	25-40 mA	recording rate	30frames/s
monochromator	Si (311)	resolution	30 mm
x-ray energy	33.3 keV		
radiation field (mm)	70 x 25 (6.5 GeV)		
radiation dose (mSV/sec)	16-48		
FWHM (keV)	0.13 keV		

Abbreviation. FWHM: full width at half maximum of the monochromatic X-ray spectrum with a peak energy level of 33.3 KeV

Ex situ ileal angiography (11 dogs) and in situ coronary angiography (10 dogs) was performed, and the images detected by either of the 3 systems described below were compared; the high-definition (HD) TV system (3), referred to as avalanche-type HDTV (New Super HARP, NHK, Tokyo) connected to a fluorescent screen with a spatial resolution of 20 mm (Figure 1), the HDTV system using charge-coupled device (CCD)(XCH 1125, SONY, Tokyo)(4) connected to the same screen and conventional TV system (XC77R, SONY, Tokyo) connected to image-intensifier (II)-(RTP9211G, Toshiba, Tokyo). The spatial resolution of the 3 detecting systems evaluated by irradiating an resolution bar chart was 30 mm, 63 mm and 170 mm, respectively.

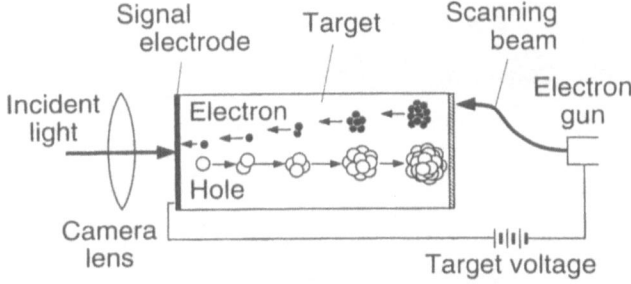

Figure 1 High-sensitivity image pick-up tube of avalanche type HDTV.

All the dogs were anesthetized with 30 mg/kg of pentobarbital (IV) and their respiration was maintained by a Harvard respirator with a flow of 1-3 l/min of oxygen. A silicon tube bypass was set between the femoral artery and superior mesenteric artery after the abdominal incision in the 11 dogs. A 15 cm length part of the ileum was hung above the abdominal wall with two surgical ties. Then iodine contrast material (2-3 ml per sec of iopamidol, Nihon Schering, Osaka) was injected into the bypass circuit via a three-way stopcock placed in the bypass for 3-4 sec while irradiating the ileum with 33.3 keV SR. *Ex situ* ileal angiography on the hung ileum above the abdominal wall (negligible tissue thickness) allow us to evaluate the spatial resolution of the detecting systems without a marked attenuation in X-ray photon density. In the latter 10 dogs, in which *in-situ* coronary angiography was performed, we evaluated the image quality with a substantial X-ray attenuation (approximately 1/30 of the original intensity) through the body with a 10 cm thickness. A coronary angiogram was taken as described for the ileal angiogram, except for a shorter injection period of 1.5-2.0 sec. In the 2 of the 10 dogs with a body thickness of 11 and 13 cm, respectively,

33 keV SR was attenuated by passing through 10 cm acrylic plate (approximately $1/2^5$) just before exposure to the dogs, in order to simulate-ray attenuation in human body with a thickness of >20 cm or more in these experiments.

RESULTS

The ileal angiograms in Fig 2 indicate the advantage of the HDTV systems for evaluating small vessels in view of their high spatial resolution. The vascular narrowing from the proximal to distal segments on the ileal wall (*vasa recta*) of the ileal artery was clearly demonstrated (arrows of the 4 different sizes in Figure 2A) and even the small segments (arrowheads in Figure 2A) communicating the adjacent *vasa recta* by the both HD video camera systems. The *vasa recta* on the ileal wall were also clearly visualized even with the conventional II-TV system (Fig. 2B), however, the vascular narrowing from the proximal to distal segments was not clear.

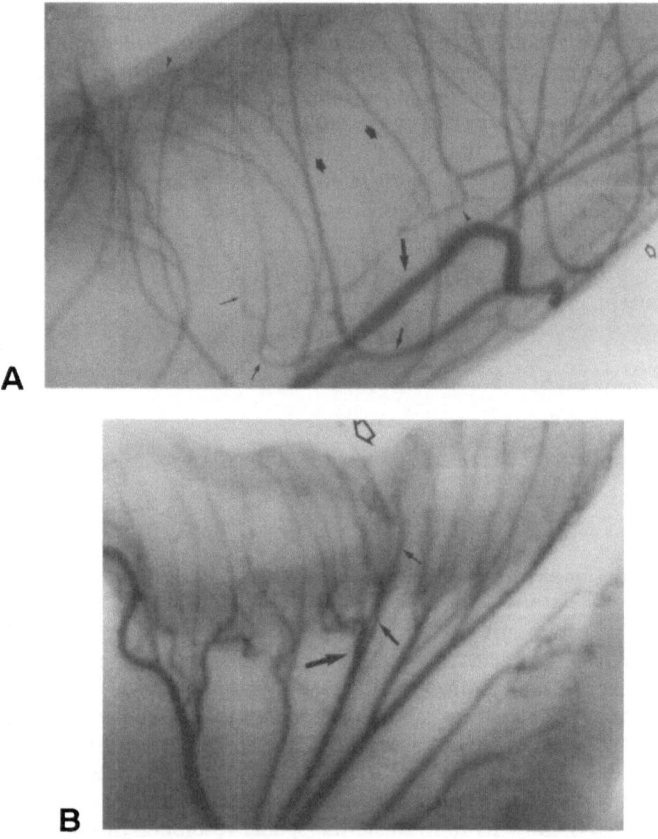

Figure 2 Ileal angiograms obtained with an avalanche-type high-definition TV system (panel A), a and a conventional II-TV system (B). The arrows of 4 different sizes (A) denote the vascular narrowing with branching, the arrowheads vascular segments communicating with the adjacent vasa recta, and the broad open arrow a copper wire with a diameter of 130 mm. These are from BME (1977)11:29-36 with permission.

In Figure 3A, penetrating transmural coronary arteries (PTA: arrow) and their branches (small arrowheads) were visualized and the vascular narrowing from the epicardial coronary artery to the penetrating transmural arteries was evident with the avalanche HDTV system, and even the fourth order intramural branches of the epicardial mother segment can be visualized (triple arrowhead). In contrast, the high-definition-TV system using a CCD failed to obtain sufficient signal to visualize coronary vessels in dogs. As shown in the Fig 3B, the PTA and their branches can be also visible in the angiogram taken by the attenuated SR (approximately $1/2^5$), although the angiographic images became darker than in Figure 3A. Thus, this system could maintain a high contrast resolution even under insufficient x-ray exposure. By applying digital processing, PTA diameter could be measured down to 95 mm and *vasa recta* to 52 mm (data not shown).

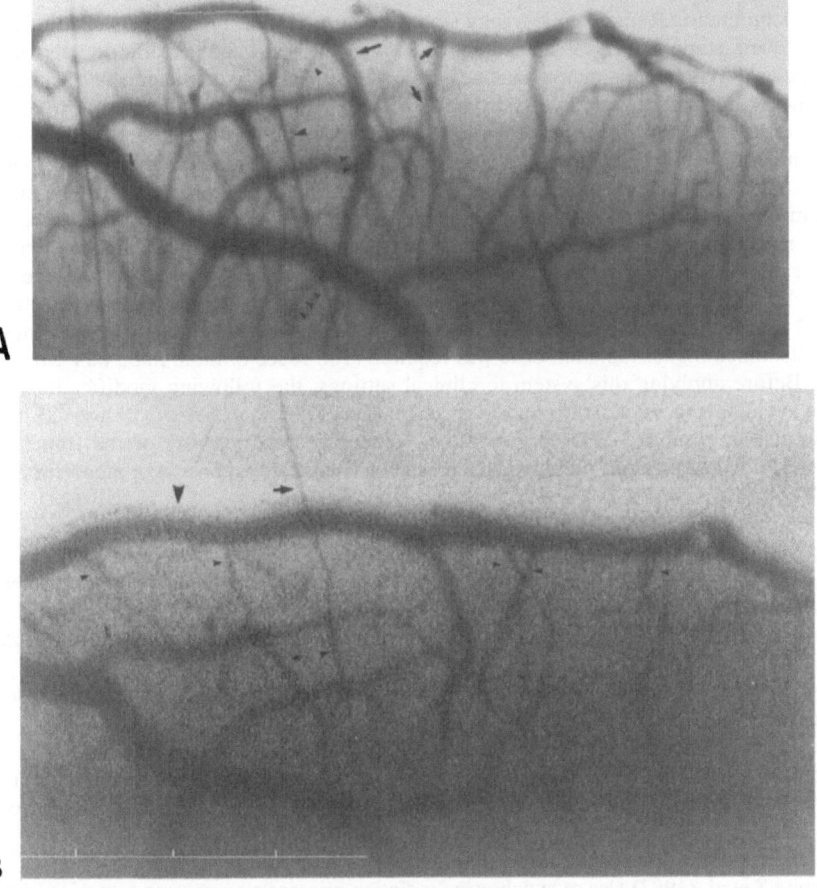

Figure 3 Coronary angiograms obtained with an avalanche-type HD TV system. The one in panel B was taken by attenuated SR with a 10 cm acrylic plate. These are from BME (1977)11:29-36 with permission.

DISCUSSION

The both the HDTV camera systems coupled to a fluorescent screen (Figure 2A) demonstrated the vascular narrowing from the proximal to the distal segments of ileal vessels under a negligible x-ray attenuation through body tissue, but conventional II-TV system did not well (Figure 2B). Only the avalanche-type HDTV camera system clearly visualized PTA and the difference in vessel diameter between PTA and epicardial coronary arteries (Fig. 3A) even under low S/N condition (3B). The CCD HDTV with a high resolution of 63 mm did not show enough sensitivity. A HDTV system generally loses its sensitivity by reducing pixel size itself. Because the number of photons per pixel becomes smaller as the pixel size decreases. The avalanche-type image pickup tube, however has a potent internal amplification system. It contains an amorphous selenium photo conductive layer, in which stable avalanche multiplication of generated carriers develops under an electric field as high as 10^{6-9} V/cm or more (3). This phenomenon increases the sensitivity to >600 times in the newest avalanche TV camera (New Super HARP); in terms of effective quantum ratio (the conversion ratio of photon to electron).

Monochromatic SR microangiography would be a useful tool for clinical evaluation of small vessel disease and angiogenesis. Visualization of PTA of the heart and perforating arteries arising from the circle of Willis or its major branches improves sufficiently the diagnosis of small vessel disease in heart and brain, such as syndrome X of the heart (5) or small cerebral infarction or obstructive disease of the Circle of Willis (6). Early detection of the atherosclerotic vascular involvement might prevent their propagation before serious clinical events. Evaluation of angiogenesis by visualizing the feeding arteries of the tumor precisely could differentiate malignant tumors from benign ones at an early stage . In near future, this system will be used to evaluate the effects of a gene therapy. Possibility of a gene therapy using anti-angiogenic substance for treatment of cancer or diabetic angiopathy is in consideration for future clinical application. A gene therapy using vascular endothelial growth factor for circulatory disorders in lower limb (7) is already in clinical trial (8). According to our recent SR angiography in goats with a similar body thickness as of human adults, much higher radiation dose was required (100 R/sec or more in 33 keV SR) than for the dogs . Before applying this system to clinical settings, the following modifications will be required to avoid an excess of x-ray exposure; conversion of continuous SR exposure (33 msec per frame) to pulse exposure (2-5 msec per frame), reducing total numbers of the frames and/or developing Gd-contrast material with higher elemental concentration with a use of monochromatic SR of >50 keV.

REFERENCES
1. Mori H, et al (1994) Visualization of penetrating transmural arteries in situ by monochromatic synchrotron radiation. Circulation 89: 863- 871
2. Mori H, et al (1996)Small vessel radiography in situ with monochromatic synchrotron radiation. Radiology 201:173-177
3. Kubota M, Kato T , Suzuki S, Maruyama H , Tanioka K. (1996) Ultrahigh-sensitivity New Super Harp camera. SPIE 2654: 325-334
4. Teranishi N (1992) Solid-state image sensor for HDTV. ITE annual convention:
5. Leikof W, Segal BL, Kasparian H. (1967) Paradox of normal selective coronary arteriograms in patients considered to have unmistakable coronary heart disease. New Engl J of Med 276: 1063-1066
6. Fisher CM (1982) Lacunar strokes and infarcts: a review. Neurology 32: 871-876.
7. Takeshita S et al. (1997) Use of synchrotron radiation microangiography to assess development of small collateral arteries in a rat model of hind limb schemia.Circulation 95:805-808
8. Isner JM et . al. (1996) Clinical evidence of angiogenesis after arterial gene transfer of phVEGF165 in patients with ischemic limb. Lancet 348:370-374

Q: It seems that they increase spatial resolution or higher sensitivity to micro-structure. Must this increase doses due to statistics ?

A: Of course one may come up with clearer images which otherwise have been invisible. Since we are using the same X-ray source as for the intravenous radiography, if we take mode of 30 frames per second, the total radiation dose could be very dangerous. By that means we have to reduce the total dose in some way down to less than 30 Roentgen. One of the major factors is reducing the number of frames per second.

Q: How can you estimate clinical application for humans and what about statistics ?

A: Maybe we would need the order of 10^4 photons/pixel/4msec=frame. So the photon flux density at the skin becomes 10^7 photons/pixel/4msec=frame when considering the x-ray attenuation of 99.9% by a body. The total flux should be at the order of 4×10^{12} photons/mm^2/sec which corresponds to 5 Roentgen of radiation dose when one takes 5 pictures per patient.

DISCUSSION ON CLINICAL LEVEL

C: We should ask the physicians what they need. The second point I'd like to add is what is the medical application. I think that it's not a medical application if you replace your sample or whatever by soft tissue and then say it is a medical application. I think this was a provocation. I think you should think what is the medical application. We would have discussion of various things related to medical applications. Let me put it in historical perspective. A few of us in this audience were in Daigo back in some years ago, 1992. When I sit, as I have, through a lot of interesting talks, nice science and technology so forth, but I keep thinking about what has happened, and changed in the field in five years. I have to admit it's not a whole lot. And that, at some level, is a bit disappointing, echoing what Rainer Dix has just said.

We have to somehow get the medical problems starting to drive the field. We have tools, we have synchrotrons, monochromators, beamlines and detectors, and everything else required. We are still hung up on angiography as sort of "the application". When people talk about medical application of synchrotron radiation, basically the only thing that come to mind is angiography. Angiography may not be what works. I don't know the answer to that.

Clearly the program in Hamburg is extremely successful, and that is probably the only real star that has risen since 1992. I don't mean to criticize the work in Japan, which has made great strides you've gone to human studies, and so forth. It has certainly progressed, but you ask yourself, "Has it developed an entire new technology to be applied to medicine ?" I don't think so. It's close. It could be.

If I think about the last five years what are the new applications we've seen ? Probably only one in five years, and that Ed Rubinstein and John Giacomini's idea of using angiography beamlines potentially to do bronchography. That's new. If you think about mammography which has been something which has risen in popularity over five years. Emilio Burattini and his people did that at Frascati years ago.

We haven't made new dramatic progress until perhaps recently we've seen Steve Wilkins comes up with new applications in phase contrast imaging and some of the stuff as you've heard we've done. We stumbled into it. We certainly didn't think about it ahead of time. And some of the Elettra work, may be that's phase contrast in a certain definition.

This field needs a new driver I think, and that new driver's got to be new ideas. It come out of medical related problems, otherwise, if we have another conference like this in five years, I'm a little bit afraid of what the results are going to be. I don't mean to be a damp on it. I think there have been a lot of exciting things happening. The technology has been advancing beautifully. We've seen new ideas here from the technical side.

But I'd like to hear more. That has to come out of medicine. Tell us what the problems are that we can try and solve with these wonderful tools that we have.

That goes to the object of medical applications Rainer just mentioned to you, and the interaction of physicians and physicists. So far, the coupling has been good. It's been dynamic in certain groups, and I would hope it would continue to be. I'd like to stir up a little controversy. I'd like to get some people talking here. We saw some beautiful images taken by Dr. Takeda and his people with aortic graphic imaging, and I tried to get response from physician in the audience. Do you really think that's important ? That's not to say it isn't wonderful work, it's beautiful work. But is it a kind of thing that's going to drive a new technology ? I've been pushing, as you know, for discussions. I have not yet in this group found a physician willing to tell me other than my colleague here from Germany. Do you need compact sources? That's a nice concept; it really is.

What was discussed today is a nice concept for a storage ring, but is it compact in the sense of a clinical tool ? What are the feelings of the physicians regarding clinical tools ? Do you want something you can put in the size of this room ? I think so.

Our physicians have been telling us recently "Without a compact tool, we are not interested." That's absolutely true. And I don't know if it's true here. I can't get anyone to tell me, and I'd like to know the answer to that.

We probably have five years or something left of the development of technology based on our large machines. Once we move beyond that. I don't have a crystal ball, but maybe a couple of research centers might work, and I'd like to hear some response to that. Please let's hear from the physicians. Let's hear from the other physicists in the audience. I have an uneasy feeling about what's going on. I would like to hear a few more comments.

C: As a physician I feel addressed by what Bill Tomlinson just said. It was very interesting for me to participate in this workshop, but what I learned is that we are pretty far away from solutions that we actually need as physicians. We need a compact source, we need some strong support, and arguments to tell administrative bosses, the insurances that we really can do it on a cost-effective base intravenous coronaary angiography (IVCAG), for example.

In Hamburg we'll finish our study within the next year at the most. We will be at a point where we'll have forty or fifty patients investigated, and we'll be able to say if this IVCAG is feasible for routine use or not. At that time we have to know if it is possible to build a compact source. That means a diameter not greater than 12 meters or 15 meters because it will be very rare if a new hospital is built with a space for a circumference of 300 meters. We need small sources.

As physicians we are used to being asked by big companies, Siemens, Phillips, and all the Japanese companies if we use this or that. They develop the technique. We even don't think about it. They have technical solutions for almost everything. Lots of things we don't need. We are not used to being involved in developing actual techniques for a solution to a medical problem, for example.

If you want to spread out synchrotron radiation on the medical applications, I think you need experts, for example, in oncology, neurology, neurosurgery and so on. Ask them what they can imagine that would be better than what they have.

In medicine, we have lots of techniques, tons of techniques. I think it is important to find people in the medical fields from really the daily routine use of medicine who will tell you what will help and what will not.

I don't really think that intracoronary angiography is an advance toward selective coronary angiography which we are doing. It's routine, daily routine. We do 410,000 selective coronary angiographies a year in Germany. So, we really have to find a technique which is cheaper, which is easier, which is outpatient service. There are probably a lots of other different applications in different fields of medicine. As a cardiologist, I have no idea, for example, what would be helpful or not in oncology. For bronchography I can't evaluate, but I think this could be something helpful for a special indication. The problem is the number of investigation enough for the high expenses which are connected with a compact source.

C: A few words about coronary angiography, we cardiologists have a very good method, that is selective coronary arteriography. If we use SR, we have to have a merit over selective coronary arteriography. We have tried IVCAG because its technique is very easy and less risky. I think the intravenous one is a good direction in the future, although it should be improved more. We cardiologists choose techniques from a practical point of view, not only quality. It should be practical. In the present we have selective coronary arteriography and we should have much more opportunities for discussion between physicians and physicists. In Japan there were only a small group of physicians who were interested in SR, so that two years ago we formed the Japanese Medical Society of SR. I am a chairman. We have tried to create the opportunities to discuss SR between physicians and physicists, and I think this is a good idea. We should pursue along this direction.

C: My question concerns coronary angiography in Japan and I understood there have been only four patients actually examined over the last few years. This is to my feeling a discrepancy. We are going to present IVCAG in two weeks at the European meeting of the Society of Cardiology. In the session again, like two months ago, at a large German Congress we presented with the competing methods of CT and MRI tomography. We have to show the best pictures. We have to convince by the pictures, by the result, and by the numbers of patients investigated. Had we only investigated 10 patients nobody would have invited us. There is no chance at all for spreading this method or addressing other cardiologists or just finding some interest.

C: It was only four patients two years ago. It does not sound continuous and not on a daily basis. The reason for this is very simple. The machine we used for the first clinical application to IVCAG belongs to a high energy physics community that has used it for boosting electrons and positrons. It is in an upgrading programme since last year, by that means just before it closed, the medical doctors, Dr. Sugishita and Dr. Itai tried getting involved, and they proceeded Japan's first clinical application. Since then we have had no beams available, particularly for that project. The question is when again we can have SR from the accumulation ring, hopefully is next February or March. After that we will be close it down for another ten months. That 's why we'd like to have our own medical facilitiy which Hyodo explained this morning.

C: I still would like to hear more back from the medical community in terms of its needs and its constraints and so forth. As I said earlier I do believe the future of the field lies with the motivation coming out of our medical colleagues, not so much any more from that of the technical side, the physicists and engineers. That's a personal opinion, and of course I could be proven wrong. But that's what I would like to get a feeling for before the meeting is completely over.

C: We cardiologists are used to work with selective CAG in movie style that is recorded in a cinema mode. Because one can see coronary arteries, which may twist and move, from many directions the cine mode has many advantages over the static style. That's a way our research does. We know that there are technical difficulties which we learned from Dr. Ando or Hyodo. But I think that the cinemode will be better in the future.

C: I understand, and I don't mean any kind of criticism. It's just very helpful if this standard question comes when and where somebody else are doing research in this field, and then I could say in Japan how many patient are being investigated, or in the U.S. so on. It is just very helpful for the method whether it is angiography or anything else. You can talk about investigations in different countries and say that different groups are working on it. It reflects a kind of interest or belief on the method.

C: I have one more comment. I am afraid it is rather dangerous to watch coronary arteries in static style; I mean from one moment of the image, because as I told you coronary arteries twist, and stenotic lesion is not uniform, not concentric sometimes. It is eccentric or only a part of the coronary artery is stenotic. I mean non-uniform, eccentric, so we should watch it in cinemode.

C: I agree. It would be very good, if we could do it in cinemode. But up to now as I understand we don't have the technique, so we started with what we are doing right now. We have two different angles, and we take four pictures per patient. I think we cover it pretty well. Right now the study is going on in our protocol that we control selective CAG every patient. We have confirmation of our diagnoses or not. Up to now we are pretty good with a confirmation rate of 84 percent.

C: In near future we'll also have a good result.

C: I think you have to make a compromise. You must decide if you only want to see two or three of the main coronary arteries, then it's OK to see these. However, if you start to want to see all three including the circumflex, then you have no chance. You can calculate from a statistical point of view. To do it in cinemode, the dose limits you. You can't. You can very easily see the right coronary artery and the LAD, because they have no superposition.

C: I was informed. Dr. Ando, you have 100 millirad per image.

C: And we have 50 times of that. Very sick persons become troubled at the circumflex. We have 15 times more photons per pixel. We have a pixel size 0.4 mm x 0.4 mm. If you have less pixel size, then it's inverse in your case.

C: Further, we are trying to reduce the radiation dose as much as possible. One way to do that is to reduce the number of frames per each second.

C: That means down to 25. Things are OK. What happens with the circumflex as you just mentioned, I have not calculated the statistics yet.

C: I think we can distinguish between the circumflex and the aorta. We need two dimensional moving images, not just a picture, or stopping mode.

C: You mean the discrimination between the left ventricle and the coronary artery ?

C: You used 100 millirad per image, and we use 5 rad per image, it is effective fifty times more. That means if we have the same pixel size, we have effective fifty times more photons, and this means in statistics only for circumflex. If you want to see the LAD, and you want to see the RCA, then you have no problem, because it's behind lung. But the problem is the circumflex, and you cannot find any angle without superposition for the circumflex,

C: We can recognize the circumflex even it is superimposed on the left ventricle. We can recognize it, because it moves over the left ventricle. We can recognize the circumflex even if it is superimposed over the left ventricle. RAO or LAO in any direction we can see coronary arteries and the left ventricle.

Q: Is that LAO ?

Q: A little bit of confusion, was this an aortic injection?

A: No. Intravenous in human. Because it moves. we can recognize it. Anyway I think cinemode is an ideal method for us, although it is a difficult technique.

C: I'd like to answer to Dr. Thomlinson. You said that intraarterial CAG is good in quality, and you asked for a comment from the cardiologist. I think it is not practical for us cardiologists, because there is no difference in technical difficulties between selective CAG and intraarterial CAG with synchrotron radiation. The intraarterial CAG is not practical, so, we do not use it. I prefer selective to intravenous CAG with SR even if it is good in quality. The selective one is good, and there is no difference in techniques.

C. At the present time the golden standard is selective CAG, but I am introducing another approach of SR to use for diagnosing coronary artery by which much clearer images are given compared to intravenous CAG. First process to insert catheter into artery is same. Direct coronary catheterization which may cause mortality is not needed in aortographic procedure. Total frequency of fatal accident in selective CAG is reported about 0.14 % in 1991, this number has not changed significantly even inspite of the improvement of catheter. In individuals more than 60 years old and less than 1 year old, the mortality rate of selective CAG is 0.25 and 1.75 %, respectively. Whereas the frequency of mortality in aortographic CAG is reported about 0.025% in 1983. Now the contrast material has been changed to non-ionic types, and material of catheter was improved, then we can use soft and small diameter of cathters from 6 - 7F to 4 - 5F. The fatal accident due to aortographic procedure could be significantly reduced now. So the technique in the aortographic procedure is not same as selective and is much safer than selective CAG accorging to the statistical reports. Also aortography is much easier to perform than selective CAG because no special training of this technique is necessary to intubate catheter into coronary artery directly. Occasionally the conventional selective coronary arteriography was not successful due to arteriosclerotic changes, but aortographic approach may not have such problems. The x-ray exposure to the operator would be greatly reduced because the catheter is placed in the aortic root, and the contrast injection can be performed by injector instead of hand injection. The pediatric cardiovascular diagnosis will be performed easily. The image quality of aortography obtained by dog experiments is thought to be sufficient for clinical diagnosis because the image of the coronary structures is clear, and even coronary branches of less than 0.2 mm in diameter and other structures of the coronary arteries are revealed even when the cardiac function is reduced. Furthermore, this aortographic arterial approach provides a means of overcoming the image overlap of the coronary arteries on the cardiac chambers. This may lead to a solution to solve the problem in intravenous CAG with SR.

C: I was just trying to stir up a little bit of conversation here.

C: I have not yet started SR research. I am a physician, and I specialize in cardiac positron emission tomography, PET now in NIRS. We have the same discussions in the PET field regarding cost effectiveness, especially in the United States. One goal is a routine clinical application. We need show people how cost effective it is, then we need to discuss how many patients we can handle per day. The second is just clinical research. I think we have to focus on the second way, even though patient numbers is very small, even though it's very expensive, or radiation dose is not small compared with conventional techniques. We may be able to obtain valuable information from this small amount of clinical research, for example, micro-circulation information or something. Even though it's very expensive, and radiation dose is not so small, the second approach is very important in clinical application.

A: The first way is a very difficult issue, cost, and patients per day, etc. for positron emission tomography, especially in the U.S.A.

Q: You must get funding, and you'll never get funding in Germany for only part of the people.

C: I believe that if we have, for example, 10,000 patients per year for one disease in a year and, even if we only perform 10 patient clinical research, then the data is very valuable, for example, for micro-circulation information. This is very helpful to understand the concept of some kinds of disease, for example cardiomyopathy. I think we should take the second way, and we should emphasize that the second way is very important. That is the best way.

C: I agree. You may be right with micro-circulation from what we learned in this meeting. But for coronary angiography it is definite that selective coronary angiography is of higher quality. We can't start saying we have to make a high investment for only a few people, because intravenous coronary angiography reveals results which we don't get with selective coronary angiography. That is not the case. The selective would be better.

C: But coronary arteriography, we can know of just 1 mm in diameter, but when we have arterial, we don't know of small arteries, 1 mm or smaller

C: That 's what I'm saying. It might be correct what you said for these very small vessels, but not what we were talking about in the high numbers of CAG patients. We have to go to the first way. We don't even think about the second way for coronary angiography, not for micro-vessel disease.

C: If you choose the first way, clinical application, then finally you need to show cost effectiveness. Your procedure is cost effective, which is very difficult.

C: Yes, that's we are talking about, cost effectiveness. This is what Dr. Dix just tried to explain with his transparency.

C: The comment you've just made is very important, and in some sense critical. We, for many years, tried to swing the emphasis at Brookhaven facility from the initially wonderful goal of absolutely pure clinical applications, which is one of the initial thrusts going back to even the days we were doing the work at Stanford SR facility there. We've always tried to temper the enthusiasm by saying that even if it's not an ultimate clinical tool, it should have a place in basic research. That's your comment. That's your type two.

We tried that, and our funding agency said "No, it's too expensive." Recently our medical support, the people who work with us, have also through their organizations, their hospitals, limited research funds. What they basically said to us is that we have to put our money elsewhere. It is just too expensive, if you can consider the overhead in bringing a patient to the Synchrotron, no matter how many patients you do a day, it's probably four or five hours of overhead on physician time, and, Dr. Dill certainly knows that's true, that that is an extraordinarily expensive research program, and recently they have said no, they just simply cannot afford that level of research. Therefore, as you have just heard, at least in Germany, and certainly in the States because we are not doing any more, really the only hope now would be class I. Nothing else but the hard fact of economics. The research budgets are limited. In the United States the clinical facilities are being forced more and more out of research, and into the clinic, just because the cost reimbursements for patient care is going down, and the time and costs are going up, and the clinical staff are required to be in the clinic far more hours. The rather inefficient use of the synchrotron for a CAG exam, even as you point out, even though it might be a wonderful research tool, and I believe it could be, I am a physicist, we've been stopped. No. we cannot do it, and it's a shame. I think your point is absolutely right. It could be a wonderful research tool . But in today's economic climate, it's failed in our country, and obviously it's also true in Germany. I hope it's not true in Japan. I'd love to see that sort of direction being taken at some level, to be saying we have two or three centers in the country, Spring-8 is coming on, and machines in Tsukuba, and elsewhere. If you could define research protocols to try and answer questions, which then could be propagated in conventional medicine away from the synchrotron. That would be wonderful. I think that's a thrust that perhaps should receive more attention than trying to propagate this as an absolute clinical tool. That's a well placed comment. I'm glad you made it.

Perspective for Medical Applications of Phase-Contrast X-Ray Imaging

Atsushi Momose[1], Tohoru Takeda[2], Yuji Itai[2], Akio Yoneyama[3], and Keiichi Hirano[4]

[1]Advanced Research Laboratory, Hitachi, Ltd., Hatoyama, Saitama 350-03, Japan
[2]Institute of Clinical Medicine, University of Tsukuba, Tsukuba, Ibaraki 305, Japan
[3]Central Research Laboratory, Hitachi, Ltd., Kokubunji, Tokyo 182, Japan
[4]Institute of Materials Structure Science, High Energy Accelerator Research Organization, Tsukuba, Ibaraki 305, Japan

SUMMARY. Interferometric phase-contrast X-ray imaging is experimentally proved to be sensitive to biological soft-tissue features without the need for staining. Radiographic and tomographic applications of this method are attractive from a diagnostic point of view. In this paper, we have presented the principle of phase-contrast X-ray computed tomography and observation results of human soft tissues. We have shown that the structures of soft structures, such as cancer, are clearly revealed. The good image quality motivated us to study the feasibility of the technique for medical applications. An important technical aim is to make an interferometer having large observation area. A two-crystal X-ray interferometer is a candidate as a device for that purpose. We expect that phase-contrast mammography might be possible with such an interferometer.

KEY WORDS: X-rays, Phase contrast, Cancer, Tomography, Mammography

INTRODUCTION

Hard X-rays are useful in nondestructively investigating structures inside thick objects. Applications to medical imaging have been studied for a long time, and many techniques are in practical use. It is also true, however, that new X-ray imaging technologies are required for more advanced diagnoses. Synchrotron sources provide us with new possibilities for exploring new medical imaging methods. In this paper, we concentrate on the possibility of phase-contrast X-ray imaging.

When X-rays travel through an object, both the amplitude and phase of the X-ray wave are modified by the object. In conventional X-ray transmission imaging, contrast is generated from the change in the amplitude. In this case, the amplitude contrast (absorption contrast) is usually insufficient for investigating soft structures in a body. This is because soft tissues are almost transparent to hard X-rays. On the other hand, phase-contrast X-ray imaging has recently been studied actively. Because the phase-shift cross section is much larger than the absorption cross section for light elements, high sensitivity to soft tissues is expected with a moderate X-ray dose.

X-ray phase information is usually missing in a transmission image behind an object. Therefore, special techniques are necessary to generate phase contrast. In the hard X-ray energy region, phase-contrast imaging methods, such as an interferometric method[1–4], a holography-like method[5–9], a Schlieren-like method[10–14], and others[15,16] are reported. Our technique is based on the interferometric method using a crystal X-ray interferometer[17] because the method was experimentally proved to be sensitive to biological soft-tissue features[3,4]. Starting from the interferometric method, we have proposed and demonstrated phase-contrast X-ray computed tomography[18]. It was shown that the sensitivity was substantial enough to depict structures inside soft tissues without staining[19–23]. In this paper, we report our recent activity on the development of phase-contrast X-ray imaging. Also, prospects for medical applications of phase-contrast X-ray imaging are discussed.

INTERPRETATION OF PHASE CONTRAST

It should be noted that the precise meaning of *phase contrast* is different depending on the method used. In the case of the interferometric method, one can observe fringes which appear every 2π phase shift. On the other hand, using the holography-like method, fringes caused by Fresnel diffraction are seen. In the case of Schlieren-like method, a part of a specific phase gradient is emphasized. Whereas such images may be useful to some extent for medical applications. However, absorption contrast is usually superposed in the phase-contrast images and information obtainable from the images is limited. Recently, we have achieved a breakthrough which enables a more sophisticated imaging method to be carried out, and this is described below.

In general, the refractive index n is written as

$$n = 1 - \delta - i\beta, \tag{1}$$

where i is the unit imaginary number. The changes in the X-ray intensity and phase on pathing through an object are related to β and δ, respectively. The projection of β corresponds to the logarithm of the X-ray intensity transmittance T; that is,

$$-\log T = \frac{4\pi}{\lambda} \int \beta dz, \tag{2}$$

where λ is the X-ray wavelength, and z is the distance in the the direction of X-ray propagation. This is a fundamental relation to understand absorption-contrast images. A relation similar to eq. (2) is found in the phase-shift process; that is,

$$\Phi = \frac{2\pi}{\lambda} \int \delta dz, \tag{3}$$

where Φ is the phase shift caused by a sample. This means that measuring the spatial distribution of Φ (phase mapping image) is analogous to the procedure of the absorption-contrast method. Furthermore, in the hard X-ray energy region, δ and β are written as

$$\delta = \frac{r_e \lambda^2}{2\pi} \sum_k N_k(Z_k + f_k^r) \quad \text{and} \quad \beta = \frac{\lambda}{4\pi} \sum_k N_k \mu_{ak}, \tag{4}$$

where r_e is the classical electron radius, and N_k, Z_k, f_k^r, and μ_{ak} are the atomic density, the atomic number, the anomalous atomic scattering factor (real part), and the atomic absorption coefficient of element k, respectively. The substitution of eq. (4) into eqs. (2) and (3) yields

$$-\log T = \int \sum_k N_k \mu_{ak} dz, \tag{5}$$

$$\Phi = \int \sum_k N_k p_k dz, \quad p_k \equiv r_e \lambda (Z_k + f_k^r). \tag{6}$$

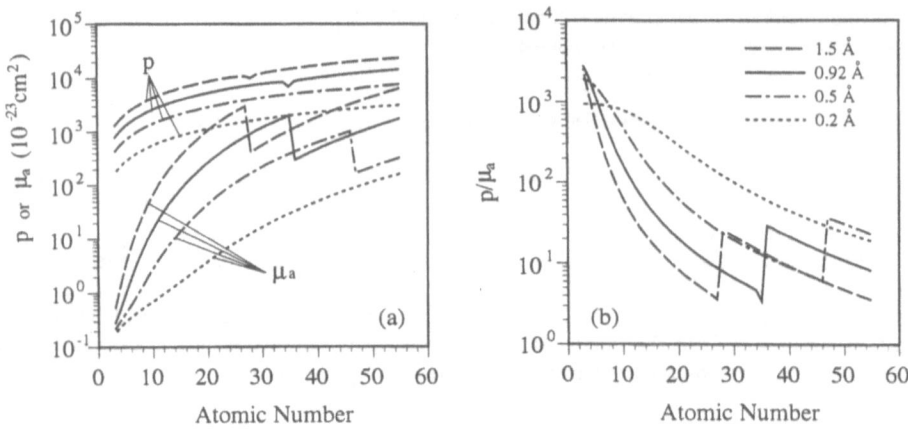

Fig. 1. (a) Calculated value of p and μ_a versus the atomic number and (b) the ratio p/μ_a.

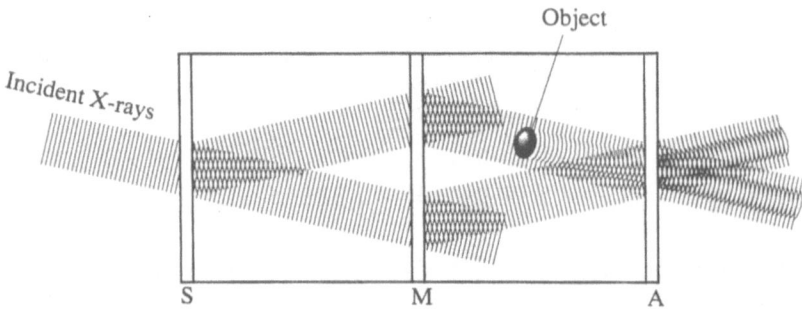

Fig. 2. X-ray interferometer and created beam paths. Wafers (S, M, A) function as X-ray half mirrors.

Thus, the difference between $-\log T$ and Φ derives from the paticular forms of μ_a and p. Figure 1(a) shows the values of μ_a and p as functions of the atomic number[24]. The ratio p/μ_a is also shown in Fig. 1(b). Curves for 8.3 keV, 13.5 keV, 25 keV, and 62 keV X-rays are shown. Thus, p is always larger than μ_a, and the ratio of the two is almost a thousand for light elements. This comparison indicates that improvement in the sensitivity is expected by the corresponding amount when the phase-mapping image is observed.

As mentioned, the phase-mapping image is different from phase-contrast images which are experimentally observable. To take advantage of the difference shown in Fig. 1, a technique is needed to obtain phase-mapping images from phase-contrast images. We used the interferometric method to measure the phase-mapping images as below.

A typical X-ray interferometer is shown in Fig. 2. The entire body of the interferometer is carved out of an ingot of silicon crystal. Three wafers formed in parallel with the same spacing function as half mirrors for X-rays when the diffraction condition is satisfied. A beam is split in to two beams behind each wafer. Consequently, X-ray beam paths shown in Fig. 2 are created.

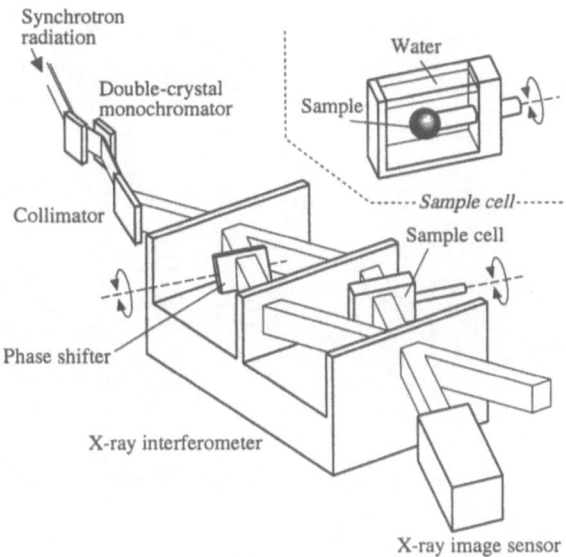

Synchrotron
radiation

Double-crystal
monochromator

Water

Sample

Collimator

⋯⋯⋯⋯Sample cell⋯⋯⋯⋯

Sample cell

Phase shifter

X-ray interferometer

X-ray image sensor

Fig. 3. Experimental setup of phase-contrast X-ray computed tomography.

When an object is placed in a beam path, an interference pattern corresponding to the phase shift caused by the object is observed in the outgoing X-ray beams from the third wafer (A).

A breakthrough was obtained by introducing the fringe scanning method for measuring the phase shift[25] which was originally developed in visible light interferometry. With this method, the phase-mapping image is calculated from several interference patterns which are obtained by changing the phase difference step by step between the two beams in the interferometer. When M interference patterns are obtained by changing the phase difference in $2\pi/M$ steps, the phase-mapping image Φ is calculated as

$$\Phi = \text{Arg}\left[\sum_{l=1}^{M} I_l \exp(-2\pi i l/M)\right], \qquad (7)$$

where I_l is the interference pattern obtained when the phase difference is $2\pi l/M$. Arg[ ] indicates the extraction of the argument. With this procedure, the influence of absorption contrast is removed, and the image contrast is quantitatively understandable. Furthermore, phase-contrast X-ray computed tomography is realized by processing the phase-mapping images obtained in different projection directions.

TOMOGRAPHIC OBSERVATION

As mentioned, both $-\log T$ and Φ are mathematically expressed in the form of projections. According to the principle of X-ray computed tomography, when input data are projections of the distribution of f which conveys structural information inside a sample, a tomogram is reconstructed as a map of f. In the case of absorption-contrast X-ray computed tomography, the spatial distribution of the linear absorption coefficient μ, which is equivalent to $4\pi\beta/\lambda$, is reconstructed, because $-\log T$ is the projection of μ. Similarly, when the phase mapping images

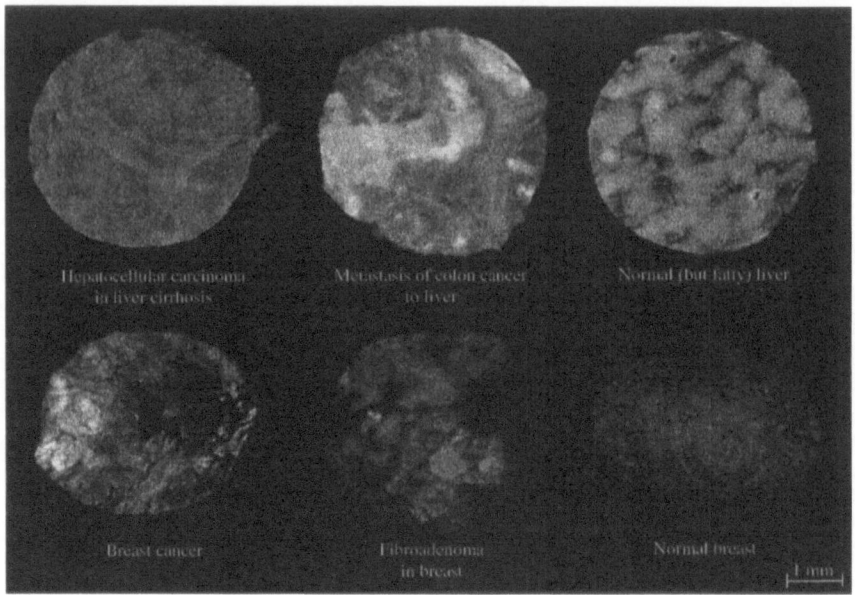

Fig. 4. Phase-contrast tomograms of human tissues.

are processed with the algorithm of tomography, a phase-contrast tomogram which maps δ is reconstructed.

Figure 3 shows an experimental setup for phase-contrast X-ray computed tomography. We installed the apparatus[20] in station BL-14B of the Photon Factory, Tsukuba, Japan, where hard X-rays from a vertical wiggler were available. X-rays of 17.7 keV were introduced to the X-ray interferometer. The thickness of the wafers of the interferometer was 1 mm, and the gap between them was 34 mm. The size of the observation area provided by the system was about 5 mm × 5 mm. A sample was rotated in a cell filled with water. A 0.5-mm thick plastic plate was rotated to vary the phase difference between the two interfering beams in order to apply the fringe scanning method. The number of the steps for the fringe scan was ten, and the sample was rotated in 0.9° steps. The X-ray intensity in front of the sample was estimated to be 5×10^5 photons/mm²/second. The exposure time to obtain one interference pattern was 6 seconds with the X-ray sensing pickup tube[26] operated at a pixel size of 12 μm × 12 μm.

We observed human tissues with phase-contrast X-ray computed tomography. Extirpated organs fixed in formalin were cut in a cylindrical shape approximately 4 mm in diameter. Structures characteristic of tissues were revealed. Carcinoma (the upper part of Fig. 4a) was differentiated from liver cirrhosis. Figure 4b shows the inside structure of a tumor appearing in a liver (metastasis of colon cancer). Necrosis was revealed with a bright contrast. Dark area in Fig. 4c corresponds to fatty tissue. Figure 4d shows the inside structure of breast cancer. Bright contrast indicates fibrous tissues in the cancer lesion. Fibroadonoma was observed as shown in Fig. 4e. The revealed structure in the tomogram is different from that in Fig. 4d. This suggests the possibility of distinguishing cancer from benign tumors. Detailed histological analyses of the tomograms are in progress.

POSSIBILITY OF MEDICAL APPLICATION

As shown in Fig. 4, many soft-tissue structures are detectable by using hard X-ray phase contrast. As a next step, we aim at applications of this technique to *in vivo* observation, and further to clinical imaging.

First, we present a guideline to interpret and predict contrast in phase-contrast tomograms. As mentioned, a phase-contrast tomogram maps the value δ inside a sample. (Strictly, the tomograms shown in Fig. 4 mapped the difference in δ between samples and water, because samples were observed in water.) According to eq. (4), δ is approximately proportional to $\sum NZ$, because f^r is negligible for light elements. This means that we can assume that δ is proportional to the specific gravity (density). Therefore, we can read phase-contrast tomograms as density maps. Although the density distribution appears in absorption-contrast tomograms to some extent, the sensitivity to the density deviation is far different from that of phase-contrast tomograms. We have estimated the detection limit of density deviation in soft tissue from the noise in our phase-contrast tomograms. The value was several milligrams per cubic centimeter[20]. When heavy elements are contained in samples, f^r is no longer negligible at their absorption edges. In such a case, we can use the relevant absorption edges to detect the distribution of the specific elements with phase contrast.

Because small density deviation is detectable with phase contrast, we can expect blood contrast without injecting contrast media. For convenience in sample preparation, the tissues observed by phase-contrast X-ray computed tomography did not contain blood. However, we have measured the refractive index of human blood with the X-ray interferometer. According to the result[27], δ of blood was about 3% larger than that of serum. This is consistent in that red blood cells are comparatively heavy among soft tissues. Therefore, it is expected that blood vessels, internal bleedings, and so on might be observable with the contrast caused by the difference in the blood density.

Finally, we point out that staining is useful even in a phase-contrast mode. It is a merit of phase-contrast X-ray imaging that many structures can be revealed without staining. However, to emphasize a specific structure, staining is necessary. Here, *staining* means the injection of materials which produce an enhanced phase shift. In this case, we are no longer restricted to using heavy materials for staining. Therefore, contrast media can be selected from a wide variety of choices. For example, by injecting physiological salt solution into blood, limited area could be emphasized with a negative contrast. Exploring contrast media for phase-contrast imaging is meaningful for applications of phase-contrast to diagnosis.

To achieve *in vivo* observation, however, we need to develop an apparatus which is suitable for objects larger than samples observed in Fig. 4. This means that a larger X-ray interferometer should be developed to generate interference with broader X-ray beams. Unfortunately, the size of the X-ray interferometer shown in Fig. 1 is limited by the size of an ingot of silicon crystal. The maximum size of observable samples is estimated to be about 2 cm. To observe objects more than 2 cm, we began examining the feasibility of an X-ray interferometer consisting of two crystal blocks shown in Fig. 5. The spacing between the blocks can be selected depending of the size of an object to be investigated. In this case, however, we have to align the two blocks and keep them stable with an accuracy corresponding to the lattice spacing of silicon to generate interference. Using a laboratory X-ray source, the interferometer was operated by Becker and Bonse[28]. There is, however, no evidence that the interferometer is suitable for phase-contrast X-ray imaging using synchrotron X-rays. Preliminarily, we studied the performance of a small

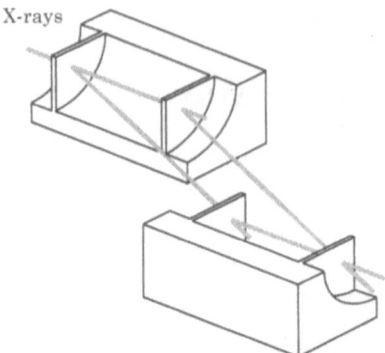

Fig. 5. Two-crystal X-ray interferometer.

(but larger than Becker and Bonse's) two-crystal X-ray interferometer at the same station as the tomographic experiments. As a result, the interferometer and the stage for the alignment of two blocks were capable of generating interference patterns of 13.5-keV X-rays with 70% fringe visibility[29]. Although we would have to develop a larger two-crystal interferometer for *in vivo* observation, the system might be a candidate as a device for such future applications.

Besides phase-contrast X-ray computed tomography, we expect radiographic applications, such as phase-contrast mammography and phase-contrast radiography. The technique for obtaining the phase-mapping images is useful even in a radiographic mode, because the images can be interpreted quantitatively. In addition, the time for the measurement can be short as required in practical radiographic applications. As shown in Fig. 4, we could depict structures in the breast tissues which did not contain any calcification. We expect phase-contrast mammography to be suitable as the first target of medical applications.

ACKNOWLEDGEMENTS

The authors are grateful for discussions with Drs. K. Nakayama and E. Seya. The experiments were performed under a proposal number 95-G349 approved by the National Laboratory for High Energy Physics.

REFERENCES

1. Bonse U, Hart M (1965) An X-ray interferometer with long interfering beam paths. Appl Phys Lett 7: 99-101
2. Ando M, Hosoya S (1972) An attempt at X-ray phase-contrast microscopy. In: Shinoda G, Kohra K, Ichinokawa T (eds) Proc. 6th International Conference of X-ray Optics and Microanalysis. University of Tokyo Press, pp. 63-68,
3. Momose A, Fukuda J (1995) Phase-contrast radiographs of nonstained rat cerebellar specimen. Med Phys 22: 375-380
4. Takeda T, Momose A, Itai Y, Wu J, Hirano K (1995) Phase-contrast imaging with synchrotron X-rays for cancer lesion. Acad Radiol 2: 799-803
5. Snigirev A, Snigireva I, Kohn V, Kuznetsov S, Schelokov I (1995) On the possibility of x-ray phase contrast microimaging by coherent high-energy synchrotron radiation. Rev Sci Instrum 66: 5486-5492

6. Snigirev A, Snigireva I, Suvorov A, Kocsis M, Kohn V (1995) Phase contrast microimaging by coherent high energy synchrotron radiation. ESRF Newsletters No. 24: 23-25

7. Cloetens P, Barratt R, Baruchel J, Guigay JP, Schlenker M (1996) Phase objects in synchrotron radiation hard x-ray imaging. J Phys D: Appl Phys 29: 133-146

8. Wilkins SW, Gureyev TE, Gao D, Pogany A, Stevenson AW (1996) Phase-contrast imaging using polychromatic hard X-rays. Nature 384: 335-338

9. Raven C, Snigirev A, Snigireva I, Spanne P, Souvorov A, Kohn V (1996) Phase-contrast micro-tomography with coherent high-energy synchrotron radiation. Appl Phys Lett 69: 1826-1828

10. Forster E, Goetz K, Zaumseil P (1980) Double crystal diffractometry for the characterization of targets for Laser fusion experiments. Kristall und Technik 15: 937-945

11. Somenkov VA, Tkalich AK, Shil'shtein SSh (1991) Refraction contrast in x-ray introscopy. Sov Phys Tech Phys 36: 1309-1311

12. Davis TJ, Gao D, Gureyev TE, Stevenson AW, Wilkins SW (1995) Phase-contrast imaging of weakly absorbing materials using hard X-rays. Nature 373: 595-598

13. Davis TJ, Gureyev TE, Gao D, Stevenson AW, Wilkins SW (1995) X-ray imaging contrast from a simple phase object. Phys Rev Lett 74: 3173-3176

14. Ingal VN, Beliaevskaya EA (1995) X-ray plane-wave topography observation of the phase contrast from a non-crystalline object. J Phys D: Appl Phys 28: 2314-2317

15. Nugent KA, Gureyev TE, Cookson DF, Paganin D, Barnea Z (1996) Quantitative phase imaging using hard X rays. Phys Rev Lett 77: 2961-2964

16. Snigirev A, Snigireva I, Bosecke P, Lequien S, Schelokov I (1997) High energy X-ray phase contrast microscopy using a circular Bragg-Fresnel lens. Opt Commun 135: 378-384

17. Bonse U, Hart M (1965) An X-ray interferometer. Appl Phys Lett 6: 155-156

18. Momose A (1995) Demonstration of phase-contrast X-ray computed tomography using an X-ray interferometer. Nucl Instrum Methods A352: 622-628

19. Momose A, Takeda T, Itai Y, (1995) Phase-contrast X-ray computed tomography for observing biological specimens and organic materials. Rev Sci Instrum 66: 1434-1436

20. Momose A, Takeda T, Itai Y, Hirano K (1996) Tomographic image reconstruction using X-ray phase information. SPIE Proc 2708: 674-684

21. Momose A, Takeda T, Itai Y, Hirano K (1996) Phase-contrast X-ray computed tomography for observing biological soft tissues. Nature Medicine 2: 473-475

22. Bonse U, Busch F (1996) X-ray computed microtomography (μCT) using synchrotron radiation (SR). Prog Biophys Molec Biol 65: 133-169

23. Momose A, Takeda T, Itai Y, Hirano K (1997) Phase-contrast X-ray microtomography: application to human cancerous tissues. In: Thieme J, Schmahl G, Umbach E, Rudolph D (eds) X-ray microscopy and spectromicroscopy. Springer-Verlag, Heidelberg, in press.

24. The values of μ_a and f^r were taken from, Sasaki S (1990) In: X-Ray Absorption Coefficients of the Elements (Li to Bi, U). KEK Report 90-16, and Sasaki S (1989) In: Numerical Tables of Anomalous Scattering Factors Calculated by the Cromer and Liberman's Method. KEK Report 88-14.

25. Bruning JH, Herriott DR, Gallagher JE, Rosenfeld DP, White AD, Brangaccio DJ (1974) Digital wavefront measuring interferometer for testing optical surfaces of lenses. Appl Opt 13: 2693-2703

26. Suzuki Y, Hayakawa K, Usami K, Hirano T, Endoh T, Okamura Y (1989) X-ray sensing pickup tube. Rev Sci Instrum 60: 2299-2302

27. Momose A, Takeda T, Itai Y, Hirano K (1995) Contrast effect of blood on phase-contrast X-ray imaging. Acad Radiol 2: 883-887

28. Becker P, Bonse U (1974) The skew-symmetric two-crystal X-ray interferometer. J Appl Crystr 7: 593-598

29. Momose A, Yoneyama A, Hirano K (1997) Operation of two-crystal X-ray interferometer at the Photon Factory. J Synchrotron Rad 4: 311-312

Q: What is the size of your block ?

A: In this preliminary study the thickness of the wafer was 1 mm and the distance between them was 35 mm.

Q: What is the size of the beam?

A: About 7 mm.

Q: What would be the size of the interferometer that you would need for mammography?

A: The beam section should be, for example, 10cm by 10cm. To produce such a beam, the distance between the wafers should be around 50 cm or 70 cm. Of course it depends on the X-ray energy. I show you the optimum energy which should be used if the thickness of the mamma is tuned to, for example 5 cm, the optimum energy is something like 30KeV.

New Methods of X-Ray Imaging based on Phase Contrast

Dachao Gao[1], Tim E. Gureyev[2], Andrew Pogany,[1] Andrew W. Stevenson[1] &
Stephen W. Wilkins[1]

[1]CSIRO Manufacturing Science & Technology, Private Bag 33, Clayton South MDC,
Victoria 3169, Australia (**e-mail**: xrsi@mst.csiro.au)
[2]CSIRO Forestry & Forest Products, Private Bag 10, Clayton South MDC, Victoria 3169,
Australia

SUMMARY. Phase-contrast X-ray images can be produced in various ways. Some aspects
of the relatively simple "in-line" method are presented which may be implemented using a
quasi-spherical X-ray wave with high spatial but not chromatic coherence. Appropriate
sources can be found in commercially-available microfocus tubes or at synchrotrons.
Compared to previous phase-contrast methods, the present one offers relatively simple
implementation, relatively high intensity and a large field of view, making it potentially
suitable for clinical applications.

KEY WORDS: Phase-contrast, imaging, radiography, refractive index, X-rays

INTRODUCTION

Towards the latter part of 1995 the world celebrated the 100th anniversary of Wilhelm Conrad
Röntgen's discovery of X-rays, for which he was awarded the first Nobel Prize for physics
in 1901. The impact of this discovery throughout the next 100 years could not possibly have
been foreseen, although Röntgen did write to his friend Zehnder on the results of mailing
reprints of his publication, including X-ray images, to scientists in various countries, "Then
hell broke loose!", and Frau Röntgen is known to have observed that "Our domestic peace
is gone".

During the past 100 years, the ability of X-rays to penetrate matter of various kinds and the
fact that different materials, such as soft tissue and bone, absorb X-rays by differing
amounts, has provided the means for imaging a great variety of objects or samples; the most
well-known field being that of medical radiography - see Röntgen's famous X-ray image of
his wife Bertha's hand [1]. Essentially all of the X-ray radiographic images recorded since
Röntgen's discovery have been collected and interpreted on the basis of absorption contrast.
This statement is equally true of the startling cross-sectional images of the human body
obtained by computerised axial tomography (CAT scanning), with which we have now
become familiar. The application of (X-ray) radiography to the non-destructive
characterisation of materials of technological importance is also very well established.

PHASE CONTRAST

The index of refraction for X-rays can be written as $n = 1 - \delta - i\beta$, where the last (i.e. imaginary) term is the one which gives rise to absorption. Recently however, several research groups around the world (see, for example, refs. 2-8) have been concentrating on ways of imaging utilising the fact that, when penetrating matter, the phase of an X-ray wave changes, as in the more familiar case of visible-light optics, leading to the possibility of refractive effects. Furthermore, the energy dependence of the two components of the refractive index is very different:

$$\beta(E) = \frac{hc}{4\pi E} \mu(E) \sim O(E^{-4})$$

$$\delta(E) = \frac{r_0 h^2 c^2}{2\pi E^2} N_0 f_R \sim O(E^{-2})$$

where E is the photon energy, μ the linear absorption coefficient, r_0 the classical electron radius, N_0 the number of atoms per unit volume, and f_R the real part of the atomic scattering factor. In particular, δ decreases much more slowly with increasing energy than does β (or μ); see Table 1.

Table 1. Comparison of absorption and phase thickness for Carbon: $t_a = 1/\mu$, $t_p = 2\pi/\phi$, ϕ being the phase difference per unit length.

E(keV)	λ(Å)	$t_a(\mu m)$	$t_p(\mu m)$
~0.25	50	1.3	1.2
~1.2	10	3.9	3.1
~12	1	4500	33
~50	0.25	420000	132

Even though $1-\delta$ differs from unity by only about one part in 10^6 for light materials, the very small value of λ means that large phase shifts can be produced even by quite moderate thickness or density variations. Nevertheless, typical refraction angles are only of the order of a few arc seconds, and quite delicate methods are required to show these refractive effects [2-8]. One such method developed in our group is illustrated schematically in Fig. 1.

The source may be either a conventional X-ray tube or a synchrotron. The first crystal provides a monochromatic, expanded plane wave for transmission through the specimen. The analyser pair selects a particular component of the transmitted wave field, selection being performed by rocking the analyser crystal pair by a small amount (< 1 arc sec). In this way bright- and dark-field components can be imaged (see, for example, Fig. 3 in ref. 2).

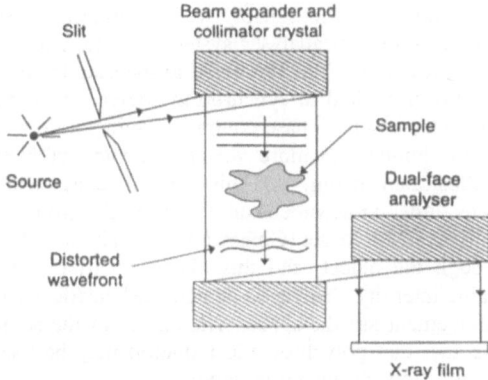

Fig. 1. Schematic diagram of the experimental arrangement, including perfect-crystal-Si monochromator (beam expander and collimator) and analyser, used to collect phase-contrast X-ray images. This method involves the X-ray beam incident on the sample being a monochromatic plane wave. After ref. 2.

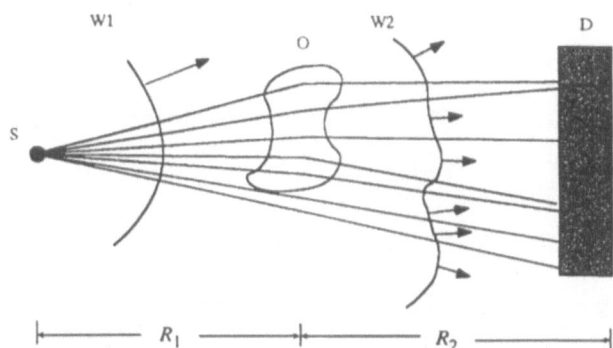

Fig. 2. Schematic diagram of the new experimental arrangement used to collect phase-contrast X-ray images. The X-ray beam incident on the object (O) is a polychromatic spherical wave (wavefront W1). A microfocus X-ray source (S) is used and the two-dimensional detector (D) intercepts the distorted X-ray wavefront (W2) transmitted through O. After ref. 9.

This and other crystal-based methods work reasonably well, within the constraints imposed by the physical size of the monochromator/analyser system, the need for high mechanical stability of components, and the low X-ray flux delivered to the sample. For these reasons, clinical medical applications appear limited to synchrotron sources. In order to overcome these and other limitations and to try to make phase-contrast imaging more widely applicable, we recently developed a much simpler and more versatile method of hard X-ray phase-contrast imaging [9,10], as illustrated in Fig. 2. This method relies on a quasi-spherical wave which can be produced by either a microfocus tube, or a synchrotron-based source with capillary concentration and a fluorescent target (Chikawa [11]). The wavefront is inevitably distorted by its passage through the object, and this distortion after further propagation manifests itself as an observable intensity change, as depicted schematically in Fig. 3. Very important aspects of this arrangement are the appropriate choice of the source size and the distances R_1 and R_2, and the fact that polychromatic radiation may be used, whereas the earlier techniques invariably use monochromatic radiation.

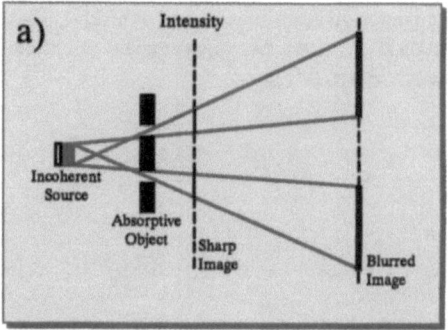

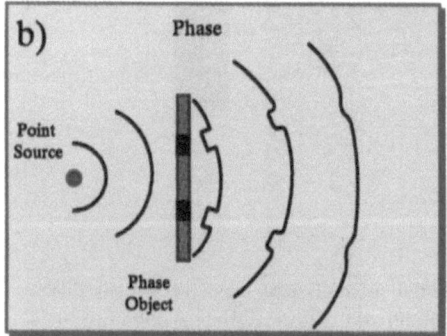
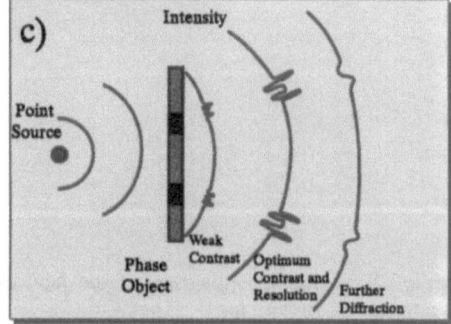

Fig. 3. (a) Geometric-optics representation of imaging of an absorptive object with an incoherent source, showing blurring due to object-image separation. (b) Wave-optics representation of imaging of a phase object with a coherent source, showing phase distortion of the wavefront. (c) As for (b), but showing observable intensity variation due to wavefront interference.

The small source size (typically 10-20 μm for commercially available microfocus tubes) can provide the sufficiently high level of spatial coherence on which the method relies. The low temporal coherence (large wavelength spread) inherent in such a source does not seriously affect this type of phase contrast. The image formed is actually a type of in-line hologram [12], and a reconstruction step is in principle required to retrieve the phase distribution introduced by the object. The relationships involved are conveniently treated in terms of spatial frequencies and intensity contrast transfer functions (CTF) (Fig. 4). Absorption

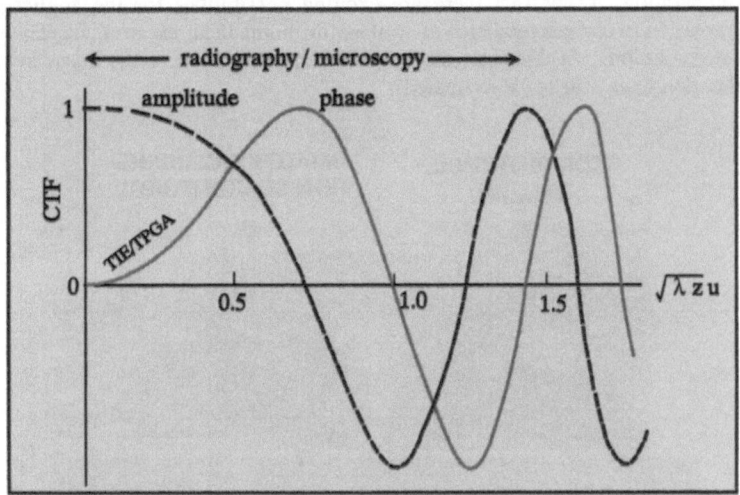

Fig. 4. Phase and amplitude contrast transfer functions (for intensity) for a point source. z is the effective object-image (radiography) distance, and u = 1/d is the spatial frequency, where d is the spatial period.

contrast can also be included naturally in this theory [13]. The absorption CTF (red curve) starts at unity for small spatial frequencies, like the more familiar modulation transfer function, but takes negative values (indicating contrast reversal) for certain spatial frequencies. On the other hand, the phase CTF (green curve) starts from zero (meaning no contrast produced by a uniform thickness homogeneous object) and increases quadratically for the small spatial frequency values typical of radiography. It can be shown that this has the effect of enhancing edge contrast in a phase object. This means that object features (e.g. anatomical details in a biological sample), especially sharp boundaries such as occur for example at the inner walls of various ducts, can be identified directly in this so-called *differential phase contrast* regime, without the need for image reconstruction. For quantitative digital image reconstruction purposes we may note that the phase and amplitude changes are then given by the projection or thin phase grating approximation, equation (5) in [9], and image reconstruction may be performed using the transport of intensity equation [14], whose validity extends roughly over the region of the curve labelled "TIE/TPGA" in Fig. 4. For higher spatial frequencies, such as may occur in microscopy, different methods will generally be required.

RESULTS

Figures 5 to 7 show various phase-contrast images collected with the basic experimental arrangement depicted schematically in Fig. 2.

Although these pictures were taken with a conventional (albeit microfocus) source, the excellent coherence properties and very high brilliance of synchrotron sources, particularly of the third generation, means that there are exciting possibilities for the application of synchrotron radiation to clinical medicine as well as for biomedical research, especially with increased time resolution. At this early stage of development however the most favourable areas of application have still to be evaluated.

CONVENTIONAL
IMAGES

IMAGES INCLUDING
PHASE-CONTRAST

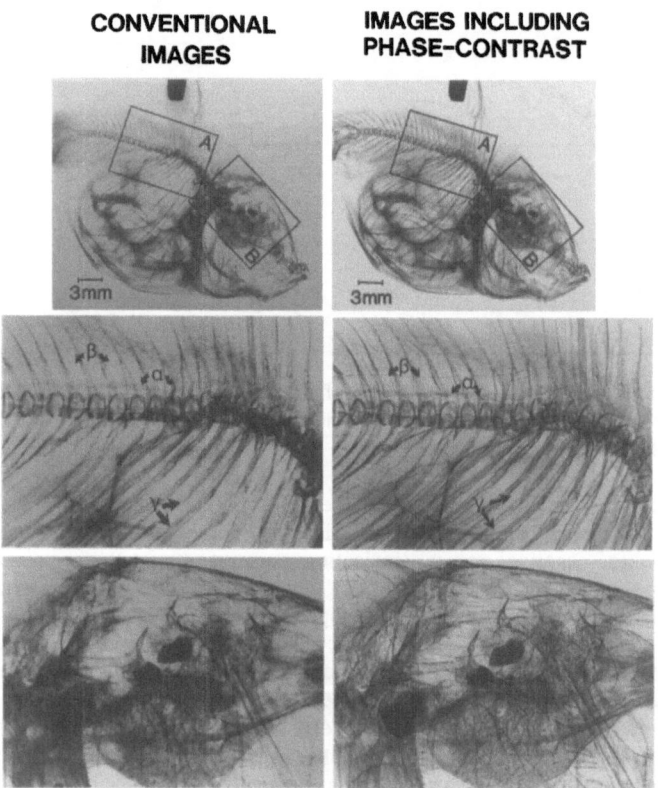

Fig. 5. Conventional and phase-contrast X-ray images for a small aquarium golfish. A microfocus source operated at 60kV was used and $R_1 = 300$mm, with $R_2 = 1$mm for the conventional image and $R_2 = 1100$mm for the phase-contrast image. Enlargements of the areas A and B are also shown in each case. The spinal cord (labelled "α"), ligament (labelled "β") and lateral line canals (labelled "γ") are particularly striking in the phase-contrast image. After, in part, ref. 9.

69

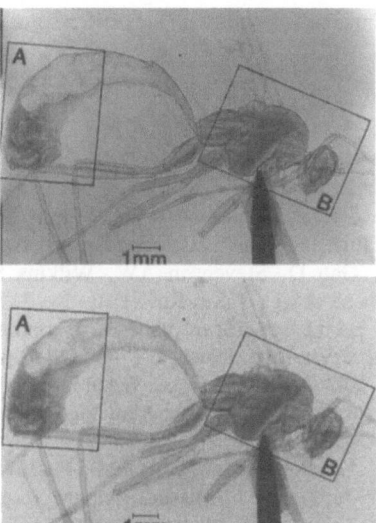

Fig. 6. Phase-contrast and conventional X-ray images for a small dragon-fly. A microfocus source operated at 65kV was used and $R_1 = 150$mm, with $R_2 = 1000$mm for the phase-contrast image and $R_2 = 10$mm for the conventional image.

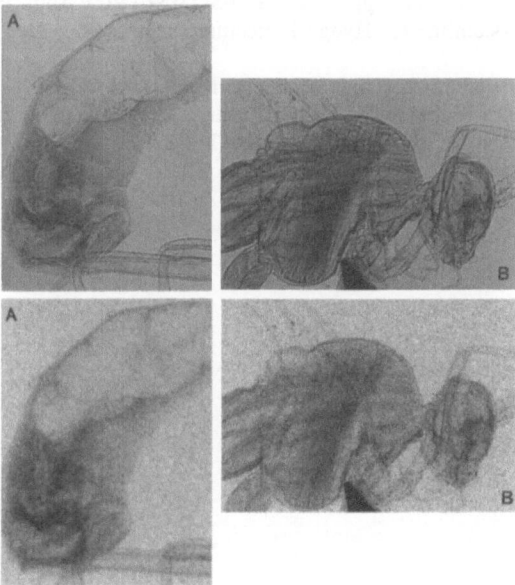

Fig. 7. Photographic enlargements of the respective regions of the images in Fig. 6.

Interest and support from Shimadzu Corporation (Japan) for some of this work is gratefully acknowledged.

REFERENCES

1. Röntgen WC (1896) On a new kind of rays. Nature 53: 274-276.
2. Davis TJ, Gao D, Gureyev TE, Stevenson AW, Wilkins SW (1995) Phase-contrast imaging of weakly absorbing materials using hard X-rays. Nature 373: 595-598.
3. Davis TJ, Gureyev TE, Gao D, Stevenson AW, Wilkins SW (1995) X-ray image contrast from a simple phase object. Phys. Rev. Lett. 74: 3173-3176.
4. Ingal VN, Beliaevskaya EA (1995) X-ray plane-wave topography observation of the phase contrast from a non-crystalline object. J. Phys. D: Appl. Phys. 28: 2314-2317.
5. Snigirev A, Snigireva I, Kohn V, Kuznetsov S, Schelokov I (1995) On the possibilities of X-ray phase contrast microimaging by coherent high-energy synchrotron radiation. Rev. Sci. Inst. 66: 5486-5492.
6. Momose A, Takeda T, Itai Y, Hirano K (1996) Phase-contrast X-ray computed tomography for observing biological soft tissues. Nature Med. 2: 473-475.
7. Nugent KA, Gureyev TE, Cookson DJ, Paganin D, Barnea Z (1996) Quantitative phase imaging using hard X-rays. Phys. Rev. Lett. 77: 2961-2964.
8. Wilkins SW (1993) Aust. Pat. Appl. PM 1519/93; (1994) PCT Appl. PCT/AU94/00480.
9. Wilkins SW, Gureyev TE, Gao D, Pogany A, Stevenson AW (1996) Phase-contrast imaging using polychromatic hard X-rays. Nature 384: 335-338.
10. Wilkins SW (1995) Aust. Pat. Appl. PN 2112/95; (1996) PCT Appl. PCT/AU96/00178.
11. Chikawa J (1996) Beamline for Hyogo Prefecture (Japanese). J. Jap. Soc. Synch. Rad. Res. 9: 462-464.
12. Gabor D (1948) A new microscopic principle. Nature 161: 777-778.
13. Pogany A, Gao D, Wilkins SW (1997) Contrast and resolution in imaging with a microfocus X-ray source. Rev. Sci. Inst. 68: 2774-2782.
14. Gureyev TE, Roberts A, Nugent KA (1995) Phase retrieval with the transport-of-intensity equation: matrix solution with use of Zernike polynomials. J. Opt. Soc. Am. A 12: 1932-1941.

Q: What kind of detector did you use to record these images ?

A: Mainly conventional high resolution X-ray film, Agfa Curix without intensifier screen, with the exception of a few images which were recorded with our home made CCD camera operating in direct mode (no intensifier screen or fibre optics).

C: You demonstrated that increasing this distance improves the phase contrast.

Q: Increasing the distance you may use a detector with more modest spatial resolution?

A: Yes, as distance from object to image plane increases (i.e.magnification), it is possible to use detectors having poorer spatial resolution. It should be emphasized that we had no crystals in the second arrangement. It was just a pure point-projection i.e. "in-line" imaging arrangement based on Fresnel diffraction.

Q: Without any crystals?

A: In the first part of the talk it was with crystals, in which case one is primarily sensitive to the gradient of the phase, but in this case the image intensities are very complicated to interpret quantitatively, and it is not easy to extract the phase directly. With the second method which I described, it is based purely on point-projection imaging and is sensitive to the second derivative of the phase, and one can retrieve the phase fairly easily in principle. A useful reference to the crystal-based imaging case is T.E. Gureyev & S.W. Wilkins Il Nuovo Cimento, Vol 19 pp545 (1997).

Diffraction Enhanced X-ray Imaging

W. Thomlinson[1], D. Chapman[2], Z. Zhong[1], R. E. Johnston[3] and D. Sayers[4]

[1]National Synchrotron Light Source, Brookhaven National Laboratory, Upton, NY 11973, USA
[2]CSRRI, Illinois Institute of Technology, 3101 South Dearborn, Chicago, IL 60616, USA
[3]Deptartment of Radiology, University of North Carolina, Chapel Hill, NC 27599, USA
[4]Department of Physics, North Carolina State University, Raleigh, NC 27695, USA

SUMMARY. Diffraction enhanced imaging (DEI) is a new x-ray radiographic imaging modality using synchrotron x-rays which produces images of thick absorbing objects that are almost completely free of scatter. They show dramatically improved contrast over standard imaging applied to the same phantoms. The contrast is based not only on attenuation but also the refraction and diffraction properties of the sample. The diffraction component and the apparent absorption component (absorption plus extinction contrast) can each be determined independently. This imaging method may improve the image quality for medical applications such as mammography.

KEY WORDS: synchrotron, mammography, diffraction enhanced imaging, DEI

INTRODUCTION

Normal medical x-ray radiography uses an area beam which, after traversing and interacting with the subject, is detected by an area detector. The interaction of x-rays with the subject is complex, involving absorption, refraction [1-2] and scattering. The scattering includes small angle scattering [3] (scattering angles less than mradians) which carries information about the subject's structure on the length scale up to microns. This information is lost in normal radiography because of its small angle nature. X-ray diffraction of perfect crystals, with its narrow reflection angular width (on the order of a few microradians) and peak reflectivity of close to unity (for Bragg diffraction), provides a mechanism for rejecting or accepting small angle scattering, thus providing additional information about the subject.

An imaging method called Diffraction Enhanced Imaging (DEI) has been reported [4] which utilizes a perfect crystal analyzer and centers around the concept of taking digital images at different analyzer positions and combining them to produce apparent absorption and refraction images of the object. It was demonstrated in experiments at the National Synchrotron Light Source that one can separate the refraction effects from the absorption by taking images at two positions on either side of the rocking curve. Objects which have different small angle scattering characteristics from their surroundings can be enhanced by taking images at suitable analyzer positions [5]. These experiments were done with standard mammography phantoms which, although suggesting the potential applicability of DEI to mammography, do not directly prove this due to anticipated differences between the phantom tumor simulation and real tumors. A new set of experiments was performed at the Advanced Photon Source (APS) to study the tissue characterization capability of DEI with biological phantoms consisting of imbedded tumors. This paper reports the preliminary results obtained in that experiment. A more detailed analysis of the results is in preparation and will be submitted for publication soon.

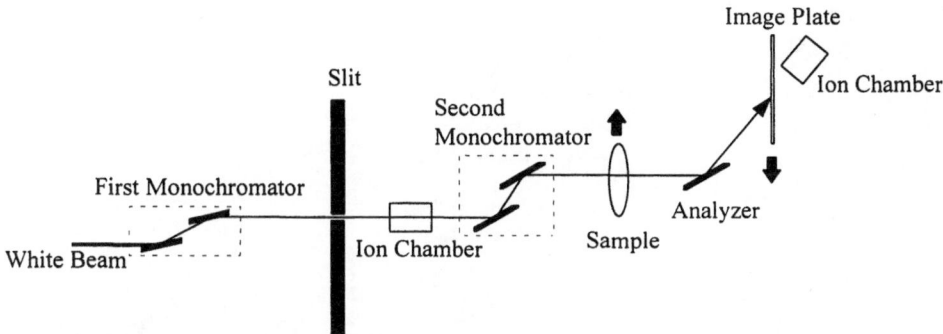

Fig.1. The setup of the experiment with an analyzer crystal

EXPERIMENTAL METHOD

The experiment was performed at the Synchrotron Radiation Instrumentation Collaborative Access Team (SRICAT) sector 1-BM-B (a bending magnet beamline) of the APS. The experimental setup is shown in Fig.1. Perfect silicon crystals in Bragg geometry were used for producing the monochromatic beam and as the analyzer. The first double-crystal monochromator was the beamline monochromator located upstream of the experimental hutch in the beamline. The [111] reflection was used for this monochromator to pre-monochromize the white beam to 18 keV and to deliver the beam into the experimental hutch. The second monochromator crystals were set to the [333] reflection. Because of the dispersion mismatch between the two monochromators and the vertical divergence of the incident beam, the tuning curve of the second monochromator unit with respect to the first monochromator was much wider than the Darwin width of the [333] reflection. Thus the beam intensity on the sample was stable against relative changes of angle between the two monochromators (which was hard to avoid in this prototype set-up due to vibrations).

The analyzer, also [333], was non-dispersive with respect to the second monochromator. The analyzer was mounted on a tangent arm with 1 meter arm length driven by a linear translator of 0.1 micrometer resolution. This provides an angular resolution of 0.1 microradians which is sufficient to tune the analyzer to any location on the analyzer rocking curve which has a FWHM of around 5 microradians for 18 keV x-rays. The tangent arm was mounted on the same optical table as the second monochromator to minimize intensity modulation due to relative angle changes between them caused by vibrations. The beam intensity at the APS was strong enough to provide a surface dose on the order of a few mGy to the sample at a sample scan speed of about 10 mm/s.

Various phantoms and biological samples were imaged. The biological samples studied included a mouse with an implanted tumor and beef tissue with an implanted subcutaneous dog tumor. Each biological sample was preserved in formalin, sealed in a plastic bag and compressed between two Lucite plates. Additional Lucite plates were added during the imaging to make the absorbing thickness on the order of 30-40 mm.

For each sample, a "normal" radiograph with the monochromatic beam at 18 keV was taken by moving the analyzer out of the beam and scanning the image plate and sample through the fan beam in the same direction and at the same speed. DEI tissue characterization studies were performed in several ways: a) With the analyzer tuned to various positions on the rocking curve, the entire phantom and the image plate were translated in opposite directions at the same speed

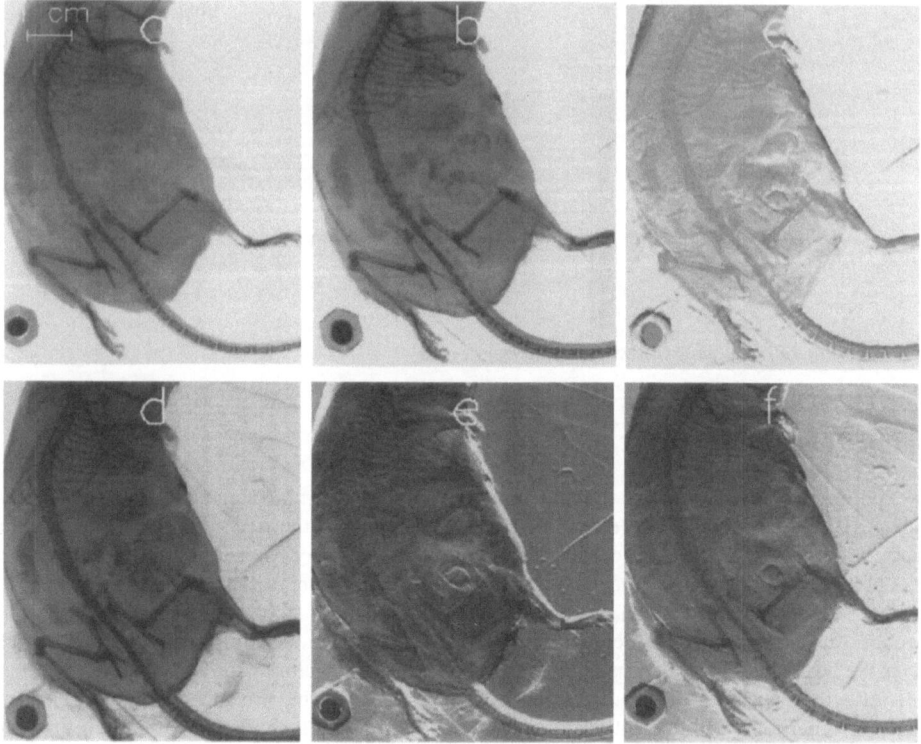

Fig. 2. Images of mouse with imbedded tumor. **a**, "Normal" radiograph taken with analyzer removed. **b**, Apparent absorption image by summing up the images taken with analyzer at ± 1.5 micro radians. **c**, Refraction image represented by the difference of the ± 1.5 micro radians images. **d**, Image taken with analyzer at the peak of the rocking curve. **e**, Image with analyzer at -3 microradians. **f**, Analyzer at +3 microradians.

through the fan beam; b) Multi-scans: with the analyzer tuned to each of a series of predefined positions on the rocking curve, a short scan of a region of sample was performed as in a). The image plate was repositioned after each scan so that images did not overlap on the image plate; c) Rocking curves through a line on the phantom were obtained by fixing the phantom in the fan beam and performing a series of exposures with incrementing analyzer position and image plate vertical position.

RESULTS AND ANALYSIS

The images of the mouse are shown in Fig.2. Fig.2a shows a "normal" radiograph. Fig.2b and Fig.2c show the apparent absorption and refraction images, respectively, of the mouse. These images are derived from the images taken at ±1.5 microradians on each side of the analyzer rocking curve. It is clear from the refraction image that the tumor (about 5 mm in diameter) has been "implanted" in the leg of the mouse. The refraction image shows the "crater" (not present in the "normal" radiograph) formed when the tumor was pushed into the tissue. Compared to the

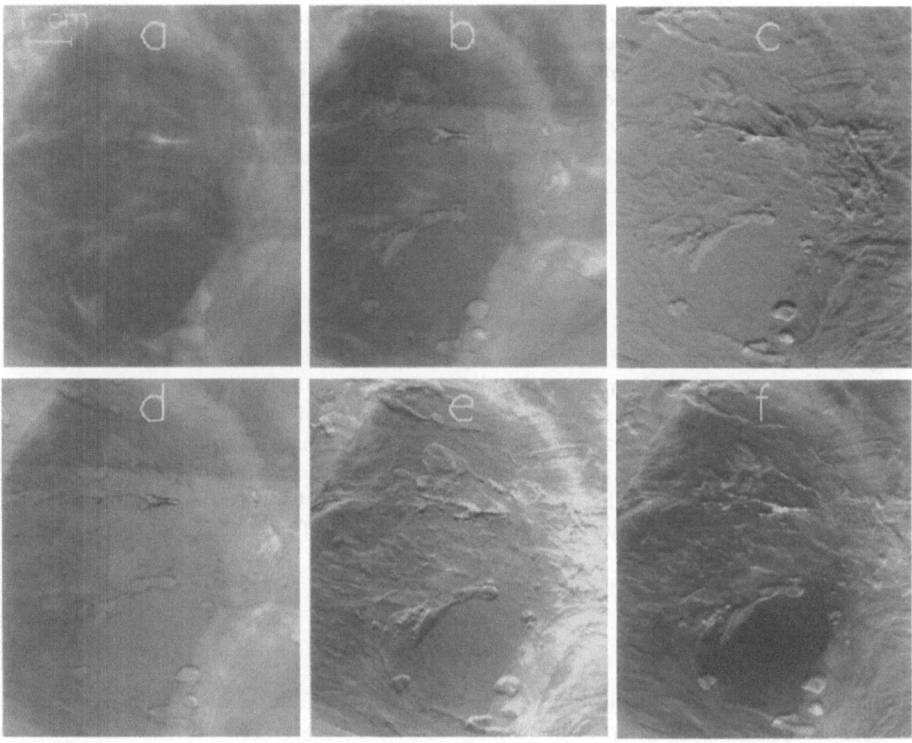

Fig. 3. Images of beef with an imbedded dog tumor. **a.** "Normal" radiograph taken with the analyzer removed. **b.** Apparent absorption image represented by sum of the images taken with the analyzer at ± 1.5 microradians. **c.** Refraction image represented by the difference of the ± 1.5 micro-radians images. **d.** Image taken with the analyzer at the peak of the rocking curve. **e.** Image with the analyzer at -3 microradians. **f.** Image with the analyzer at +3 microradians.

"normal" radiograph, the apparent absorption image (Fig.2b) shows more contrast for the tumor. This demonstrates DEI's ability to enhance tissues whose small angle scattering is different than the surrounding tissues. Fig.2e and 2f show images taken further in the wings of the analyzer rocking curve at plus/minus 3 microradians.

The images of the beef with the imbedded dog tumor are shown in Fig.3. Fig.3a shows a "normal" radiograph. The tumor is the roughly circular object with about 2 cm diameter close to the bottom of the image. Fig.3b and Fig.3c show the apparent absorption and refraction images, respectively. It is clear from the refraction image that the tumor has been "implanted" in the beef. The refraction image shows the "crater" formed when the tumor was pushed into the tissue. The crater is not present in the "normal" radiograph. This clearly demonstrates DEI's ability to enhance edges of features in biological objects. Since DEI is not sensitive to refraction when the analyzer is on top of the peak, the apparent absorption image (Fig.3b) is comparable to the image taken with the analyzer at the peak of the rocking curve (Fig.3d). Figs.3e and 3f show images taken farther out on the wings of the analyzer rocking curve at ± 3 micro-radians. It appears that the dog tumor may have a lack of small angle scattering and a lack of complex refraction at large analyzer rocking curve angles due to smoother morphology of the tumor as compared to beef tissue. There is a reversal in the contrast of the tumor relative to the beef when the analyzer angle is changed from the peak (Fig.3d) to +3 (Fig.3f) micro-radians. This is due to the different relative small angle scattering distributions of the tumor and the beef, and suggests that the tumor can be selectively highlighted. This indicates that DEI may be sensitive to the extinction and refraction contrast in cancerous tissue. In all cases, it is clear that new information is obtained by the DEI technique and that DEI at different analyzer positions on the rocking curve can enhance different features of the sample.

DISCUSSION

The consequence of the two sources of contrast (refraction and extinction contrast) is of importance to mammography and medical imaging in general. These contrast sources are largely energy independent effects as opposed to absorption. Conventional radiography depends on the absorption of x-rays by an object to create the radiograph, thus a compromise must be made between the contrast, signal to noise ratio and the absorbed dose. Refraction and scattering is expected to remain the same as the imaging energy is increased. This raises the possibility of successfully applying this technique at higher x-ray energies. This will be the focus of further investigation.

ACKNOWLEDGMENTS

We would like to thank Fuji Medical Systems for the loan of the AC3 image plate reader system and technical support in setting up and operating the unit. We would like to also thank the staff members at APS SRICAT for technical support and beamtime. This work was supported in part by US ARMY grant DAMD17-96-1-6143 and at the National Synchrotron Light Source by US Department of Energy Contract DE-AC02-76CH00016 and ARPA contract AOB227.

REFERENCES

1. Bushuev VA, Ingal VN, Belyaevskaya EA (1996) Dynamical theory of images generated by noncrystalline objects for the method of phase-dispersive introscopy. Crystallography Reports 41(5): 766-774
2. Podurets KM, Somenkov VA, Shilstein SS (1989) Neutron radiography with refraction contrast. Physica B 156&157: 691-693
3. Guinier A, Fournet G, Walker CB Yudowitch KL (1955) Small-angle scattering of x-rays. Wiley, NewYork.
4. Chapman D, Thomlinson W, Arfelli F, Gmür N, Zhong Z, Menk R, Johnston RE, Washburn D, Pisano E, Sayers D (1996) Mammography imaging studies using a Laue crystal analyzer. Rev Sci Instrum 67(9): CD-ROM
5. Chapman D, Thomlinson W, Johnston RE, Washburn D, Pisano E, Gmür N, Zhong Z, Menk R, Arfelli F, Sayers D (1997) Diffraction enhanced x-ray imaging. Phys Med Bio, Accepted for publication

Q: I want to ask you about the total flux used for normal contrast and off-peak small angle scattering contrast.

A: Off hand I can't give you the flux. We always work within the range of conventional mammography, that is, if you look at some of those numbers you saw, and in fact lower, we are always in the range of 50 to 100 millirads of effective absorbed dose. You have to understand that's obvious where that comes from. When you use film or an image plate, image quality depends on literally the exposure to the detector. So, what really determines the dose you're going to deliver is the exposure required, optimal exposure for basically the dynamic range of the detector you're using. Since we are using mammography film, and image plates aren't dramatically different, about a factor of two in terms of where you'd like to work. So, the exposures for a 45 mm thick sample is really equivalent to that of a mammography examination.

Q: If you change the angle from 3 microrad to 6 microrad, can you optimize the angle depending on the sample?

A: If you looked at the wood, for example, wood has a scattering distribution that goes up millirads. The material in our ACR phantom went out to some number of about 10 microrad. You get dramatic differences in the small angle scattering profile. Exactly where you want to see it, depends on the small angle micro scattering of background material versus the material of interest. You like to see it where you're optimizing material of interest relative to the other material. It could be at the peak for certain materials, it could be the reverse.

Q: There is still another thing when you try to understand the small angle scattering when you use an analyzer crystal. The analyzer crystal has one property, namely, its own thermal diffuse scattering which gives wings, so that the apparent small angle scattering that you see is always more than the true one.

A: I agree. But in the case of wood, it does not matter. I showed you the difference between the calculated and measured, and that's almost certainly it. It is one of our ideas.

Q: How about applying a sort of combination of more than two kinds of technique like a combination of computer tomography with a phase contrast imaging technique ?

A: It is an obvious thing to try and do.

Q: How does this effect your contrast , or effect your images?

A: This work is much too young for us to have gotten to that level of detail. In fact polarization is something to be dealt with. At least we are now beginning to understand the fundamentals of this apparent absorption we've seen, and then there are other second order effects like the fact that diffractive index effects are not totally separated out from the apparent absorption. Now whether that is important in particular materials of geometry. We don't know yet. That is the approximations we have made. Similarly polarization effects could in fact effect particular material and be very important.

Phase Contrast Imaging in the Field of Mammography

M. Di Michiel (1), A. Olivo (1)*, G. Tromba (3), F. Arfelli (3), V. Bonvicini (1), A. Bravin (1), G. Cantatore (1), E. Castelli (1), L. Dalla Palma (2), R. Longo (1), S. Pani (1), D. Pontoni (1), P. Poropat (1), M. Prest (1), A. Rashevsky (1), A. Vacchi (1), E. Vallazza (1).
(SYRMEP - SYnchrotron Radiation for MEdical Physics - Collaboration)

(1) Dipartimento di Fisica - Università di Trieste and INFN - Sezione di Trieste
(2) Istituto di Radiologia - Università di Trieste
(3) Sincrotrone Trieste SCpA
* corresponding author

SUMMARY. It is very well known that imaging low contrast details in soft tissues is the main limitation of conventional X-ray radiology. Phase contrast imaging overcomes this limitation. Up to now, however, all the applications of this technique required high radiation doses, raising several questions about its utilisation in medical radiology.

The first low dose phase contrast X-ray images were obtained by the SYRMEP Collaboration at ELETTRA, the Trieste synchrotron radiation facility. We produced high contrast resolution images of phantoms and of a specimen of human breast tissue with doses comparable to those used in standard mammography by introducing an intensifier screen behind the X-ray film. Our theoretical simulations and experimental tests not only demonstrate how the ELETTRA bending-magnet beam is suitable for phase contrast imaging, but also show that the source size requirements are not very stringent. This opens the way to widespread applications of this simple and effective technique to medical radiology and to other fields.

KEY WORDS: mammography, phase-contrast

Introduction

Phase contrast imaging can solve some of the basic problems of conventional radiographic X-ray imaging, which encounters severe difficulties with objects containing details having small differences in absorption. A source with sufficient spatial coherence makes it possible to detect the effects of the phase perturbations caused by the objects, even if absorption is negligible.

This image sharpening technique is based on the observation of the interference patterns produced by spatial variations of the refractive index. The method has been tested by Snigirev et al. [1,2] and by Wilkins et al. [3] on different organic samples: their experimental set-up and detectors, however, needed very high radiation doses, preventing application to medical radiology.

Our approach solves this problem and we propose here the first application of phase contrast imaging to medical radiology, specifically to mammography. An intensifying screen enabled us to obtain high contrast mammographic images at doses fully compatible with medical applications.

Our theoretical simulations and experimental results also show that the constraints on the source are not stringent. At our source to sample distance, a source size not larger than 200 - 250 μm is suitable. This source size is also available at a few second generation synchrotron sources. Furthermore, almost no wavelength filtering is required [3].

Experimental method

A simulation based on Fresnel-Kirchoff diffraction integrals [4] was developed. Taking into account the energy range from 8 to 35 keV for the incident radiation, the angular range within which interference takes place ranges from 10 to 100 µrad. The interference pattern is not detectable immediately behind the object, and increasing the distance between the detector and the object makes it possible to convert a small angle into a detectable length. Therefore imaging tests were performed at the SYRMEP beamline choosing a sample to detector distance ranging from 0.7 m to 2.5 m. Fig. 1 shows the SYRMEP beamline layout and ref. [5] provides a detailed description of the beamline. The monochromator is based on a monolithic channel-cut Si(1,1,1) crystal delivering energies ranging from 8 to 35 keV, the beam cross section in the experimental area is equal to ~100x3mm2.

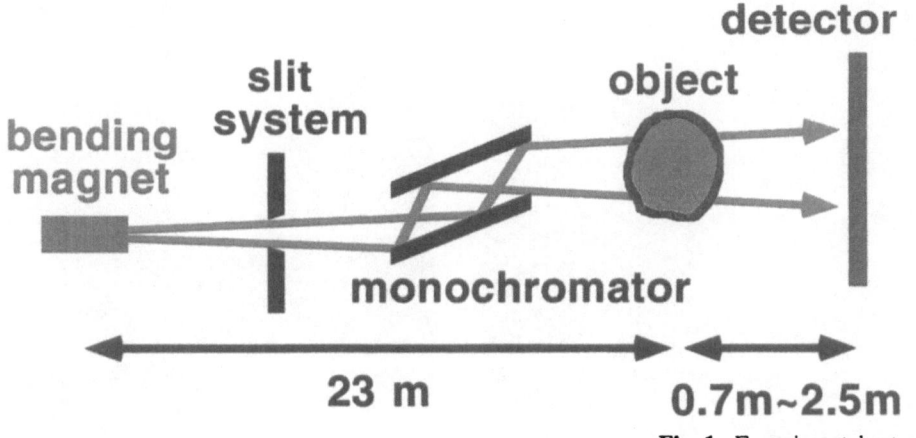

Fig. 1 Experimental set-up

High resolution Kodak X-ray films and conventional Kodak mammographic film-screen systems were used to detect the X-rays. Images were obtained by scanning object and detector through the laminar beam.

Theoretical simulations performed at 17 keV show that the angular distance between the first interference maximum and the first minimum is of the order of 10 µrad. This means that, in order to preserve spatial coherence, the source size must be smaller than ~230 µm for our source to sample distance of 23 m, and that larger source to sample distances would allow wider sources.

Images of a bar pattern test object taken at different sample-to-detector distances gave us the possibility of estimating the dimensions of our source. Since these dimensions are 1100 µm x 140 µm (FWHM), we expect sharp interference patterns in one direction and blurred ones in the other. Image analysis confirmed the theoretical expected value of ~10 µrad for the angle between the first minimum and the first maximum of the interference pattern, and therefore the requirements for the source size.

Results and discussion

Images of different samples of organic fibres, insects, flowers, etc. were recorded with high resolution Kodak X-ray films. Fig. 2 shows six nylon wires embedded in a glue drop, imaged both with the conventional absorption geometry (detector a few cm from the sample) and with the phase contrast geometry (detector to sample distance of ~1 m). Fig. 3 shows images of a mimosa flower: phase contrast images exhibit a large enhancement in contrast resolution compared to conventional absorption ones.

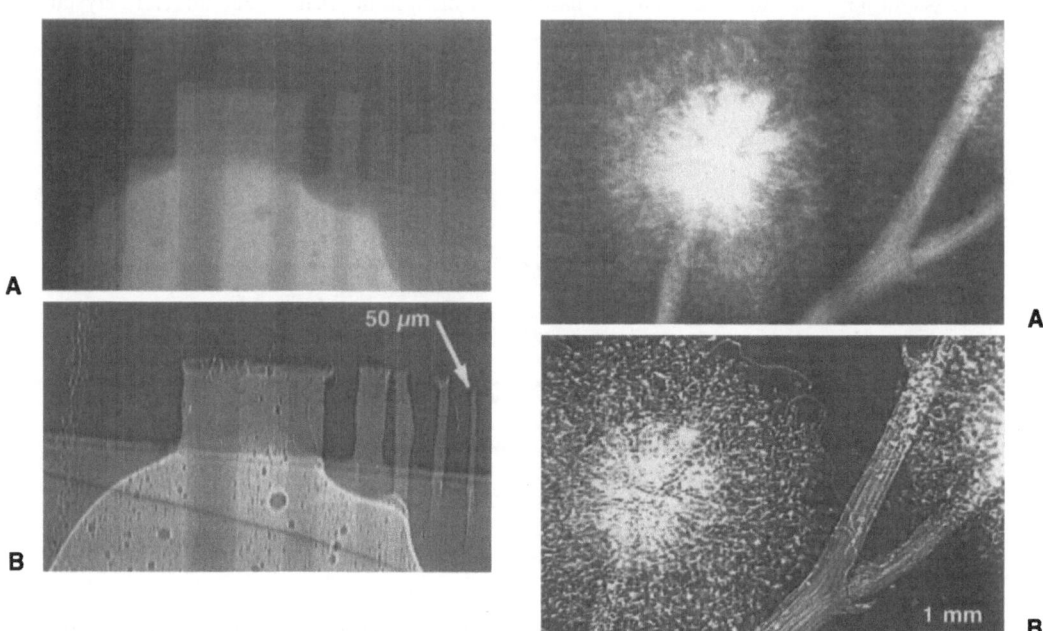

Fig. 2: Images of six nylon wires - diameters ranging from 50 μm to 800 μm - embedded in a glue drop, recorded on high resolution X-ray film. Fig. 1A shows the conventional absorption image, Fig. 1B the phase contrast one. The beam energy for both images was 10 keV.

Fig. 3: Images of a mimosa flower, recorded on high resolution X-ray film. Fig. 3A shows the conventional absorption image, Fig. 3B the phase contrast one. The beam energy for both images was 10 keV.

The delivered dose for these first pictures was, however, very high - about 50 times higher than conventional mammography. To increase the detection efficiency in order to reduce the delivered dose and make the technique suitable for medical radiology, we evaluated the effects of an intensifying screen. The interference pattern is convolved with the film-screen system point spread function, and a certain loss in spatial resolution occurs. Images, however, still exhibit a remarkable enhancement in contrast resolution due to the high intensity of the interference peaks.

With this method images of mammographic test objects, insects and specimens of human breast tissue were recorded using both imaging geometries on conventional film-screen systems, delivering a dose comparable to that of a standard mammography. Fig. 4 and 5 show images of the head of a bee and of a specimen of human breast tissue respectively. In both cases, even with the negative side effects of the intensifying fluorescent screen, the phase contrast technique strongly improves the image quality, especially in terms of contrast resolution. In particular, in Fig. 6 the visibility of the internal structures of the tissue is greatly enhanced in the phase contrast image.

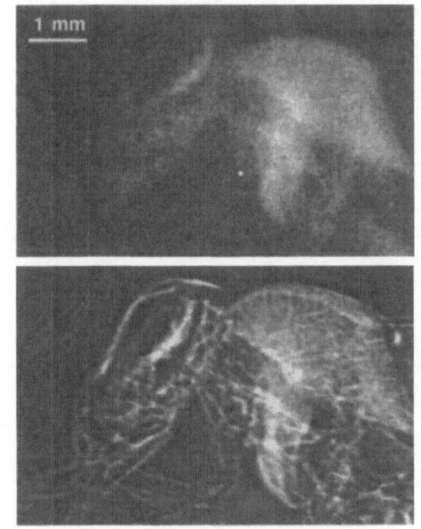

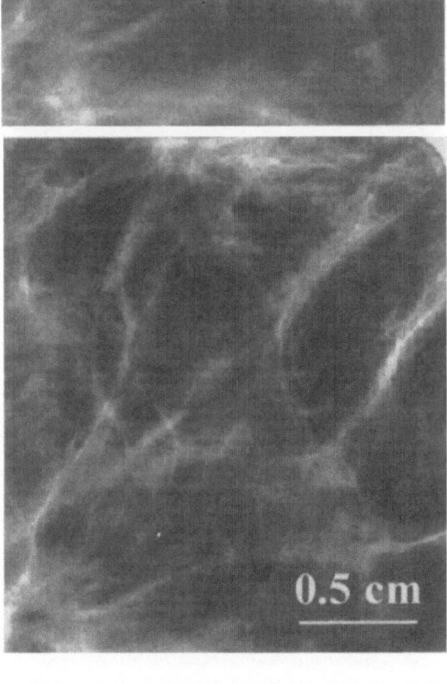

A

B

Fig. 4: Images of a bee recorded with a conventional film-screen system. Fig. 5A shows the absorption image, Fig. 5B the phase contrast one. The beam energy for both images was 17 keV.

Fig. 5: Images of a specimen of human breast tissue recorded with a conventional film-screen system. Fig. 5A shows the absorption image, Fig. 5B the phase contrast one. In this last figure visibility of the internal structures of the tissue is highly enhanced. The beam energy for both images was 17 keV.

In conclusion, phase contrast imaging can be achieved with low doses, fully compatible with conventional mammographic examinations, while preserving a substantial enhancement in contrast resolution. Furthermore, both simulations an experimental results tests show that, with proper source to sample distance, sources larger than 200 μm can be used. High coherence sources like ELETTRA or ESRF appear desirable but not strictly necessary.

References

1 A. Snigirev, I. Snigireva, V. Kohn, S. Kuznetsov, I. Schelokov, Rev. Sci. Instrum. 66 (12), (1995).
2 A. Snigirev, I. Snigireva, A. Suvorov, M. Kocsis, V. Kohn, E.S.R.F Newsletter reports. 22, 20 (1994)
3 S. W. Wilkins, T. E. Gureyev, D. Gao, A. Pogany, A. W. Stevenson, Nature 384, (1996)
4 M.Born and E.Wolf, Principles of optics: electromagnetic theory of propagation, interference and diffraction of light, (Pergamon Press, Oxford, 1975)
5 F. Arfelli et al., Rev. Sci. Instrum. 66 (2), (1995)

MAMMOGRAPHIC IMAGING USING A HARPICON-BASED IMAGE DETECTOR

Keiji Umetani[1], Hironori Ueki[1], Tohoru Takeda[2], Yuji Itai[2], Masayoshi Akisada[3,4] and Yasuhito Sasaki[5,6]

[1] Central Research Laboratory, Hitachi, Ltd., Kokubunji, Tokyo 185, Japan
[2] Institute of Clinical Medicine, University of Tsukuba, Tsukuba, Ibaraki 305, Japan
[3] Tama Health Management Center, Tachikawa, Tokyo 190, Japan
[4] Department of Radiology and Information Science, International University of Health and Welfare, Ohtawara, Tochigi 324, Japan
[5] Faculty of Medicine, University of Tokyo, Bunkyo-ku, Tokyo 113, Japan
[6] National Institute of Radiological Sciences, Inage-ku, Chiba 263, Japan

SUMMARY. A high-spatial resolution imaging system employing lens coupling between a fluorescent screen and a HARPICON™ camera was evaluated as a digital mammographic imaging device. A mammographic image on the fluorescent screen is focused on the photoconductive layer of the high sensitivity HARPICON tube by lenses. The limiting spatial resolution in the 1024×980 pixel mode of the camera is about 60 μm at an input field of 50×50 mm on the screen. Images of a standard mammographic phantom were taken at the monochromatized X-ray energy of 20 keV. The images showed smaller specks of microcalcifications and tumor masses than those discernible in images obtained with a conventional screen-film mammography unit.

KEY WORDS: Mammography, HARPICON camera, Digital imaging, Fluorescent screen

INTRODUCTION

Mammography is an effective technique for taking images of tumor masses and microcalcifications in the early examination of breast cancer. However, small breast masses and microcalcifications are not reliably detected with conventional screen-film mammography because of limitations on image contrast and spatial resolution. Digital imaging systems provide advantages in image quality over conventional screen-film systems. Digital mammographic imaging systems with a small field of view have been investigated using a charge-coupled-device (CCD) optically coupled to a fluorescent screen [1]. Furthermore, commercially available systems have been produced for stereotactic breast needle biopsy [2].

On the other hand, synchrotron radiation (SR) has been applied to monoenergetic X-ray mammography for a high signal-to-noise ratio that results in high-contrast images with a low X-ray dose to the patient [3,4]. In the experiments, a conventional mammographic screen-film system was used for imaging and a photostimulable-storage-phosphor plate was also used for digital imaging. Using SR's inherently highly collimated and tunable radiation with better patient-detector geometry, monoenergetic X-ray mammography should obtain high-quality radiographs of soft-tissue lesions.

We performed preliminary experiments to obtain high-quality mammographic images at the Photon Factory in Tsukuba. For the imaging, a high-spatial-resolution image detector using a HARPICON-camera fluorescent-screen lens-coupling approach was used to detect smaller microcalcifications than that detected by conventional screen-film mammography and monochromatized X-ray was used to take images of smaller tumor masses [5,6].

IMAGING METHOD

The X-ray imaging system in Fig. 1 was placed at superconducting vertical wiggler beamline BL-14C at the Photon Factory. The SR beam is monochromatized and expanded horizontally by an asymmetrically cut silicon <311> crystal. An X-ray image on the screen is focused on the photoconductive layer of the HARPICON tube by lenses with high numerical aperture. The field of view on the screen is 50 × 50 mm. Images on this area are detected in the 1024 × 980 pixel mode of the camera. The equivalent pixel size projected onto the screen is 50 μm.

The HARPICON is a pickup tube with an amorphous selenium photoconductive target and is characterized by its internal amplification system which uses stable avalanche multiplication of photo-generated carriers under a strong electric field in the photoconductive layer. Image signals from the camera are converted into digital format by an analog-to-digital converter with 12-bit resolution and are stored in a frame memory with image format of 1024 × 980 pixel corresponding to the camera's 1050 scanning-line mode. After image acquisition, images are transferred to a workstation and image-processing operations are performed. The system routinely uses an image processing procedure which corrects the raw image for signal nonuniformities due to local variations in X-ray intensity and sensitivity of the image detector.

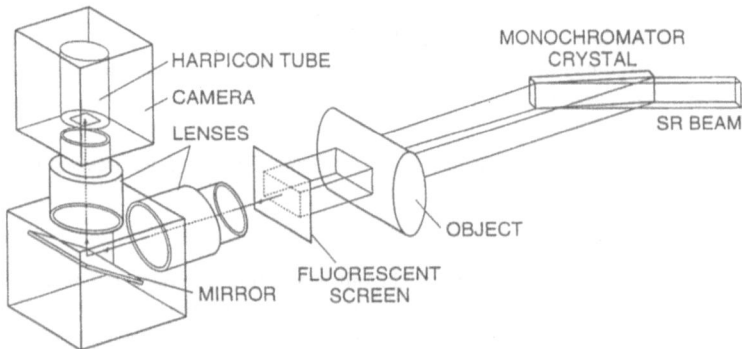

Fig. 1. Schematic of whole experimental setup of X-ray imaging system.

EXPERIMENT AND RESULTS

An X-ray spatial-resolution chart was placed on the detector input plane to examine the detector's resolution. The limiting spatial resolution obtained by the image in Fig. 2 is 8 line-pairs/mm (about 60 μm), which is less detailed than that defined by the equivalent pixel size of 50 μm because of resolution limitation caused by the fluorescent screen at the monochromatized X-ray energy of 20 keV. The 20-keV X-rays are mainly absorbed in the front surface side of the screen layer but the transformed light photons are emitted at the opposite surface. If a thin-phosphor-layer screen is used, the spatial resolution will be improved.

Images of the standard mammographic phantom (Model 11, CIRS, Inc., Virginia) which has the thickness of 4 cm and consists of microcalcifications, masses, stepwedge, fibrils and line-pair test target were taken with a dose of about 4 mSv/image at the X-ray energy of 20 keV. Though the field of view is 50 × 50 mm on the screen, the X-ray beam has a rectangular cross-section of 25 × 35 mm (width × height). This is because the asymmetrically cut silicon <311> crystal is made for use in angiography at the X-ray energy of 33.3 keV. Partial images of the phantom are shown in Fig. 3. On the image, small specks of microcalcifications and simulated tumor masses are discernible.

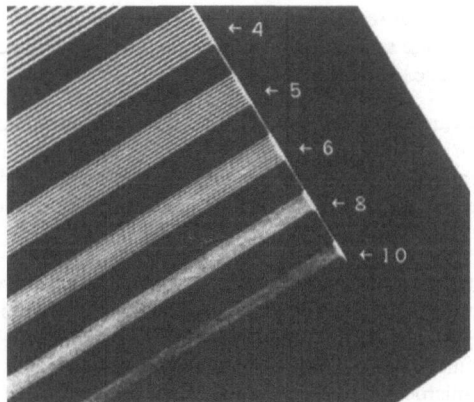

Fig. 2. X-ray image of spatial resolution chart taken in this system. The spatial frequencies are, from bottom to top, 10, 8, 6, 5, 4 and 3 line-pairs/mm.

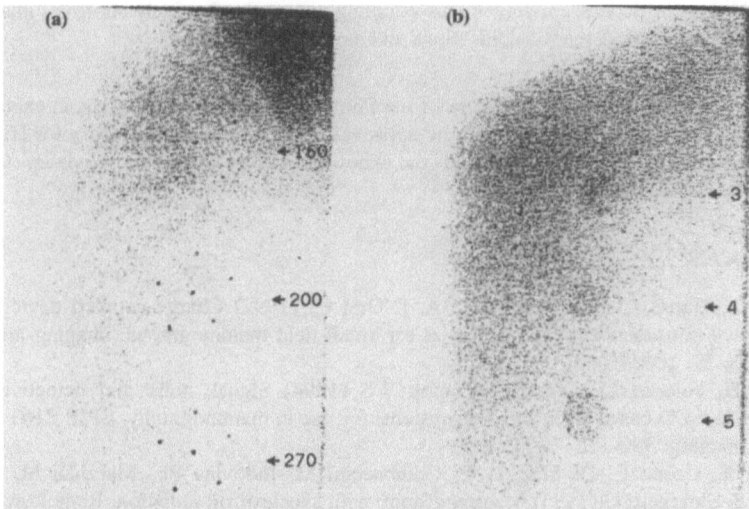

Fig. 3. X-ray images of standard breast phantom. a) 3 groupings of subcutaneous microcalcification with largest at 270 μm diameter and smallest at 160 μm. b) 3 simulated tumor masses ranging from 5 to 3 mm in diameter.

DISCUSSION

In the experiment, an HR-4 intensifying screen (Fuji Medical Systems Co. Ltd., Japan) was used to transform the X-ray image into a visible image. If an HR-3 screen that is the highest-spatial-resolution screen of Fuji Medical Systems's products is applied, the spatial resolution of 10 line-pairs/mm will be obtained [7] because the phosphor layer of the HR-3 are thinner than that of the HR-4 and MTF (modulation transfer function) of the HR-3 at 2 line-pairs/mm is about 20% higher than that of the HR-4. The spatial resolution of 10 line-pairs/mm and the field of view of 50 × 50 mm on the screen have nearly the same performance as those of the commercially available digital-imaging systems for stereotactic breast needle biopsy [2].

The mammographic image can be viewed just after the X-ray exposure in our system but real-time imaging is not needed for mammographic imaging. For mammographic digital imaging, the photostimulable-storage-phosphor plate system and a film-image digitizing system for the conventional film-screen combination will be also available if spatial resolution of these system is improved.

The standard breast phantom is usually used to adjust a conventional screen-film mammography unit at the Institute of Clinical Medicine, University of Tsukuba. On the phantom image taken by the conventional mammography unit, the grouping of microcalcification with 160 μm diameter and the simulated tumor mass with 3 mm diameter were not detected. However, the present system could detect these microcalcifications and the tumor mass.

Digital imaging systems are expected to provide advantages over conventional screen-film radiography in image quality by performing image processing. Furthermore, inherently highly collimated monochromatized X-ray with better patient-detector geometory and with less scattered X-ray from the patient can produce high-contrast images. The combination of monochromatized X-ray obtained from SR and the high-spatial-resolution digital imaging system using the HARPICON-camera fluorescent-screen lens-coupling approach effectively improves image quality to allow detection of small microcalcifications and small tumor masses.

The authors thank Dr. Osamu Shimomura of the Photon Factory for the support in experiments at BL-14C. This work was performed with the approval of the National Laboratory for High Energy Physics (acceptance No. 95-Y005) and the Photon Factory Program Advisory Committee (proposal No. 95-G290).

REFERENCES

1. Karellas A, Harris LJ, Liu H, Davis MA, D'Orsi CJ (1992) Charge-coupled device detector: performance considerations and potential for small-field mammographic imaging applications. Med. Phys. 19: 1015-1023
2. Roehrig H, Fajardo LL, Yu T, Schempp WS (1994) Signal, noise and detective quantum efficiency in CCD based x-ray imaging systems for use in mammography. SPIE 2163 Physics of Medical Imaging: 320-332
3. Burattini E, Cossu E, Di Maggio C, Gambaccini M, Indovina PL, Marziani M, Pocek M, Simeoni S, Simonetti G (1995) Mammography with synchrotron radiation. Radiology 195: 239-244
4. Johnston RE, Washburn D, Pisano E, Burns C, Thomlinson WC, Chapman LD, Arfelli F, Gmur NF, Zhong Z, Sayers D (1996) Mammographic phantom studies with synchrotron radiation. Radiology 200: 659-663
5. Umetani K, Ueki H, Ueda K, Hirai T, Takeda T, Doi T, Wu J, Itai Y, Akisada M (1996) High-spatial-resolution medical-imaging system using a HARPICON camera coupled with a fluorescent screen. J. Synchrotron Rad. 3: 136-144
6. Takeda T, Umetani K, Doi T, Echigo J, Ueki H, Ueda K, Itai Y (1997) Two-dimensional aortographic coronary arteriography with above-K-edge monochromatic synchrotron radiation. Acad. Radiol. 4: 438-445
7. Umetani K, Ueki H, Takeda T, Itai Y, Mori H, Tanaka E, Uddin-Mohammed M, Shinozaki Y, Akisada M, Sasaki Y (1998) High-spatial-resolution and real-time medical imaging using a high-sensitivity HARPICON camera. J. Synchrotron Rad. to be published.

Specific Element Imaging by Monochromatic X-ray CT Using Synchrotron Radiation

Yasuaki Nagata[1], Hironao Yamaji[1], Kazuo Hayashi[1], Katsuhiro Kawashima[2], K. Hyodo[3] and M. Ando[3]

[1]Process Technology Research Laboratories, Nippon Steel Corp., 20 − 1 Shintomi, Futtu − shi, Chiba, 293 Japan
[2]Tokyo Engineering University, 1404 − 1 Katakura, Hachioji − shi, Tokyo, 192 Japan
[3]Photon Factory, National Laboratory for High Energy Physics, 1 − 1 Oho, Tukuba, Ibaraki 305, Japan

SUMMARY. We have developed a high energy, high resolution monochromatic x-ray CT system using Synchrotron Radiation. At the present stage, we have achieved the production of monochromatic x-rays up to 75 keV and succeeded in taking the CT images of materials up to 50 keV with large absorption coefficients that are difficult to image by conventional methods. We have produced three-dimensional CT images of a sintered iron ore specimen with a pixel size of about 7 μm with a slice thickness of 20 μm. The three-dimensionally reconstructed images of the sintered iron ore provide such information on the inside of sinter that is not obtainable by conventional surface observation alone. To evaluate the contrast resolution using the K-edge subtraction method we have investigated iodine and gadolinium solutions from the subtraction CT images. These results showed that the SR-CT system can quantitatively and nondestructively measure the trace distribution of a given element in the object by selecting the monochromatic x-rays corresponding to the K-edge energy of the element. The developed SR-CT will become a powerful tool to evaluate a wide variety of materials, including in vivo tissues and ferrous materials.

KEY WORDS: X-ray computed tomography, K-edge subtraction method, Three-dimensional imaging

Introduction

X-ray computed tomography (CT) can observe cross sections of objects without destroying them and thus is widely used in industry as well as in medicine. In industry, x-ray CT plays a very important role as a nondestructive evaluation tool in detecting flaws in objects, measuring the internal structure and the density of objects. At present, research and development are under way for improving the spatial resolution and contrast resolution of x-ray CT.

Recent years have seen active research on synchrotron radiation (SR) as a source, because it has by far a higher brilliance than x-rays produced by x-ray tubes and can be collimated with a divergence angle of a few milliradians. Since SR has a wide frequency band, monochromatic x-rays in a few keV to 100 keV can be produced. The continuous production of monochromatic x-rays has become possible for the first time with SR; conventional monochromatic x-ray CT had used isotopes [1]. The x-rays can be optimally selected to suit the material and size of objects and the quality CT images can be improved. Additionally, when CT images are taken with monochromatic x-rays below and above the K-absorption edge of a particular element and the CT images subtracted, the distribution of the element can be obtained and related works were reported[2-13]. Furthermore, recently to achieve a higher resolution new imaging technique has been developed such as a phase-contrast x-ray CT[14] and x-ray CT using diffraction method[15].

To allow the widespread application of CT to materials, we developed a CT system that can utilize radiation from a vertical wiggler beam line (BL14C) at the Photon Factory (PF) of the National Laboratory for High Energy Physics (KEK) [16]. As can be seen from the spectral characteristics shown in Fig. 1, such an insertion device can produce SR of higher brilliance in a higher energy region than conventional bending magnets. A crystal monochromator was designed and developed to yield high energies up to 75 keV, unobtainable in the past [17-19]. Enlargement of projected images and production of monochromatic x-rays were simultaneously achieved by the use of asymmetric Bragg reflection of crystals to improve spatial resolution and contrast resolution. This paper introduces the experimental system, and we evaluate the CT images taken and the performance of the SR-CT system.

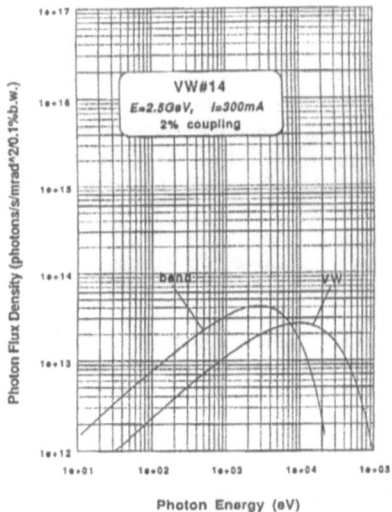

Fig. 1. Intensity spectra for the vertical wiggler.

SR-CT System

Outline of System

The imaging of a given element by the K-edge subtraction method requires a monochromatic x-ray beam of sufficient intensity and energy resolution, and a mechanism for high accuracy adjustment to any desired K-absorption edge energy value of the element, among other factors. Our system is designed to utilize monochromatic x-rays in the high energy region, extend the K-edge subtraction method to heavy elements, and improve contrast resolution by increasing the intensity of monochromatic x-rays.

The SR-CT system is schematically illustrated in Fig. 2. The system consists of a specimen scanner, crystal monochromator, x-ray detector, and signal processing unit. Enlargement of projected images and production of monochromatic x-rays are simultaneously achieved by the use of asymmetric Bragg reflection of crystals to improve spatial resolution and contrast resolution. The SR is collimated by slits and irradiated onto the rotating specimen. The x-ray beam transmitted through the specimen is passed through the crystal monochromator and measured with a one-dimensional or two-dimensional x-ray detector that consists of a phosphor and a CCD array detector. In the case of a two-dimensional x-ray detector, projected images can be demagnified using a lens corresponding to the size of the specimen. The mechanical components are all driven by stepping motors. These system components as well as the specimen operating section are controlled by a dedicated controller and a microcomputer. The main components of the system are described below.

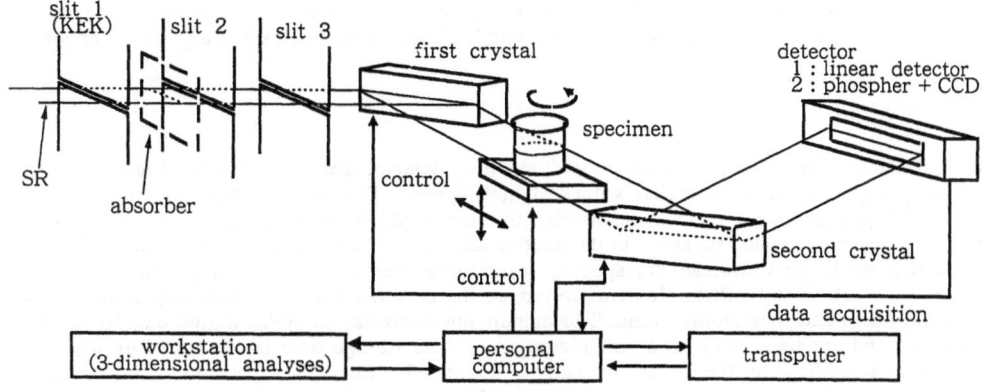

Fig. 2. Schematic diagram of SR-CT.

Crystal Monochromator

We have adopted the two-crystal method for our system to select monochromatic x-rays over a wide band according to the material of samples and to completely eliminate higher-order harmonics.

In addition, to obtain CT images with high resolution simultaneously, Bragg asymmetric reflection from a single crystal was used to enlarge the projected x-ray image, and the images were detected with a detector of high spatial resolution[20].

The variation in the lattice spacing of the first crystal with the heat load of low energy x-rays contained in SR must be reduced to improve the stability of the monochromatic x-ray beam over time. The first crystal is fixed in a copper block, and cooling water whose temperature is controlled to high accuracy is circulated through the copper block. The copper block and first crystal are bonded by thin films of gallium to enhance the conduction of heat between the water-cooled copper block and first crystal. The SR-CT system is equipped with a cooling water recirculating device that can control the temperature of the water bath to ± 0.01 °C in view of the effect of the surrounding environment.

To prevent the surface oxidation of the first crystal, the water-cooled copper block and first crystal are installed in a sealed container constructed with a Kapton film (Du Pond polyimide film), and the container is filled with inert He gas.
Each crystal is equipped with a six-axis mechanical drive unit corresponding to the X axis, Z axis, rough rotation, fine rotation, swivel to back and forth, and swivel to right and left. All axes can be driven by a stepping motor. The accuracy of movement varies from axis to axis. The minimum angle of rotation is 0.01 second of arc for the axis of fine rotation used for the high accuracy adjustment of monochromatic x-ray energy when the K-edge subtraction method is applied, for example.

Specimen Scanner

To obtain cross-sectional images with high spatial resolution, it is necessary to collimate SR to micron order with high accuracy and to set the axis of rotation of the specimen normal to the collimated beam.

In the specimen scanner shown in Fig. 2, Slits 2 and 3 are parallel and are pre-adjusted so that the axis of rotation of the specimen stage is normal to the plane formed by the slits. A precision micrometer with graduations of 0.1 μm is used to set a slice thickness of about 10 μm to a few tens of micrometers by the two slits to high accuracy. An ionization chamber is installed after each slit to adjust the slit with respect to the axis of SR with high accuracy. Each slit is adjusted to about 10 μm.

X-ray Detector

The SR-CT system adopted an x-ray photodiode array detector that has high spatial resolution and can read projection data as digital values at high speed. The detector has 200 μm thickness $Gd_2O_2S \cdot Tb$ phosphors coupled by optical fiber to the photodiode array and is sensitive to x-rays in an energy region of 10 to 100 keV. In the photodiode array, 512 elements, each measuring 2.5 mm by 36 μm, are linearly arranged at a spacing (center-to-center) of 50 μm. The photodiode array is cooled to -30 °C by Peltier elements to reduce the dark current output and to provide a wide dynamic range and long storage time. The outputs are converted to 16-bit digital data by an A/D converter and are transferred to a microcomputer. The storage time is controlled by the same computer according to the x-ray intensity. Figure 3 shows the schematic illustration of two-dimensional detector. In this case CCD array detector and phosphor sheet are used.

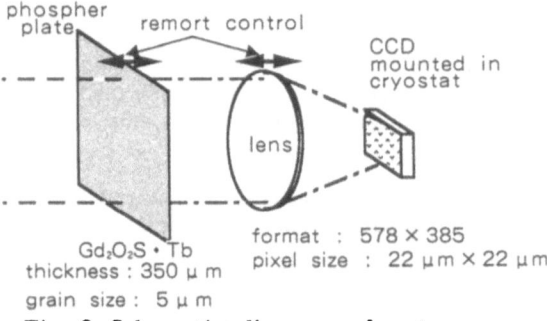

Fig. 3. Schematic diagram of a two – dimensional detector.

Data Collection and Image Reconstruction

As the specimen is rotated by a given angle, the x-ray beam transmitted through the specimen is stored as an electric charge proportional to the intensity of the transmitted x-ray beam over a given time. Then, the projected data of the preset number of pixels (256 or 512 pixels) are converted from analog to 16-bit digital data and are transferred to the microcomputer. These operations are repeated to collect projection data for the given angle change and store them in a hard-disk memory.

The measured projection data are preprocessed for logarithmic transformation, detector dark current correction and other operations, using nine transputers that are high-speed parallel coprocessors, and reconstructed into a CT image. A filtered back projection (FBP) method is employed for CT image reconstruction. The CT image reconstruction time is about 4 min for 512 × 512 pixels. If three-dimensional display of CT images are required, a workstation is used.

Experimental Results and Discussion

Figure 4 shows the schematic illustration of a sintered iron ore and vertical section of its three-dimensional CT image. The three-dimensional CT image was reconstructed from 40 sections, and the CT image of each section was taken with a slice thickness of 20 μm. This image provides such information on the inside of sintered iron ore that is not obtainable by conventional surface observation alone.

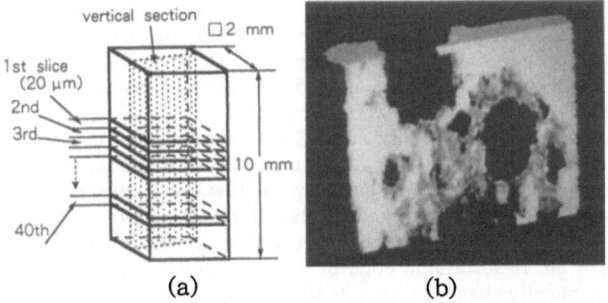

(a)   (b)

Fig. 4. (a) Schematic illustration of a sintered iron
ore and (b) vertical section of its CT image.

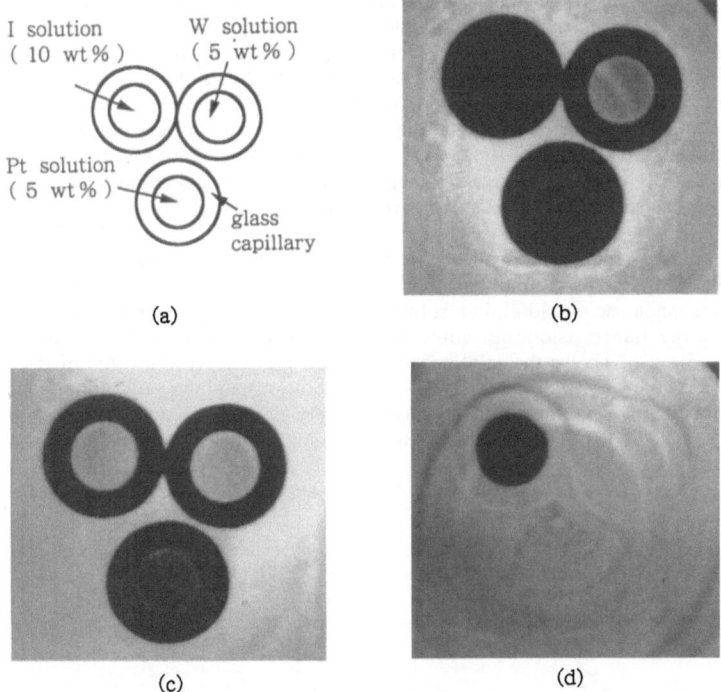

(a)   (b)

(c)   (d)

Fig. 5 K-edge subtraction method applied to an iodine solution.
(a) Cross-sectional drawing of the sample. (b) CT image
at 33.21 keV above the absorption edge. (c) CT image at
33.13 keV below the absorption edge. (d) CT image obtained
by subtracting (b) from (c).

Figure 5 shows the results obtained when the K-edge subtraction method was applied to an iodine solution. Iodine is used as contrast medium in angiography in which x-rays are utilized to obtain information on blood vessel form and blood flow in living organisms. The K-edge subtraction method is applied to iodine because an improvement in contrast resolution is in strong demand[21]. The specimens are assumed to be living organisms such as mice or rats of about 5 to 10 mm in size, and the enlargement ratio is correspondingly lower, with a 25 μm pixel size designed. In this case the <333> and <440> Ge crystals were used. Figure 5(a) shows the shapes of the specimens. Three glass capillary tubes, each measuring 1.6 mm in outside diameter and 1.0 mm in inside diameter, were bundled together. One tube was filled with 10 wt% iodine solution, and the other two were filled with a 5 wt% tungsten solution and a 5 wt% platinum solution, respectively, for the purpose of comparison. The pixel size was 25 μm, the slice thickness 200 μm, the storage time per projection 1 s, and the total collection time about 3 min 30 s for 200 sets of projection data over 180°. Figure 5(b) shows the CT image taken at an energy above the K-absorption edge of iodine, and Fig. 5(c) shows the CT image taken at an energy below the K-absorption edge of iodine. Figure 5(d) is the CT image obtained by subtracting the CT image (c) from the CT image (b). The images of platinum and tungsten are eliminated because their absorption coefficients are very similar below and above the K-absorption edge of iodine. Iodine is clearly imaged because its absorption coefficient drastically changes across its K-absorption edge.

The determination of iodine concentrations was investigated from the subtraction CT images obtained by the K-edge subtraction method. Three glass capillary tubes were bundled together as in the above experiment. The tubes were filled with iodine solutions of different iodine concentrations. The CT images were taken under the following conditions: pixel size of 25 μm, slice thickness of 40 μm, storage time of 2 s per projection, and total collection time of about 7 min for 200 sets of projection data over 180 degree. Figure 6 shows the relationship between the relative CT value of the subtraction image (with respect to the CT value of a 1 wt% iodine solution) and the iodine concentration. It is evident from the graph that the correlation between the iodine concentration and the CT value is good and that iodine concentration can be quantitatively determined to about 0.1 wt%. These results suggest that the SR-CT system can quantitatively and nondestructively measure the distribution of a given element in the specimen.

The SR-CT system can generate monochromatic x-rays in a high energy region. This is considered as the reason that the K-edge subtraction method can also be applied to elements of high atomic number. We have made use of gadolinium solutions. Since gadolinium has its K-edge at 50.2 keV, it can improve x-ray transmission and allow the radiation dose to be reduced compared to the iodine[22, 23]. Figure 7 shows the relationship between the relative CT value of the subtraction image (with respect to the CT value of a 1 wt% iodine solution) and the gadolinium concentration. The concentration of gadolinium could be quantitatively determined to about 3 wt% from the subtraction CT images with a pixel size of about 24 μm and with a slice thickness of 240 μm.

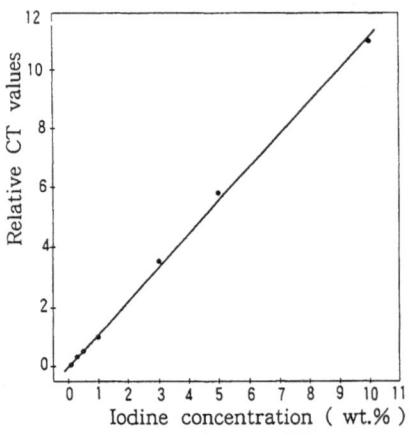

Fig. 6. Relative CT value vs iodine concentration.

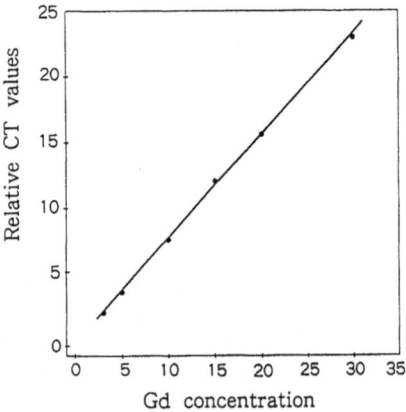

Fig. 7. Relative CT value vs Gd concentration.

Finally, important considerations for improving the resolution and quality of CT images are discussed. The CT image of a specimen is reconstructed from a set of projection data [Eq. (1)] taken while the specimen is rotated. The following dark current correction and logarithmic

93

transformation are performed on the projection data set, and the CT image of the specimen is reconstructed by the filtered back projection (FBP) method.

$$P(X,\theta)=\ln\left[\frac{I(X,\theta)-d(X)}{I_0(X)-d(X)}\right],\tag{1}$$

where I $(X,\ \theta)$ is the x-ray detector output obtained when the specimen is rotated through the angle θ, X is the position of the detector element, $d(X)$ is the dark current of the x-ray detector, and I_0 (X) is the x-ray detector output without the specimen.

The factors considered to affect the quality of CT images are: ① time-dependence of the x-ray intensity distribution, ② time-dependence of the detector dark current, and ③ time-dependence of the detector sensitivity. The change with time of the dark current of the detector is sharply reduced when the x-ray detector is cooled by Peltier elements, and the change with time of the sensitivity of the x-ray detector is not large enough to pose any problem. However, in future it is necessary to stabilize the sensitivity more or to adopt a higher quality detector. At present, the quality of CT images is restricted by the change with time of the x-ray intensity distribution. It would be useful to study the processing and data collection methods to allow for the decay of SR with time.

REFERENCES

1.   Tonner PD, Tosello G (1986) Computed tomography scanning for location and sizing of cavities in valve castings. Materials Evaluation 44: 203-208
2.   Grodzin L (1983) Optimum energies for X-ray transmission tomography of small samples. Applications of synchrotron radiation to computerized tomography I. Nucl. Instrum. Method. 206: 541-545
3.   Grodzin L(1983) Critical absorption tomography of small samples. Proposed applications of synchrotron radiation to computerized tomography II. Nucl. Instrum. Method. 206: 547-552
4.   Thompson AC, Llacer J, Finman LC, Hughes EB, Otis JN, Wilson S, Zeman HD(1984) Computed tomography using synchrotron radiation. Nucl. Instrum. Method. 222: 319-323
5.   Flannery P, Deckman HW, Roberge WG, D'Amico KL (1987) Three-dimensional X-ray microtomography. Science. 237: 1439-1444
6.   Kinney JH, Johnson QC, Bonse U, Nichols MC, Saroyan RA, Nusshardt R, Pahl R, Brase JM (1988) Three-dimensional x-ray computed tomography in materials science. MRS Bulletin. 13: 13-17
7.   Engelke K, Lohmann M, Dix WR, Graeff W (1989) A system for dual energy microtomography of bones. Nucl. Instrum. Method. A274: 380-389
8.   Hirano T, Usami K, Sakamoto K (1989) High resolution monochromatic tomography with X-ray sensing pickup tube. Rev. Sci. Instrum. 60: 2482-2485
9.   Dilmanian FA, Garrett RF, Thomlinson WC, Berman LE, Chapman LD, Hastings JB, Luke PN, Oversluizen T, Siddons DP, Slatkin DN, Stojanoff V, Thompson AC, Volkow ND, Zeman HD (1991) Computed tomography with monochromatic X-rays from the National Synchrotron Light Source. Nucl. Instrum. Method. B56/57: 1208-1213
10.   Zeman HD, Dilmanian FA, Garrett RF, Berman LE, Chapman LD, Hastings JB, Oversluizen T, Siddons DP, Stojanoff V, Thomlinson WC (1991) An X-ray monochromator for dual-energy computerized tomography using synchrotron radiation. Nucl. Instrum. Method. B56/57: 1218-1222
11.   Graeff W, Engelke K (1991) Microradiography and microtomography. In: Ebashi S, Koch M, Rubenstein E (eds) Handbook on Synchrotron Radiation Vol. 4, North-Holland, Amsterdam, pp361-406
12.   Takeda T, Akatsuka T, Hyodo K, Sato M, Yoshioka H, Ishikawa N, Nemoto H, Hiranaka Y, Akisada M (1990) Synchrotron radiation computed tomography for biomedical use. Photon Factory Activity Report 8: 348
13.   Dolbnya IP, Gavrilov NG, Mezentsev NA, Pindyurin VF (1992) Development of an x-ray microscopy and microtomography station at the VEPP-3 storage ring. Rev. Sci. Instrum. 63(1): 609-610

14. Momose A, Takeda T, Itai Y (1995) Phase-contrast x-ray computed tomography for observing biological specimens and organic materials. Rev. Sci. Instrum. 66(2): 1434-1436

15. Raven C, Shigirev A, Snigireva I, Spanne P, Souvorov A, Kohn V (1996) Phase-contrast microtomography with coherent high-energy synchrotron x-rays. Appl. Phys. Lett. 69(13): 1826-1828

16. Ando M, Satow Y, Kawata H, Ishikawa T, Spieker P, Suzuki S (1986) Design of beamline 14 for the PF vertical wiggler and its operation. Nucl. Instrum. Method. A246:144-148

17. Nagata Y, Yamaji H, Kawashima K, Hyodo K, Kawata H, Ando M (1992) High energy high resolution monochromatic X-ray computed tomography using synchrotron radiation. Nondestr. Test. Eval. 7: 299-307

18. Nagata Y, Yamaji H, Kawashima K, Hyodo K, Kawata H, Ando M (1992) High energy high resolution monochromatic X-ray computed tomography using the photon factory vertical wiggler beamline. Rev. Sci. Instrum. 63(1): 615-618

19. Nagata Y, Yamaji H, Kawashima K, Hyodo K, Ando M (1992) High energy high resolution monochromatic X-ray computed tomography system. Res. Nondestr. Eval. 4: 55-78

20. Matsushita T, Hashizume H (1983) X-ray monochromators. In: Koch EE(eds) Handbook on Synchrotron Radiation, Vol. 1A, North-Holland, Amsterdam, pp261-314

21 Hyodo K, Nishimura K, Ando M (1991) Coronary angiography project at the Photon Factory using a large monochromatic beam. In: Ebashi S, Koch M, Rubenstein E (eds) Handbook on Synchrotron Radiation Vol. 4, North-Holland, Amsterdam, pp55-94

22. Zeman HD, Siddons DP (1990) Contrast agent choice for intravenous coronary angiography. Nucl. Instrum. Method. A291: 67-73

23. Zeman HD, Di Bianca FA, Thomlinson WC (1991) A kinestatic charge detector for intravenous coronary angiography using synchrotron radiation x-rays. IEEE Trans. Nucl. Sci. 38(2): 641-647

Synchrotron Radiation Computed Tomography applied to the Brain : Phantom Studies at the ESRF Medical Beamline

A.M. Charvet[1], C. Lartizien[1], F. Estève[1], G. Le Duc[1], A. Collomb[1], H. Elleaume[1], S. Fiedler[2], A. Thompson[2], T. Brochard[2], U. Kleuker[2], H. Steltner[2], P. Spanne[2], P. Suortti[2], J.F. Le Bas[1].

[1]Rayonnement Synchrotron-Recherche Médicale, Université Joseph Fourier de Grenoble, at ESRF
[2]European Synchrotron Radiation Facility (ESRF), BP 220, 38043 Grenoble, France

SUMMARY: A monochromatic computed tomography (CT) system for clinical studies in brain pathology is part of the medical beamline ID17 at the ESRF (European Synchrotron Radiation Facility). We have carried out preliminary phantom studies to determine the minimum detectable iodine and gadolinium concentrations by the K-edge subtraction technique as well as the minimum detectable change in potassium concentration by dual-energy quantitative CT.

KEY WORDS: X-ray - brain - computed tomography - contrast agents

INTRODUCTION

Computed tomography (CT) applied to brain pathology was approved as a research program on the medical beamline ID17 at the European Synchrotron Radiation Facility (ESRF). Both medical imaging and computing techniques have considerably improved in the past twenty years. Fast methods such as signal processing and reconstruction techniques are now available allowing very accurate studies of anatomic slices of the human body. The contrast obtained for a given tissue depends on signal variations, and thus is linked to the physical parameter measured. It is then possible to define a contrast semiology for each technique (X-ray, γ-ray, Magnetic Resonance Imaging (MRI), Ultrasound) correlated to anatomic information and tissue characterization. Nowadays, efforts are concentrated to extend the usefulness of these techniques beyond anatomic mapping and contrast approach to obtain functional or metabolic information (cerebral blood flow, oxygen consumption, glucose consumption, uptake and behaviors of particular metabolites like neuromediators or drugs). This kind of information appears essential especially in the neurosciences to understand physiopathology and to guide therapeutic choices. Despite an excellent spatial and temporal resolution, CT scan has known few developments in functional imaging until now (i.e. Xenon-CT to measure cerebral blood flow) [1]. Actual limits for clinical CT systems are well-known: artefacts due to diffuse scattering, beam hardening due to the polychromaticity of the X-ray source, source size, etc. Nevertheless, CT still remains the only quantitative technique available with the same absolute scale everywhere (Hounsfield units) justifying further investigations with another X-ray source. The X-ray source provided by synchrotron radiation in general and the ESRF in particular exhibits interesting properties to minimize these problems, allowing for example experiments with a monochromatic beam. Thus, using synchrotron radiation, new investigations in clinical research are now possible [2] such as our monochromatic CT project at the medical beamline ID17 [3],[4],[5], which follows the work of A. Dilmanian [6], [7]. This project is focused on brain pathologies (tumors, ischemia and epilepsy), with a predominant aim of answering the following questions:
1-Is it possible to obtain selective concentration measurements of contrast agents (like gadolinium and iodine) at clinical concentrations by using a synchrotron radiation monochromatic CT scanner ? Accessing concentration measurements of intravenous contrast agents, i.e. accessing blood distribution is one of the central purpose of our program to characterize the blood brain barrier (BBB) rupture phenomenon, endothelial permeability and the tumor angiogenesis process.
2-Is it possible to access concentration measurements of endogenous elements such as potassium and to study tissue ionic modifications ? These modifications are the keys to understanding and predicting metabolic behavior after epilepsy crisis or ischemic injuries.
More generally, these goals are correlated to local clinical research directions which are already investigated with others imaging techniques such as biomedical MRI.

The medical beamline ID17 at the ESRF provides synchrotron radiation X-rays in the 20-100 keV range for three main programs, coronary angiography, computed tomography applied to the brain and microbeam radiation therapy. Two energy-selective imaging methods, K-edge subtraction CT (KES-CT) and dual-energy quantitative CT (DEQCT), will be implemented in the clinical system to improve contrast resolution and provide quantitative images.

MATERIALS AND METHODS

In the present paper, we report on preliminary measurements carried out on phantoms during the spring and early summer of 1997 to evaluate the limits of both techniques.
DEQCT is investigated to detect brain lesions of altered elemental concentrations, such as potassium. It is based on the dependency of the Compton and photoelectric part of the attenuation coefficient on the energy and the atomic number Z. Tissues are mainly constituted of two groups of elements: low Z and intermediate Z elements. X-ray transmission is measured at two widely separated energies. The data are processed to produce two quantitative images of the effective average density of each group of elements, with an improved contrast resolution compared with a single energy CT image [8].
The KES technique is mainly dedicated to small cerebral tumour imaging and ischemia analysis. This technique uses the sharp rise in the photoelectric component of the attenuation coefficient of gadolinium or iodine at the binding energy of the K electron [9],[10]. Two images are taken in turn, immediately above and below the K-edge. The resulting subtracted image is quantitative for the contrast agent and we expect a significantly higher contrast resolution than in a conventional CT image.
The CT setup uses a fixed fan-shaped monochromatic X-ray beam of 1.5 mm height and 120 mm width and a subject rotating around a vertical axis. The monochromator consists in two bent (111) silicon crystals, operated in Laue mode and mounted in a fixed exit configuration [11]. It is tuneable from 20 keV to 90 keV. Distance between source and object is approximately 155 m, between object and detector 5 m. Attenuation is measured using a current integrated multipixel cooled Germanium detector. The detector itself is a single slab of Germanium, 2 mm thick, with 2 rows of 432 pixels of 0.35 mm width each, deposited on the crystal by photolithography. A single row was used in the work presented here. The X-ray detector is followed by 864 channels of 16 bit current-integrating electronics. The instrumentation used during the measurements and briefly described above is part of the clinical system, and was in an early commissioning phase at the time of the experiments. The patient positioning system was not available; electromechanical translation and rotation stages were used to position and rotate the phantoms instead. Similarly, the triggering system for fast data acquisition -1 line every millisecond- was not available, leading to acquisition times of the order of 30 minutes per image, or even longer at the beginning, whereas the clinical system is expected to take an image in 2 to 5 seconds. Problems with the CT system included monochromator drifts, and a rather large number of bad pixels (~ 20 in 864 pixels) in the detection system. The former has been largely eliminated, by implementing gravity water cooling of the crystals, better tuning procedures for the monochromator, and faster data acquisition. The latter has been traced to the bonding on the Germanium detector crystal and is being addressed.
DEQCT was carried out using Plexiglas tubes and a Plexiglas and aluminium head phantom of diameter 10 cm containing solutions of KOH at several concentrations. The average potassium concentration in the cerebral tissue is on the order of 3 mg/cm^3. Preliminary experiments were performed with high concentrations (10 to 50 mg/cm^3) to test the feasibility. Then, lower concentrations (0.3 to 10 mg/cm^3) were used to reach physiological levels. Data were obtained at 40 keV and 80 keV, for different radiation doses. Similar phantoms filled with Gd and I solutions of different concentrations (0.1 to 3 mg/cm^3) were imaged at their respective K-edges (50.239 keV for Gd and 33.169 keV for I). For the experiments discussed here, dosimetry parameters were chosen close to classical brain examination in conventional CT, i.e. a dose equivalent to a skin-entry dose of 5 cGy per image pair.

RESULTS

The results of potassium concentrations measurements using DQECT are summarized in fig. 2 and 3 below. Figure 1 illustrates the subtraction technique on a set of 7 Plexiglas tubes filled with varying KOH concentrations in solution. The density image shows decreasing gray scales for decreasing concentrations as expected.

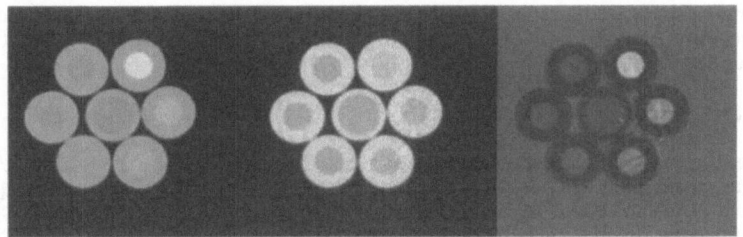

Fig. 1: Potassium phantom images showing reconstructed images at 42 keV, 87 keV and density image.

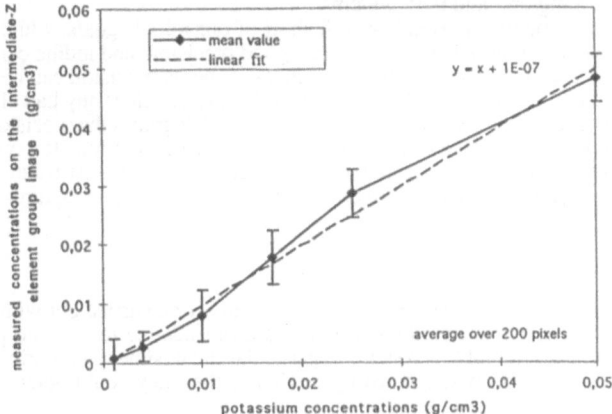

Fig. 2: Measured potassium concentrations versus actual concentrations for the 7 tubes-phantom filled with physiogically high concentrations. Voxel size was 0.35x0.35 mm².

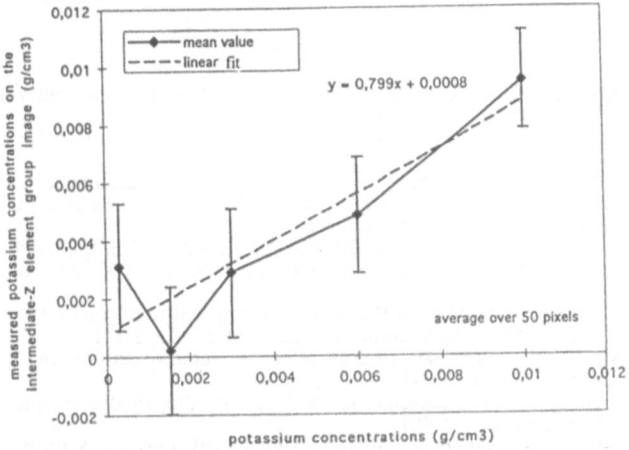

Fig. 3: Measured potassium concentrations versus actual concentrations for the 10 cm diameter head phantom. Voxel size was 0.35x0.35 mm².

Figure 2 shows a plot of measured concentrations vs actual concentrations for the phantom shown in fig. 1. Figure 3 is a similar plot obtained in the case of the 10 cm diameter head phantom filled with solutions of potassium with concentrations below 10 mg/cm³. A quantitative analysis of the data indicates that we are presently able to measure a concentration of 6 mg/cm³ of potassium with an error of the order of 30% for clinical radiation doses in a voxel of about 3x3x2 mm³.

Under the same dosimetry conditions, the measurements on the 10 cm diameter head phantom show that we can quantify 1mg/cm³ (±10%) of I or Gd in a 6 mm diameter detail and 2 mg/cm³ (±10%) in a 3 mm diameter detail.

DISCUSSION

As stated above, average potassium concentration in healthy cerebral tissue is about 3 mg/cm³. In the case of contrast agents, iodine concentration in the blood vessels for normally injected quantities is about 4 mg/cm³. Concentrations of gadolinium in the blood vessels using a product such as Gado-butrol (developed by Schering) could reach 1.3 mg/cm³. In healthy brain tissue, this would lead to concentrations of iodine and gadolinium of respectively 0.2 mg/cm³ and 0.07 mg/cm³. However in the case of the breakdown of the BBB, we expect concentrations of iodine and gadolinium respecti-vely on the order of 1.5 mg/cm³ and 0.45 mg/cm³.

The preliminary measurements reported here fall short of our initials goals, which were to measure changes in potassium concentrations of 100% with a good precision, and iodine concentrations of 1.5 mg/cm³ (with a good precision as well). However, measurements precision can be improved by fine tuning the instrumentation, in particular the X-ray detection system since any bad channel on the solid state detector leads to artefacts in the reconstructed images and degrades the precision in concentration meaurement. We were also sensitive to long term drifts in the monochromator system, drifts which have since been improved but will be irrelevant in any case when the fast rotation system (patient positioning device) is routinely available. We expect to win factor 2 or 3 by optimizing the set-up.

CONCLUSION

The measurements presented here were only preliminary and were carried out with a system still in a commissioning phase. Further measurements are therefore needed to test the potential limits in quantification of a clinical cerebral CT system. In particular the dosimetry conditions we had imposed were quite severe and it has been suggested by clinicians that they could potentially be relaxed in certain cases.

This work was supported by a grant from Région Rhône-Alpes where UJF, LETI-CENG, INSA Lyon, CHU-Grenoble and ESRF were partners. Results were obtained thanks to beam time at ESRF.

REFERENCES

1. Nambu K, Suzuki R, Hirakawa K (1995). Cerebral blood flow: measurement with Xenon-enhanced dynamic helical CT. Radiology 195: 53-57.
2. Thomlinson W. (1992). Medical applications of synchrotron radiation. Nucl Instr and Meth in Phys Res A319: 295-304.
3. ESRF Home Page, World Wide Web: http://www.esrf.fr. ID17 Page ,"Beamlines" section.
4. Elleaume H, Charvet AM, Le Bas JF (1997). The synchrotron beam, a new dimension for contrast media research? Acta Radiologica 38, Supplement 412: 29-41.
5. Moulin-Elleaume H (1997): ESRF Beamline Handbook, Edited by R. Mason, Grenoble.
6. Dilmanian FA (1992). Computed tomography with monochromatic X-rays. Am J Physiol Imaging 3/4: 175-193
7. Dilmanian FA, Garrett RF, Thomlinson WC (1991). Computed tomography with monochromatic X-ray from the NSLS. Nucl Instr and Meth in Phys Res B56-57: 1208-1213.
8. Alvarez RE, Macovski A (1976). Energy-selective reconstructions in X-ray computerized tomography. Phys Med Biol 21: 733-744.
9. Riederer SJ, Mistretta CA (1997). Selective iodine imaging using K-edge energies in computerized x-ray tomography. Med Phys 4: 474-481.
10. Thompson AC, LLacer J, Campbell Finman L, Hughes EB, Otis JN, Wilson S, Zeman D (1984). Computed Tomography using Synchrotron Radiation. Nucl Instr and Meth in Phys Res 222, 319-323.
11. Suortti P, Schulze C (1995). Fixed-Exit Monochromators for High-Energy Synchrotron Radiation. J Synchotron Rad 2:6-12.

IODINE-FILTER IMAGING SYSTEM FOR SUBTRACTION ANGIOGRAPHY AND ITS IMPROVEMENT BY FLUORESCENT-SCREEN HARPICON DETECTOR

Keiji Umetani [1], Tohoru Takeda [2], Hironori Ueki [1], Ken Ueda [1], Yuji Itai [2], Izumi Anno [2], Teiichi Nakajima [3] and Masayoshi Akisada [3, 4]

[1] Central Research Laboratory, Hitachi, Ltd., Kokubunji, Tokyo 185, Japan
[2] Institute of Clinical Medicine, University of Tsukuba, Tsukuba, Ibaraki 305, Japan
[3] Tama Health Management Center, Tachikawa, Tokyo 190, Japan
[4] Department of Radiology and Information Science, International University of Health and Welfare, Ohtawara, Tochigi 324, Japan

SUMMARY. Our initial studies in animal experiments using K-edge energy subtraction transvenous coronary angiography at the Photon Factory were undertaken using an iodine filter for energy switching combined with an X-ray image intensifier. In vivo subtracted images of coronary arteries in dogs were obtained in the form of motion pictures. However, the image quality was not good for medical examinations because the contrast material was highly diluted. A new image detector with a fluorescent-screen lens-coupling approach has been developed to take high quality images. By using the new detector in place of the X-ray image intensifier, image quality has markedly increased in coronary angiography.

KEY WORDS: Coronary angiography, Energy subtraction, Digital imaging, HARPICON

INTRODUCTION

After Rubenstein and his coworkers reported dual-energy digital subtraction transvenous coronary angiography using a monochromatized X-ray in 1981 [1], several groups around the world have developed various imaging systems for diagnosing coronary artery disease. American and German groups have improved the dual-energy imaging system to the point where it can be tested in human studies [2, 3]. In Japan the first human studies of transvenous coronary angiography using a single-energy approach were performed in May 1996.

A group of researchers from Hitachi, Ltd. and the University of Tsukuba began studying of coronary artery diagnosis in 1987. Studies in dogs were performed using an iodine-filter method for K-edge subtraction transvenous angiography. In this method, the real-time subtracted images of dog's coronary arteries were obtained [4, 5]. A new image detector was then developed to improve the image quality using a HARPICON™ camera and a fluorescent screen in place of an X-ray image intensifier [6]. The avalanche multiplication type HARPICON camera is 32 times more sensitive than a conventional SATICON™ camera.

IMAGING METHODS

The X-ray imaging system was placed at the superconducting vertical wiggler beamline BL-14C. The SR beam was monochromatized and expanded horizontally by an asymmetrically cut silicon <311> crystal. In the iodine-filter imaging system shown in Fig. 1(a), the angle of the crystal was adjusted until the energy band of the monochromatized X-ray was centered at the iodine K-edge. A set of the iodine- and aluminum-filtered images, corresponding respectively to the low- and high-energy images in conventional dual-energy imaging, was sequentially taken by synchronizing the timing of the mechanical movement of the filters into and out of the SR beam. The X-ray image detector consisted of the X-ray image intensifier, an optical system with an oscillating mirror and the SATICON camera. The X-ray image intensifier's output of the iodine- and aluminum-filtered images were focused side-by-side on the photoconductive layer of the camera tube by the oscillating mirror. After image acquisition, the energy-subtracted image was produced.

A high-spatial-resolution detector using a fluorescent-screen lens-coupling approach was developed to improve image quality [6, 7]. In Fig. 1(b), an X-ray image on the screen was focused on the photoconductive layer of the high-sensitivity HARPICON camera by lenses with high numerical aperture.

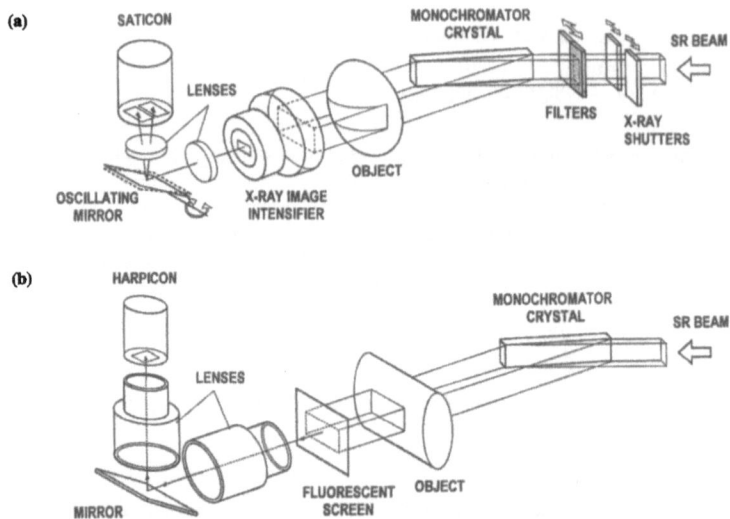

Fig. 1. Schematic drawing of the imaging systems: a) the iodine-filter imaging system with the X-ray image intensifier and b) the fluorescent-screen HARPICON detector system.

EXPERIMENTS AND RESULTS

The spatial-resolution-chart images taken in the 512×460 pixel-matrix mode are shown in Fig. 2. Though the image contrast of the bar pattern at 2 line-pairs/mm is 3-5% in the iodine-filter imaging system, it is around 50% in the fluorescent-screen HARPICON detector system.

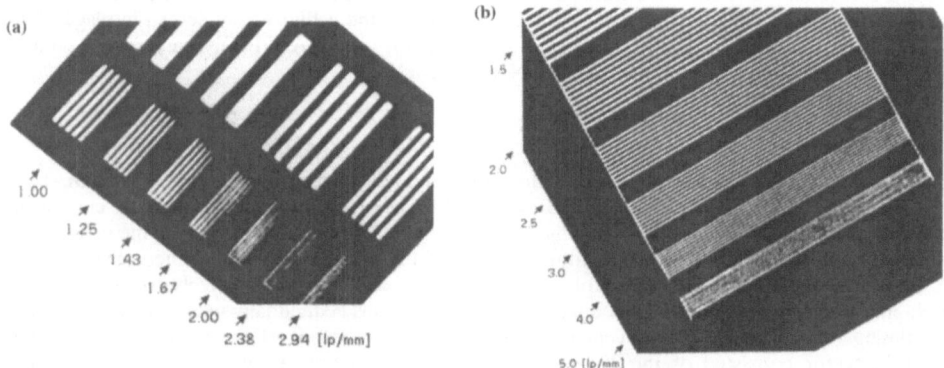

Fig. 2. X-ray images of resolution chart taken by a) the iodine filter method with the X-ray image intensifier and by b) the fluorescent-screen HARPICON detector.

101

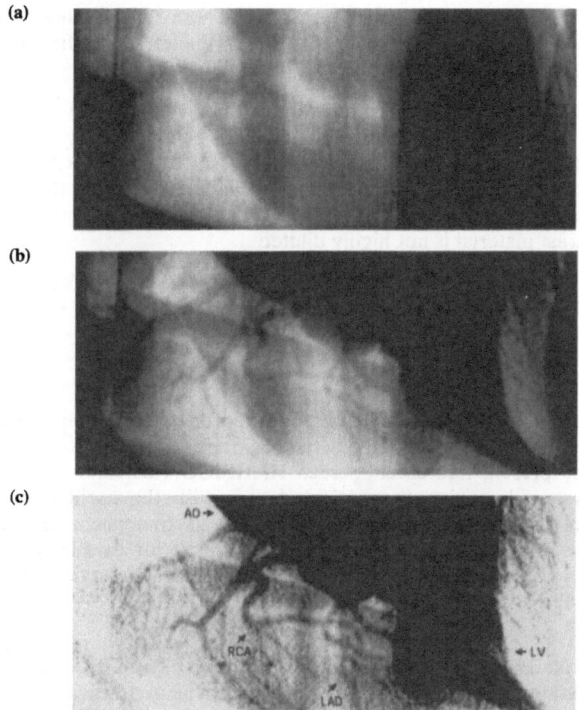

Fig. 3. A set of dog's heart images, obtained after transvenous injection using the iodine-filter method: a) iodine-filtered image, b) aluminum-filtered image and c) subtracted image.

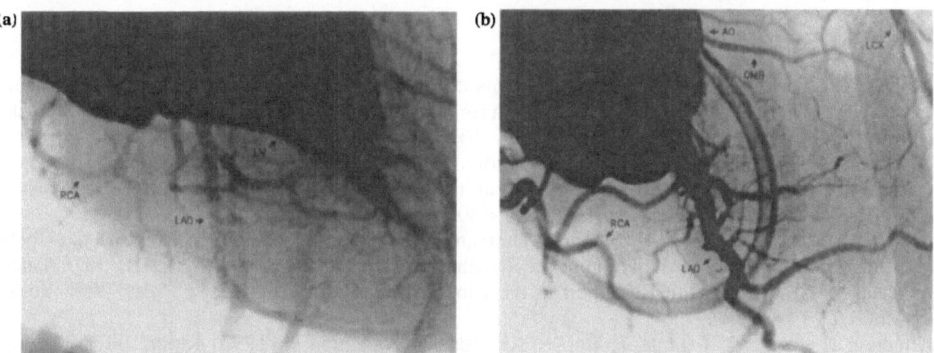

Fig. 4. Heart images of dogs, obtained using the fluorescent-screen HARPICON detector. Images were taken by injection into a) the inferior vena cava and b) the aorta.

In vivo imaging by injection into the inferior vena cava using the iodine-filter method was performed on dogs weighing about 12 kg. The set of three images in Fig. 3 was taken for dual-energy digital subtraction angiography using the iodine-filter method in 1991. The bottom image was obtained by the subtraction operation using a) the iodine-filtered image and b) the aluminum-filtered image. In vivo imaging by injection into the inferior vena cava and the aorta using the fluorescent-screen HARPICON detector were then performed on dogs. The set of two images in Fig. 4 was taken in 1995 using just above the iodine K-edge energy X-ray, corresponding to the high-energy X-ray in conventional dual-energy imaging. These images show the left anterior descending artery (LAD), the right coronary artery (RCA), the left circumflex artery (LCX), the obtuse marginal branch (OMB), the left ventricle (LV) and the aorta (OA).

The image after the contrast material injection into the inferior vena cava in Fig. 4(a) is of higher quality than that of the aluminum-filtered image in Fig. 3(b) and the energy-subtracted image in Fig. 3(c). A higher contrast image is obtained by the fluorescent-screen HARPICON detector than that by the iodine-filter method using the X-ray image intensifier. Moreover, the image in Fig. 4(b) taken by contrast material injection into the aorta is of much higher quality than that of all above images because the contrast material is not highly diluted.

The experiments were approved by the Medical Committee for the Use of Animals in Research of the University of Tsukuba, and conformed to the guidelines of the American Physiological Society.

DISCUSSION

Image quality in the iodine-filter method for subtraction coronary angiography will be improved by using the fluorescent-screen HARPICON detector in place of the X-ray image-intensifier SATICON detector. The present fluorescent-screen HARPICON detector can be applied to the iodine-filter imaging system by using the optical device with the oscillating mirror and the mechanical device for movement of the filters. Furthermore, as an application of the iodine filter method, the fluorescent-screen lens-coupling approach is suitable for an energy-selective detector that can take the high- and low-energy images at the same time. A detailed description of this detector has been presented elsewhere [6].

The authors thank Ms Rika Baba and Mr. Tomoharu Kajiyama of the CRL, Hitachi, Ltd., for their support in image processing and image analysis. This work was performed with the approval of the National Laboratory for High Energy Physics (acceptance Nos. 87-Y002, 88-Y003, 89-Y015, 90-Y001, 91-Y005, 92-Y006, 93-Y003, 94-Y001 and 95-Y005) and the Photon Factory Program Advisory Committee (proposal Nos. 87-189, 89-167, 91-231, 93-G238 and 95-G290).

REFERENCES

1. Rubenstein E, Hughes EB, Campbell LE, Hofstadter R, Kirk RL, Krolicki TJ, Stone JP, Wilson S, Zeman HD, Brody WR, Macovski A, Thompson AC (1981) Synchrotron radiation and its application to digital subtraction angiography. SPIE 314 Digital Radiography: 42-49
2. Thomlinson W (1994) Medical applications of synchrotron radiation at the National Synchrotron Light Source. In: Chance B, et al. (eds) Synchrotron Radiation in the Biosciences. Oxford University Press, New York, pp 674-680
3. Dix WR, Graeff W, Hamm C, Heuer J, Hultschig H, Kupper W, Lohmann M, Rust C (1994) Coronary Angiography at the Hamburger Synchrotronstrahlungslabor (HASYLAB). In: Chance B, et al. (eds) Synchrotron Radiation in the Biosciences. Oxford University Press, New York, pp 666-673
4. Umetani K, Ueda K, Takeda T, Itai Y, Akisada M, Nakajima T (1993) Iodine filter imaging system for subtraction angiography using synchrotron radiation. Nucl. Instr. and Meth. A335: 569-579
5. Takeda T, Itai Y, Yoshioka H, Umetani K, Ueda K, Akisada M (1994) Synchrotron radiation cine K-edge energy subtraction coronary arteriography using an iodine filter method. Med. & biol. Eng. & Comput. 32: 462-468
6. Umetani K, Ueki H, Ueda K, Hirai T, Takeda T, Doi T, Wu J, Itai Y, Akisada M (1996) High-spatial-resolution medical-imaging system using a HARPICON camera coupled with a fluorescent screen. J. Synchrotron Rad. 3: 136-144
7. Takeda T, Umetani K, Doi T, Echigo J, Ueki H, Ueda K, Itai Y (1997) Two-dimensional aortographic coronary arteriography with above-K-edge monochromatic synchrotron radiation. Acad. Radiol. 4: 438-445

Development of a Monochromatic X-ray Computed Tomography with Synchrotron Radiation for Functional Imaging

Tohoru TAKEDA, Masahiro KAZAMA, *Tsutomu ZENIYA, *Tetsuya YUASA, *Masahiro AKIBA, *Akira UCHIDA, **Kazuyuki HYODO, *Takao AKATSUKA, **Masami ANDO, Yuji ITAI

Institute of Clinical Medicine, University of Tsukuba, 1-1-1 Tennodai, Tsukuba-shi, Ibaraki 305 Japan
*Department of of Electrical and Information Engineering, Yamagata University
**Photon Factory, KEK

SUMMARY

X-ray CT with synchrotron radiation (SR) is being developed to detect very low concentrations of contrast material for functional evaluations of regional blood flow and metabolism of organs corresponding with their anatomical structures. The theoretical detectability of iodine contrast material is expected to be about 35 μg iodine / g with 0.2-mm spatial resolution at a 1-mm slice thickness. However, the minimal detectable iodine concentration of this system is about 200 μg/ml on the above K-edge image due to the poor dynamic range of x-rat detector. The use of a CCD detector cooled by liquid nitrogen is planned to improve the dynamic ranges of the detector.

KEYWORDS: Monochromatic x-ray CT, Synchrotron radiation, Functional imaging

INTRODUCTION

Conventional x-ray computed tomography (CT) is widely used to diagnose many kinds of disease in clinical practice, and to image cerebral blood flow by stable xenon inhalation [1-2]. Whereas, monochromatic x-ray CT with synchrotron radiation (SR) is being used to analyze the fine structures of material in scientific research because of its sufficient x-ray flux and the tunability of energy spectrum for visualization of the spatial distribution of specific elements [3-11]. Biological experiments with SR were performed by Thompson (dog heart with iodine contrast material) in 1984 [12], Borodin (lymph node) in 1986 [13], Engelke (bone imaging) in 1989 [14-15] and Takeda (rat skull) in 1994 [16]. Recently very fine images of bony structures were obtained [17-19]. In Brookhaven National Laboratory, Dilmanian et al are developing a high sensitive SR x-ray CT system to map low and intermediate Z-elements (i.e. P, S, Cl, K, Ca, and Fe) for neurological diagnosis[20-23].

We are constructing a biomedical SR x-ray CT system to detect very low concentrations of contrast material (a few μg iodine /g) for functional evaluations of regional blood flow and metabolism of the organs corresponding with their anatomical structures [24-28]. Fig.1 shows SPECT image of a brain after cerebral infarction. The spatial resolution of this system is about 11 mm, but the infarcted area in the left front-temporal lobe was demonstrated as reduced perfusion. Preliminary study using the commercially based x-ray CT, 50 μg/ml iodine solution and 50 μg/ml gadolinium solution could be detected clearly and quantitatively in a brain phantom using a 10-mm slice thickness (Fig.2) [25]. As SR x-ray CT has great advantages to improve image contrast, image with much better spatial resolution than SPECT will be obtained. The theoretical detectability of contrast material, and the experimental results by SR x-ray CT are described in this paper.

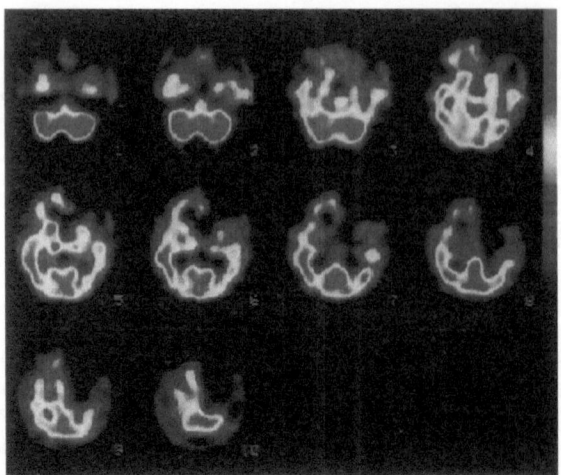

Fig.1 SPECT image of the brain with IMP

The infarcted area on left front-temporal lobe is demonstrated as reduced perfusion.

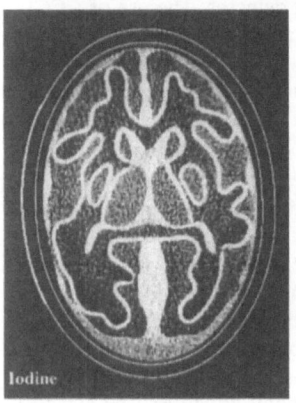 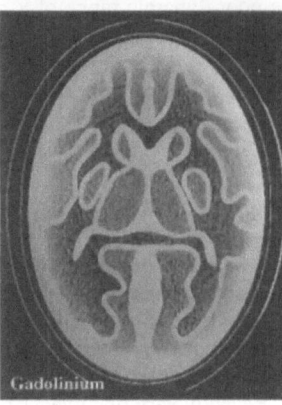

Fig.2 Phantom image obtained by conventional x-ray CT
(GE CT9800 HiLight)
A: CT image of brain phantom
 left; iodine (80 kp, 300mA)
 right; gadolinium (120 kp, 140mA)
B: CT value of brain phantom
 Area corresponding to thalamus and cortex contain contrast agents, whereas white matter contains water. The parts of cortical surface and basal ganglion are well enhanced. Images of gadolinium has much better contrast than those of iodine. Good statistical uniformity of image is obtained in Gd contrast agent.

A

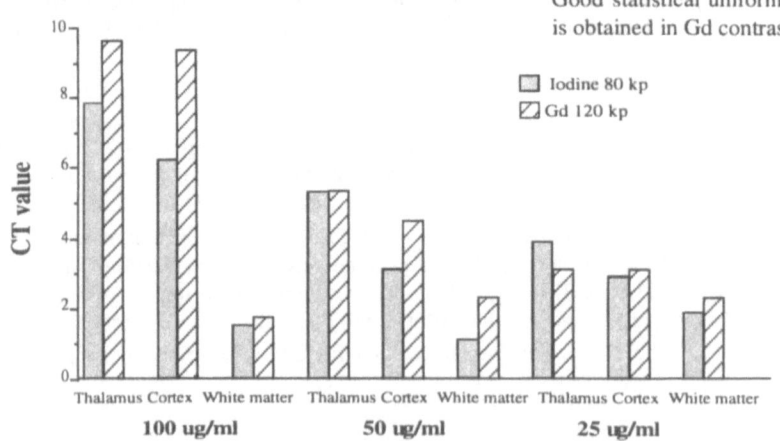

B Concentration of contrast material

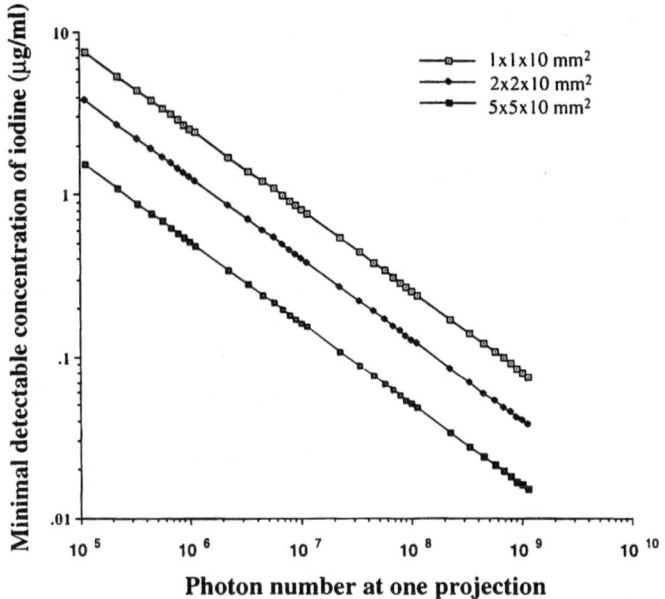

Fig.3 The relationship between the minimal detectability of iodine and photon flux

MINIMAL DETECTABILITY OF CONTRAST MATERIAL

In the ideal state without scatter radiation, the minimal detectability of contrast element can be calculated by the noise due to photon counting statistics in CT [29]. The signal-to-noise (S/N) ratio (σ^2/μ^2) is defined by the equation below:

$$\frac{\sigma^2}{\mu^2} = \frac{\Pi^2 \int_{-\infty}^{\infty} k^2 |W(k)|^2 dk}{m^2 \mu^2} \sum_{j=1}^{m} \left(\frac{1}{N_j}\right)$$

where μ is the true value of the attenuation coefficient and σ^2 is the variance of the measured attenuation at a given point. The value of m is the number of projections, N_j is the photon flux density [photons/mm^2] of the unscattered photons that have passed through the element of interest and detected in the jth projection, and W(k) is the window function of the corrective filter for the reconstruction.

Using the above equation, the relationship between the minimal detectability of iodine and photon flux density is calculated (Fig.3). The theoretical minimal detectable concentration of iodine is 35.3 µg/ml in this experiment ; μ = 177.0 [cm^{-1}] (above K-edge energy), m = 180, N_j = 1.0 x 10^6 photons/mm^2/projection (7.0 x 10^7 [photons/mm^2/sec] x 0.04 [sec] x exp(-0.33 x 3)), 0.2-mm spatial resolution, and 1-mm slice thickness. For human studies using 5-mm spatial resolution with 10-mm slice thickness like a PET study, 450 ng iodine /g is expected to image at 180 projections and 10^6 photons/mm^2/projection.

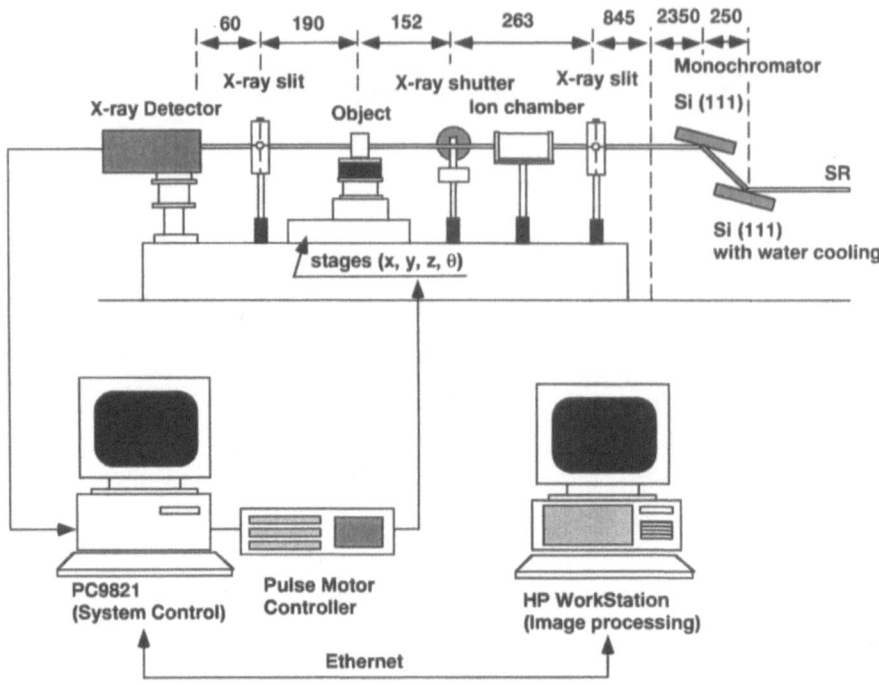

Fig.4 Schematic diagram of SR x-ray CT system

MATERIALS & METHODS

SR-CT system

The SR x-ray CT system is constructed at the beam line BLNE5A of the Tristan Accumulation Ring in KEK (6.5 GeV, 20-40 mA, 1 T bending magnet). This system consists of a rotating x-ray shutter, a silicon (111) double crystal monochromator, an x-ray slit system, a rotating object table, an ionization chamber, an x-ray linear array detector, and a computer (Fig.4).

a) Monochromator

The double crystal monochromator containing two silicon (111) crystals generates a monochromatic x-ray beam almost parallel to the incident white x-ray beam. The x-ray energy is set at just above and below the K-edge of iodine (33.2 and 33.0 keV), and the x-ray energy is slightly detuned to eliminate the high-order x-ray contamination (99 keV). The monochromatic x-ray beam size is 65 mm in width by 3 mm in height. The incident and monochromatic x-rays are collimated to decrease the scatter radiation by the slit system. The first crystal radiated by the incident white x-rays is water cooled to reduce the heat effect of white x-rays.

b) X-ray detector

The x-ray linear array detector (Hamamatsu Photonics Ltd., Japan) consists of a Gd_2O_2S scintillator coated on a glass fiber optical plate and a silicon photodiode array. The detection area is 51.2 mm in width and 3.2 mm in height, with 256 channels (1 element = 0.2 mm x 3.2 mm). The x-ray intensity data are digitized by a 16-bit analog-to-digital converter. The theoretical dynamic range of this detector is about 60000 : 1 (6 x 10^9 electrons : 1 x 10^3 electrons).

c) System control

The monochromatic x-ray CT system is controlled by a personal computer and a pulse motor controller. The x-ray detector is also controlled by the personal computer through a direct-memory access interface board. The well organized system control allows CT data to be obtained automatically.

Objects

A cylindrical acrylic phantom 35-mm in diameter with small holes (1, 1.5, 2, 3, 4, 5mm) was filled by iodine. A rat brain filled with iodine microspheres was imaged. The exposure time of each projection was 40 msec. The slice thickness of objects was set at 1 mm, 180 projection data was obtained at 1 degree rotation step.

Image reconstruction

Projection data entered into the personal computer were sent to an engineering work station (HP9000 model 725/75 : Hewlett-Packard) through the ethernet. As the monochromatic x-ray intensity declines exponentially owing to the decrease in the ring current, the correction of x-ray intensity is performed by an ionization chamber. Reconstructions are carried out using filtered back-projection in real space, and a Shepp and Logan filter.

RESULTS

In the contrast-resolution phantom images obtained at 1-mm slice thickness, the above K-edge, below K-edge and K-edge energy subtraction are shown in Fig.5. On the above K-edge image, the minimal concentration of iodine contrast material was 200 µg/ml. On the K-edge energy subtraction images, it was 500 µg/ml. The image quality of the above K-edge image was better than that of the K-edge energy subtraction image.

The K-edge energy subtraction image of the rat brain containing iodine microspheres demonstrated the distribution of iodine microspheres (Fig.6). The cerebral arteries filled with iodine microspheres were clearly revealed, and the ischemic regions at the right temporal lobe and frontal lobe were shown as non-vascular regions.

DISCUSSIONS

The minimal detectable iodine concentration of this system is about 200 µg/ml on the above K-edge image and 500 µg/ml on the K-edge energy subtraction image. The contrast resolution on the above K-edge energy image is about 2 times higher than that on the K-edge energy subtraction image because of increased image noise by the subtraction process. However, the measured minimal detectable concentration of iodine on the above K-edge image is about 6 times higher than that expected in this experiment, which was calculated to be 35.3 µg/ml by Chesler's equation.

In the experiment, the contrast resolution is determined by the quantum noise of x-ray photons, the contamination of scatter radiation, the dynamic range of the sensor, and the dynamic range of the analog-to-digital converter. The most important contributor to insufficient contrast resolution in this SR x-ray CT system might be the poor dynamic range of the sensor system. The planned dynamic range of x-ray linear array detector was 60000 : 1, but the actual dynamic range was very poor (150 : 1) due to significant dark currents. Using this detector in the above K-edge energy, the contrast resolution was calculated to be about 220 µg/ml at one projection. Consequently, the limited dynamic range of the x-ray detector is thought to be the most serious drawback of this SR x-ray CT system. At present, we are planning to use a new CCD detector which is cooled by liquid nitrogen. In this CCD, the dynamic range of the sensor is expected to exceed 6000:1.

Above K-edge

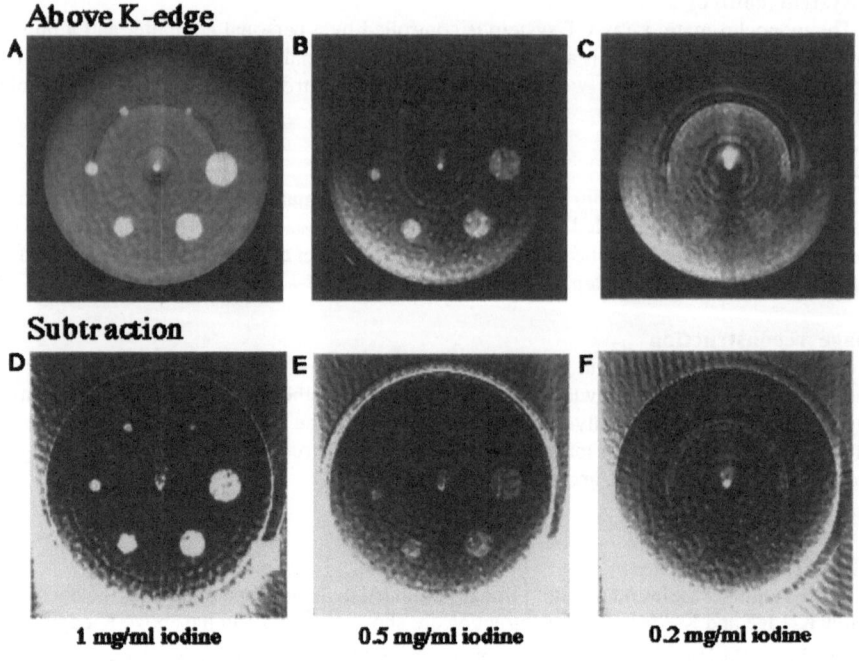

Subtraction

1 mg/ml iodine   0.5 mg/ml iodine   0.2 mg/ml iodine

Fig.5 SR x-ray CT image of phantom filled by iodine
   The size of hole is 1, 1.5, 2, 3, 4 and 5 mm respectively.

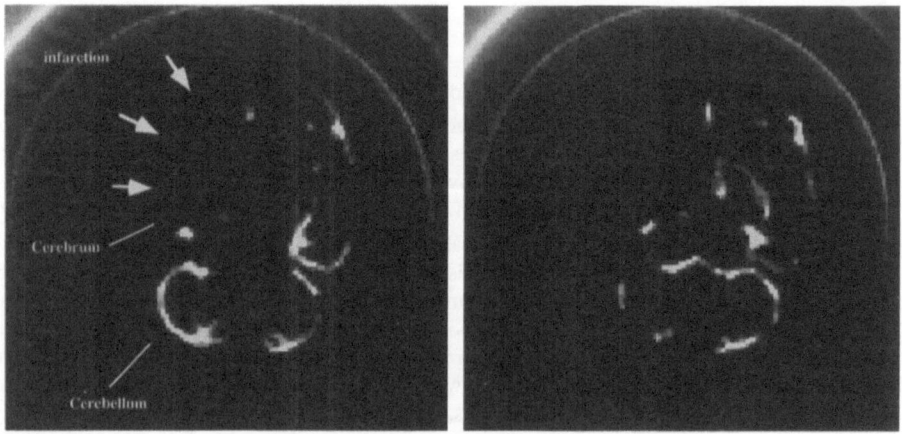

Fig.6 Iodine K-edge energy subtraction image of rat skull containing iodine microspheres
   The cerebral arteries were clearly revealed, and the ischemic regions at the right temporal lobe
and frontal lobe were shown as non-vascular regions.

Acknowledgement
This study has performed under the approval of the National Laboratory for High Energy Physics (proposal No. 90-074, 92G248, 94G304). This research was partially supported by Grants-in-aid for Scientific Research #05404037, #08407024 and Developmental Science Research #06507002 from the Ministry of Education, Science and Culture, Japan.

REFERENCES

1. Meyer JS, Hayman LA, Yamamoto M, Sakai F, Nakajima S (1980) Local cerebral blood flow measured by CT after stable xenon inhalation. AJR 135: 239-251
2. Winkler SS, Sackett JF, Holden JE, Flemming DC, Aleznder SC, Madsen M, Kimmel RI (1977) Xenon inhalation as an adjunct to computerized tomography of the brain: preliminary study. Invest. Radiol. 12:15-18
3. Grodzins L (1983) Optimum energies for x-ray transmission tomography of small samples. Application of synchrotron radiation to computed tomography I. Nucl. Instr. Meth. 206:541-545
4. Grodzins L (1983) Critical absorption tomography of small samples. Proposed application of synchrotron radiation to computed tomography II. Nucl. Instr. Meth. 206:547-552
5. Flannery BP, Deckman HW, Roberge WG, D'Amico KL (1987) Three-dimensional x-ray microtomography. Science 237:1439-1444
6. Hirano T, Usami K, Sakamoto K (1989) High resolution monochromatic tomography with x-ray sensing pickup tube. Rev. Sci. Instrum. 60:2482-2485
7. Kinney JH, Johnson QC, Nichols MC, Bonse U, Saroyan RA, Nusshardt R, Pahl R (1989) X-ray microtomography on beamline X at SSRL. Rev. Sci. Instrum. 60:2471-2474
8. Nubhardt R, Bonse U, Busch F, Kinney JH, Saroyan RA, Nichols MC (1991) Microtomography : a tool for nondestructive study of materials. Synchrotron Radiation News 4:21-23
9. D'Amico KL, Dunsmuir JH, Furguson SR, Flannery BP, Deckman HW (1992) The Exxon microtomography beam line at the National Synchrotron Light Source. Rev. Sci. Instrum. 63:574-577
10. Nagata Y, Yamaji H, Hayashi K, Kawashima K, Hyodo K, Kawata H, Ando M (1992) High energy high resolution monochromatic x-ray computed tomography using the Photon Factory vertical wiggler beamline. Rev. Sci. Instrum. 63:615-618
11. Nagata Y, Yamaji H, Hayashi K, Kawashima K, Hyodo K, Kawata H, Ando M (1992) High energy, high resolution monochromatic x-ray computed tomography radiation system. Res. Nondestr. Eval. 4:55-78
12. Thompson AC, Llacer J, Campbell Finman, Hughes EB, Otis JN,Wilson S, Zeman HD (1984) Computed tomography using synchrotron radiation. Nucl. Instr. Meth. 222:1208-1213
13. Borodin Y, Dementyev EN, Dragun GN, Kulipanov GN, Mwzentsev NA, Pindyurin VF, Sheromov MA, Skrinsky AN, Sokolov AS, Ushakov VA (1986) Scanning x-ray difference microscopy and microtomography using synchrotron radiation of the storage ring VEPP-4. Nucl. Instr. Meth. A 246:649-654
14. Engelke K, Lohmann M (1989) A system for dual energy microtomography of bones. Nucl. Instr. Meth. A 274:380-389
15. Graeff W, Engelke K (1991) Microradiography and microtomography. Handbook on synchrotron radiation 4 pp361-405, North-Holland.
16. Takeda T, Itai Y, Hayashi K, Nagata Y, Yamaji H, Hyodo K (1994) High spatial resolution CT with a synchrotron radiation system. J. Comput. Assist. Tomogr. 18(1):98-101

17. Bonse U, Busch F, Gunnewig O, Beckmann F, Pahl R, Delling G, Hahn M, Graeff W (1994)
    3D computed x-ray tomography of human cancellous bone at 8 μm spatial and 10^{-4} energy
    resolution. Bone and Mineral 25:25-38
18. Bonse U, Busch F (1996) X-ray computed microtomography(μCT) using synchrotron radiation
    (SR). Prog. Biophy. Molec. Biol. 65 No 1/2:pp133-169.
19. Salome M, Peyrin F, Cloetens P, Baruchel J, Spanne P, Suortti P, Laval-Jeantet AM (1997)
    Assessment of bone micro-architecture using 3D computed microtomography.
    ESRF News letter 28:26-28
20. Dilmanian FA, Garrett RF, Thomlinson WC, Berman LE, Chapman LD, Gmur NF,
    Lazarz NM, Luke PN, Moulin HR, Oversluizen T, Slatkin DN, Stojanoff V, Thompson AC,
    Volkow ND, Zeman HD (1991) Computed tomography with monochromatic x rays from
    the National Synchrotron Light Source. Nucl. Instr. Meth. B56/57:1208-1213
21. Nachaliel E, Dilmanian FA, Garrett RF, Thomlinson WC, Chapman LD, Gmur NF,
    Lazarz NM, Moulin HR, Rivers ML, Rarback H, Stefan PM, Spanne P, Luke PN, Pehl R,
    Thompson AC (1992) Monochromatic computed tomography of the human brain using
    synchrotron x-rays:technical feasibility. Nucl. Instr. Meth. A319:305-310
22. Dilmanian FA (1992) Computed tomography with monochromatic x rays.
    Am. J. Physiol. Imaging 3/4:175-193
23. Dilmanian FA, Wu XY, Parsons EC, Ren B, Kress J, Button TM, Chapman LD, Coderre JA,
    Giron F, Greenberg D, Krus DJ, Liang Z, Marcovici S, Petersen MJ, Roque CT, Shleifer M,
    Slatkin DN, Thomlinson WC, Yamamoto K, Zhong Z (1997) Single- and dual-energy CT with
    monochromatic synchrotron x-rays. Phys. Med. Biol. 42:371-387
24. Takeda T, Akatsuka T, Hyodo K, Itai Y, Hiranaka Y, Zeniya T, Yuasa T, Sato M, Wu J,
    Ishikawa N, Nemoto H (1990) Synchrotron radiation computed tomography for biomedical use.
    PF Activity Report 8:348
25. Takeda T, Akatsuka T, Hyodo K, Hiranaka Y, Zeniya T,Yuasa T, Sato M, Wu J, Ishikawa N,
    Itai Y (1992) Synchrotron radiation computed tomography to detect tracer material.
    Medical Imaging Technology 10:299-300
26. Itai Y, Takeda T, Akatsuka T, Maeda T, Hyodo K, Uchida A, Yuasa T, Kazama M, Wu J,
    Ando M (1995) High contrast tomography with synchrotron radiation.
    Rev. Sci. Instrum. 66(2):1385-1387
27. Zeniya T, Takeda T, Hyodo K, Yuasa T, Maeda T, Uchida A, Wu J, Hiranaka Y, Akatsuka T,
    Itai Y (1997) Detecttability of trancer materials in synchrotron radiation x-ray computed
    tomography: Perliminary experiments using a prototype system with imaging plate as a detector.
    Medical Imaging Technology 15:121-137 (abstract in English)
28. Kazama, M, Takeda T, Akiba M, Yuasa,T, Hyodo K, Ando M, Akatsuka T, Itai Y (1997)
    Performance study of monochromatic synchrotron x-ray computed tomography using a linear
    array detector. Medical Imaging Technology 15:615-624
29. Chesler DA, Riederer SJ, Pelc NJ (1977) Noise due to photon counting statistics in computed
    x-ray tomography. J. Comput. Assist. Tomogr. 1:64-74

Contrast Analysis in Coronary Images using 2D Monochromatic X-rays for Optimized Dedicated Synchrotron IVCA System

Yasunari Oku[1,2], Kazuyuki Hyodo[1,3], Masami Ando[1,3], Zhong Zhong[4] and William Thomlinson[4]

1 The Graduate University for Advanced Studies, 1-1, Oho Tsukuba, Ibaraki 305, Japan
2 Kawasaki Heavy Industries, Ltd., 118, Futatsuzuka, Noda, Chiba 278, Japan
3 Institute of Materials Structure Science, KEK, 1-1, Oho Tsukuba, Ibaraki 305, Japan
4 NSLS, Brookhaven National Laboratory, Long Island, NY 11973, U.S.

SUMMARY. The intravenous SR coronary angiography is so simple and safe that its application to screening looks promising. In the case of the 2D imaging method, scattered x-rays may cause deterioration of image quality because of the wide exposure area. The third higher harmonic diffracted by a single monochromator is also harmful. Therefore, deterioration of image contrast due to these causes and its improvement by x-ray grids were investigated by a newly developed simulation program and experiments using synchrotron radiation at NSLS, BNL. The experiments were performed using an acrylic phantom with a hole which imitates a coronary artery and contains iodine diluted by water. By these processes, the SR source specifications to provide sufficient image quality for diagnosis have been fixed so that a practical synchrotron IVCA system was designed.

KEY WORDS: Coronary angiography, 2D imaging, Scattered x-rays, 3rd higher harmonic, Image contrast, Simulation program, Dedicated SR source

INTRODUCTION

Intravenous SR coronary angiography is relatively simple and safe. Construction of a dedicated compact radiation source at a hospital would be needed for its application to screening examination. Therefore, design of a practical SR source system dedicated to intravenous coronary angiography is valuable. Dynamic imaging using a two-dimensional imaging system (Hyodo K. et al., 1991) is very useful to see not only stenosis but also the blood flow through coronary arteries on the heart. However, it has been pointed out that the exposure area covering the whole heart is so wide that scattering of x-rays from a patient's body may cause a deterioration of the image contrast and visibility. X-ray grids which are commonly used in hospitals are effective for suppressing scattered x-rays, when x-ray examinations are performed. The x-ray grid is a plate piled up with thin wood and lead alternately, which stops the scattered x-rays by the lead but allows the primary x-rays to pass through the wood. A realistic intravenous coronary angiography system using SR, which is based on investigations of deterioration of image contrast due to scattered x-rays and the third higher harmonic (Konishi K. et al. 1985), and its improvement by x-ray grids, will be needed, if this method is adopted as a screening process. A compact radiation source (Oku Y. et al. 1993, Oku Y. et al 1994) will make this method practical.

SIMULATION OF IMAGE CONTRAST

A simulation program using the Monte Carlo method has been developed, in order to study the influence of the scattered x-rays and the third higher harmonic on images for medical diagnosis and the effect of suppressing scattered x-rays by x-ray grid insertion. The phantom comprises an acrylic block with a hollow tube analogous to a coronary artery filled with iodine diluted by water. The monochromatic incident x-rays are primarily 33.17 keV and 99.51 keV as the third higher harmonic, and uniformly distributed as a two-dimensional beam. The x-ray grid, if it is used, is inserted between the phantom and the detector. Coherent scattering, incoherent scattering, the photoelectric effect, and fluorescence x-ray generation by the photoelectric effect were considered. This program gives location, photon energy and attenuation by the photoelectric effect of each photon arriving at the detector. The number of these photons are added to the digital matrix data corresponding to each pixel, and thus two-dimensional simulation images are generated.

EXPERIMENTS FOR VERIFICATION OF THE SIMULATION PROGRAM

An experiment was performed at the X-17 B1 beamline of the NSLS in Brookhaven National Lab. (BNL) in order to verify the image contrast made by the simulation program. An asymmetric lapped silicon (311) crystal was used as a monochromator. An acrylic block with a hole, which imitates a coronary artery whose diameter was from 1 to 5 mm, containing iodine diluted by water was used. Its thickness was 100 mm, the distance between the acrylic and the detector was 10 mm and the concentration in weight of diluted iodine was 5 %. An II (Image Intensifier) used as a detector was the same type as the one used in the clinical application of two-dimensional SR coronary angiography (Hyodo K. et al. to be published, Ohtsuka S. et al. to be published), RTP9211G-G10 made by TOSHIBA. The experimental images were recorded by an 8 mm video recorder. The analog data of video tapes were transferred to digital data, and analyzed on a personal computer. Figure 1 shows an example of the image profile, and contrast against the background is expressed as (a-b)/(a-c). The simulations under the same conditions were carried out considering the II response vs. the photon energy. The contrast was compared between the simulation and the experiment in both cases of without the grid and with the grid. Figure 2 shows good agreement of contrast between simulations and experiments for various artery diameters.

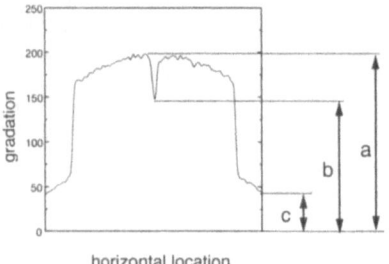

Fig. 1. An example of profile of the image. The artery shadow depth is (a-b). The contrast of artery is (a-b)/b. The contrast of artery against the background is (a-b)/(a-c).

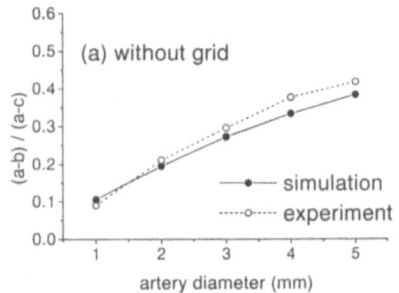
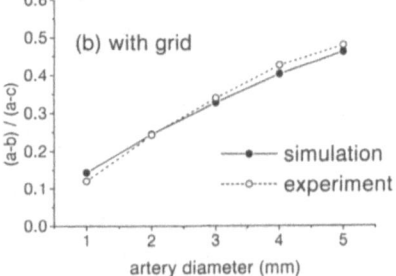

Fig. 2. Comparison between simulation and experiment of the contrast of the artery against the background expressed as (a-b)/(a-c) as a function of the artery diameter. (a) without grid (b) with grid

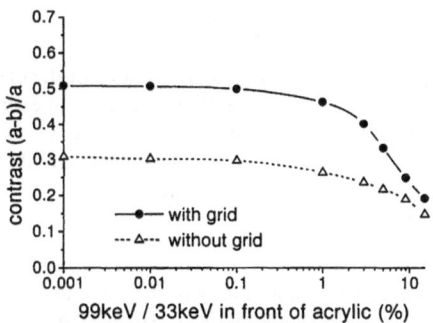

Fig. 3. Artery contrast ((a-b)/a), as a function of the ratio of the third higher harmonic photon flux against 33.17 keV photons in front of the phantom in the case of the 150 mm×150 mm beam required by medical doctors. The acrylic thickness is 160 mm, the distance between acrylic and the detector is 100 mm, the artery diameter is 5 mm, and the concentration of iodine in weight is 5%.

DESIGN OF THE STORAGE RING

The quantum noise per signal should be sufficiently smaller than the contrast of the artery images. The minimum value of the ratio of the artery shadow depth with 1 mm of the diameter and 1% concentration of iodine in weight (a-b in Fig. 1), against the standard deviation of quantum noise, was chosen to be 2. The S/N ratio was determined based on the ratio to be 60. From it, the necessary photon flux (I) of 3600 into a pixel was obtained. The necessary total photon flux at 33.17 keV, the iodine K-edge energy, in front of the detector was obtained from the above I and the ideal exposure area of 150 mm×150 mm for coronary angiography; it was 2.0×10^9 photons/image considering a pixel size of 0.2 mm. On the other hand, the contrast deterioration of the images due to 99.51 keV photons, the third higher harmonic, was investigated. The analyzed artery contrast, ((a-b)/a in Fig. 1) against the ratio of 99.51 keV to 33.17 keV photons in front of the phantom is shown in Fig. 3. The incident x-ray beam size was 150 mm×150 mm. The acrylic thickness was 160 mm, the distance between the acrylic and the detector was 100 mm, the artery diameter was 5 mm, and the concentration of iodine in weight was 5%. The contamination ratio of the third higher harmonic should be 0.1%, because the contrast when using an x-ray grid was saturated at that point.

At a radiation source, the necessary total photon flux at 33.17 keV is 9.7×10^{11} photons/image per 4 msec and the allowed contamination of the 99.51 keV photons against the 33.17 keV photons is 0.18%, considering attenuation due to passing through a beamline with three elements such as a beryllium filter with a total 1 mm thickness, an aluminum filter with a 1 mm thickness and across 4 m of air, and the diffraction process at the monochromator. A maximum photon critical energy of 9.0 keV was obtained from the above allowed contamination of 99.51 keV of 0.18%. A stored electron beam current of 500 mA and the number of poles of a superconducting wiggler of 5 were determined as reasonable values under the current technologies. From the values of the critical energy, the beam current and the number of the wiggler poles, the electron beam energy to obtain the necessary photon flux at 33.17 keV was determined to be 1.5 GeV. The magnetic field of the wiggler was determined to be 6.0 T by the critical energy and the beam energy.

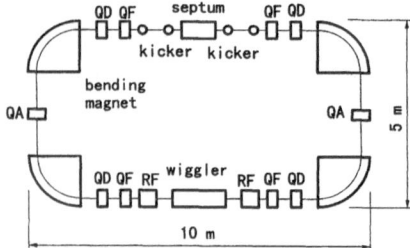

Fig. 4. The lattice of the electron storage ring for IVCA. The beam energy is 1.5 GeV. The beam current is 500 mA. The magnetic field of the wiggler and the bending magnet are 6 T and 4T.

An electron storage ring dedicated to coronary angiography to meet the above basic specifications, was designed using the program SAD of KEK (Oide K. et al. since 1986). The Chasman-Green type was adopted as a lattice, because dispersion suppression on the insertion device was easily avoidable of so much emittance growth by exciting the insertion device. Superconducting bending magnets with a field of 4 T were adopted. The lattice of the storage ring is shown in Fig. 4. The size of the ring is about 10 m × 5 m.

CONCLUSIONS

The necessary photon flux was calculated by comparing the standard deviation of quantum noise with artery image contrast using the developed program. Characteristics of image contrast and its improvement by x-ray grids against the contamination of the third higher harmonic were investigated by the simulation program, and the allowable contamination limit was determined. The required specifications of the radiation source for SR coronary angiography were obtained from the necessary photon flux and allowed contamination of the third higher harmonic, and a conceptual design of the SR source system for coronary angiography was carried out. (Oku Y., 1997)

ACKNOWLEDGMENTS

The authors would like to greatly thank Professor Hitoshi Kanamori, Dr. Nobuyuki Nakamori of Kyoto Institute of Technology, Professor Hideo Hirayama and Dr. Yoshihito Namito of KEK for their kind advice on the simulation methods and their information about x-ray attenuation data. The authors also would like to acknowledge Professor Susumu Kamada and Dr. Kazufumi Ohmi of KEK for their advice on the design method of the synchrotron radiation source and instruction in the use of the storage ring design code. Last but not least, they would like to thank Dr. Akira Iwata of Kawasaki Heavy Industries, Ltd. for his encouragement and support throughout this study.

REFERENCES

Hyodo K., K. Nishimura, and M. Ando, in Handbook on Synchrotron Radiation, edited by
    S. Ebashi, M. Koch, and E. Rubenstein (Elsevier, Amsterdam, 1991), **4**, p 55.
Hyodo K., et al.: To be published in Journal of Synchrotron Radiation.
Konishi K., F. Toyofuku, K. Nishimura, M. Ando, K. Hyodo, A. Maruhashi, M. Akisada, S.
    Hasegawa, A. Suwa and E. Takenaka; Jpn. J. Med. & Inf. Sci. **2**, p113 (1985).
Oide K. et al.; A computer program complex for accelerator design developed in KEK (since 1986),
    Home page address; http://www-acc-theory.kek.jp/SAD/sad.html.
Ohtsuka S. et al.; To be submitted.
Oku Y., K. Aizawa, S. , M. Ando, K. Hyodo, and S. Kamada, IEEE Proceedings of the 1993
    Particle Accelerator Conference, **2**, p. 1468 (1994).
Oku Y., K. Aizawa, K. Hyodo and M. Ando; Rev. Sci. Instrum. **66**, No.2, Part 2, p1451 (Feb. 1995).
Oku Y.; Ph. D thesis, The Graduate University for Advanced Studies (1997).

Q: Scattering is only in one direction ?

A: Scattering is 2D and a cross-grid is two dimensional, too.

Q: I just wondered if you simulated the merits of the scatter grid along the detector.

A: Yes. It is effective, but this penumbra is harmful. It is due to the finite light source size. In the case of AR clinical application, this light source size is small. However, in the case of a dedicated ring, this L1 will be shorter while this light source size is larger in order to store a higher current.

Q: What was your source size in your simulated light source ?

A: About 8 mm because the emittance is so high.

Q: What happens if you increase L2. Do you reduce background ? How does the background reduction compare to using scatter grid ? If you increase L2, you'll get less background.

A: If this L2 is big, this penumbra width becomes bigger, so, it is very harmful for the image.

Q: Was there any reason why wood was used ?

A: If this is, for example, aluminum, the scatter may become small, but direct X-ray is attenuated too much. For example, this length is 3.75 mm, but if this was aluminum, it would be less than 30 percent.

C: Yes. on the other hand these aluminum insertions can be made thin, and structure supported otherwise, so that the lead could be relatively thick and the aluminum thin in the middle.

Q: The Monte Carlo Code includes a correct description of the polarization and the radiation in all phases of scattering ? Did you use Stokes parameters ? How did you include polarization in your calculation because that certainly has an effect on multiple scattering.

A: We haven't taken into account the polarization because that effect is very small and almost negligible

DICUSSION ON IMAGING

Ch: Are there an other general comments that any one would like to make regarding what we have heard so far or the future applications of synchrotron radiation. There was a comment this morning regarding prostate cancer for example. We also heard a comment regarding the potential imaging of the lymph system or other potential programs that people have been thinking about.

Q: Is it difficult to constitute dynamically three dimensional structure of the biological body by angiography? For instance, confocal microscopy is a very powerful method, but in confocal microscopy only very small material can be seen. In the same sense, is it difficult to construct dynamically the three-dimensional structure ?

A: Presently only three dimensional structure comes from computer tomography, micro-computer tomography. I don't think there's the equivalent set of the confocal microscope, although I am not sure about the phase contrast work. Maybe Dr. Wilkins will address some of that in terms of whether you can get depth profile information, and therefore three dimensional process. I don't understand it well enough, perhaps you can address it in his talk, or perhaps now.

A: Phase contrast is direct analogy between the phase and the linear attenuation coefficient curve. What you can do with absorption in terms of tomography you can equally do with phase contrast to the extent that you preserve coherence in the sample. If you lose coherence too badly, then you're in trouble.

A: That's right. Because in what we do, we have absolutely no coherence at any point in our study, and therefore, all we get is an integral through the sample. We have no depth information whatsoever.
A: While still using very ordinary absorption rays for coronary angiography, if we will be able to have two instant monochromatic beams by any means, like installing two storage rings at the same time, of course, it is very costly, but I think basically this could lead to 3D reconstruction of coronary arteries by a technical method using a stereoscopic.

C: That stereoscopic possibility was studied at some length by Clemence Schultz in his thesis some years ago. He thought how this information, actually some experiment on phantom the famous Frank was done at Brookhaven just by taking two separate views from different angles. He was able to construct the arteries and have arterial lumen along the artery from the reconstruction. I think that is really the maximum information which you can get on the conditions of the arteries if that can be done.
Basically, it would be possible to do it like the inter-line scan type angiography, if you have two detectors, two sets of monochromators, so basically it is a question of money. There is a little question of dosage but perhaps not very crucial. If one of the imaging systems is taken as the principle system and other one giving just the space or the third dimension, and the geometrical information, it might well work. The way the facility at ESRF is built, the hutch is high enough to take another beam. Also there is an option for including another monochromator using different reflection, so that the two beams, or two pairs of beams, could be crossing at the patient and then detected behind the patient. We have the top option open but at this moment it's in the freezer, meaning that we don't have the money.

C: Being an optimist and idealist, I would like to try to look a little bit ahead beyond the immediate techniques that people are using now, because I think there are actually some very exiting possibilities that we can develop for medical imaging. When I was talking about phase contrast imaging, I really didn't get into some of the advantages, potential advantages. One of the key advantages of the point-projection method is that you are not tied to an absorption edge. You can immediately go to higher voltage, higher energy X-rays than the iodine absorption edge.

The other feature of phase contrast imaging in the point projection method, is that it is essentially edge sensitive, so when we talk about something like an artery overlying some other feature, if you are doing edge detection, you are only picking up an edges of organs and arteries. Therefore, one artery overlies some other feature, you are not being blocked out by that other feature, because all you are tracing potentially are the edges of the feature. Therefore, the overlying problem need not be so serious.

The other things from what Professor Chikawa said, there are exiting possibilities for changing the whole mind-set in terms of imaging, normally you think of a synchrotron as producing monochromatic or being used to produce highly monochromatic parallel beams. To change the view point from going from parallel beam to divergent beams, it has tremendous advantages. You can readily change geometry. You can change field of view. The demands on detector is not so stringent. You can use much lower resolution detectors, and still get high resolution information, because you are automatically got a magnification factor. There are all sort of things to open up new opportunity for imaging. That as we tune, improve the techniques, the instrumental techniques, the medical applications will flow very rapidly but I'm naive in a lot of thing.

There are a great number of potential advantages in phase contrast imaging. It means you can think in a different way about contrast agents. It may open up a whole new range of contrast agents. I know there are another problems, but they may be simpler in some ways. You also have the feature that to a large extent, you don't need monochromatic radiation. To a first approximation you can use broadly polychromatic radiation, especially for thinner objects. You have this freedom to vary voltage as you are looking at the objects. This means you can reduce the absorbed dose to the patient. That's an immediate advantage. You've got all the other advantages. You can reduce scatter in the image, because you've got a potentially large distance between the object and the recording media. Basically there are a whole range of advantages from these sort of techniques. The question that sticks in my mind is what sort of fluxes can be obtained, at the patient or at the object by these fluorescent techniques. I think that is something that needs to be worked on and clarified. If you look at an image in normal from the point projection method gives you an edge enhanced images which is essentially a second derivative of the intensity distribution. It's done by physical means not fancy numerical processing. It is immediately bringing out certain features which are easy to recognize, and can help in interpretation. You always have the option, the potential of going back from this differentiated image back to a more true image of the object in terms of electron density.

Conceptual design of a medical application radiation source

E.Levichev, N.Mezentsev
Budker INP, 630090 Novosibirsk, Russia
A.Iwata, S.Kamiya
KHI, 118 Futatsuzuka, Noda, Chiba, 278 Japan

Abstract

The main goal of the project is to develop a rather compact but low emittance SR facility with the electron energy of 2÷2.4 GeV. Low emittance ($\varepsilon_x < 10$ nm) together with the insertion devices allow to perform medical experiments otherwise available only at 6÷8 GeV light sources which are much larger and costly than that presented below.

1 Introduction

At present world-wide interest is growing to the possibility of medical application of unique SR properties to create new tools for medical research, diagnosis, and treatment.

Most of the current research areas for medical applications which involve SR are as follows: *imaging* (angiography, limphography, bronchography, monochromatic X-ray computed tomography, multiple-energy computed tomography, mammography); *micro-imaging* (X-ray microscopy, micro-tomography, secondary X-ray source microscopy); *in-vitro medical research* (X-ray refraction microscopy, structural biology, EXAFS, fluorescent trace element analysis); *radiotherapy* (photon activation therapy, microbeam radiation therapy).

The required spatial resolution of image for the coronary angiography is 0.1 mm. To obtain this value, a high spectral brightness in the photon energy range $10 \div 100$ keV is necessary. And as the brightness is inversely proportional to the horizontal emittance ε_x, the later is the parameter of large importance. Considering the geometry of the angiography experiment one can estimate the required emittance to reach the resolution mentioned above as $\varepsilon_x \sim 10$ nm-rad.

According to [1], an exposure time of 2 ms per image is required. Assuming a 2-D imaging system with the exposure area $\simeq 150 \times 150$ mm^2, the total flux at the monochromator has to be $> 4 \times 10^{14}$ phot/s for 33 keV photons.

Following conditions were considered when defining the working energy of the medical storage ring: low manufacturing and maintenance cost; circumference minimization; high spectral brightness for the $5 \div 100$ keV spectral range; possibility of installing high field IDs; optimal flux ratio first/third radiation harmonics; possibility of using mini-undulators without the lifetime reduction.

A superconducting $7.5 \div 8$ T wavelength shifter provides the spectral range up to 120 keV for three beamlines.

A scanning superconducting 20-pole wiggler is proposed to increase the flux for fast 2-D imaging. It radiates the uniform photon flux in the cone of 10×10 mrad^2 and satisfies the time resolution requirement.

To choose the electron energy, in Fig.1 33 keV photon flux and the ratio of photon flux at 33 keV and 99 keV are shown. The later is an important parameter for X-ray imaging using the K-edge subtraction method. One can see that for lower energy the photon flux drops down, but for higher energy the first/third harmonics ratio decreases, especially for a 3-pole superconducting shifter. Taking it into account and making the optimization of the beam emittance, an undulator and wigglers radiation we have compromised the required storage ring energy as $E = 2.2$ GeV.

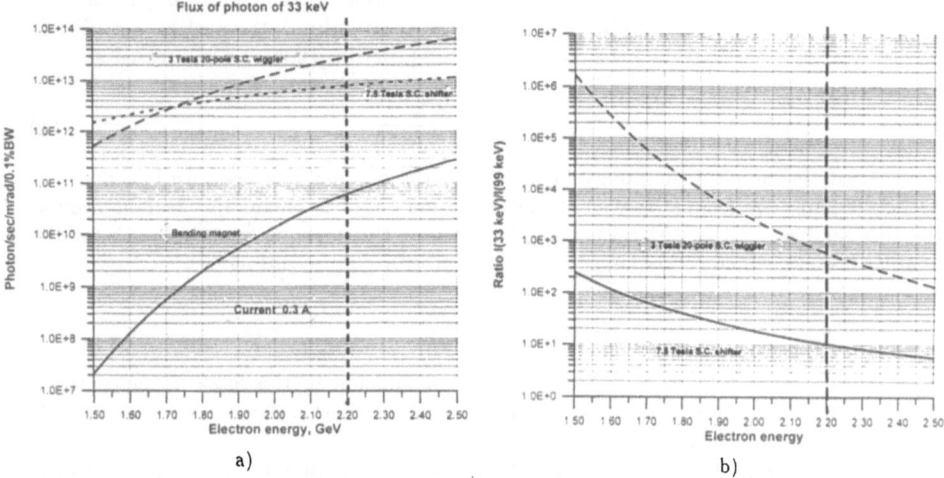

Fig. 1 a) 33 keV photon flux integrated over vertical angle per mrad of horizontal angle in 0.1% BW vs. electron energy; b)33 keV/99 keV flux ratio vs. beam energy for an electron current of 0.3 A.

At present days a mini-undulator (MU) seems to be rather promising for generating high flux and brightness photon beams within the fundamental energy range of $5 \div 10$ keV, being installed at relatively low electron energy rings ($2.0 \div 2.5$ GeV). Higher harmonics of an MU can extend the radiation energy up to $20 \div 40$ keV and may be successfully used for various clinical applications. Promising experiments with the MU were performed at the NSLS X-ray ring [2].

We fixed the minimum gap of in-vacuum mini-undulator as $1.5 \div 2$ mm and optimized its period length λ_0 relating to the fundamental photon energy and radiation spectral flux.

For small λ_0, the fundamental energy grows up, but the photon flux drops down. Especially drastically it goes for third and fifth harmonics. The flux ratio for 5 mm and 7 mm periods is $\sim 10^{-2}$ for third harmonic and $\sim 10^{-4}$ for fifth harmonic. Finally we chose for further estimations $\lambda_0 = 7$ mm and the pole gap $g = 2$ mm ($K_{max} = 0.568$).

2 Lattice design

Mini-undulators do not require dispersion-free straight sections and use of non-traditional lattice seems quite reasonable. After some studies we chose a basic low emittance cell with a triple non-achromatic bend TB(NA) that is a compact cell consisting of three dipoles and two quadrupoles. Horizontal dispersion is not matched to zero at the cell ends and provides inside the dipoles good conditions for emittance minimization. Two quadrupole dublets are used between the basic low emittance cells to adjust beta-functions for the mini-undulator accommodation.

To find a particular lattice solution we need to define values of the lattice functions in the straight sections. Small-gap undulator provides a serious vertical aperture limitation and may reduce the beam lifetime, which depends on the value of β_z here.

A main process limiting the beam lifetime in the presence of small-gap undulator is the elastic scattering on residual gas atoms. It leads to an angular kick on the betatron motion, and if the induced amplitude exceeds the aperture limit, the particle get lost. In practical units for N_2 ($Z = 7$) the elastic scattering lifetime (hours) is expressed as

$$\tau_s = 10^7 \frac{E^2}{p} \frac{a_z^2}{\beta_{z0} < \beta_z >}, \tag{1}$$

where E is the electron energy in GeV, p is the residual gas pressure in $nTorr$, a_z is the aperture limit equal to 1/2 of undulator gap, $< \ >$ means the average around the ring, and β_{z0} is the vertical envelop function at the aperture limit azimuth (at the undulator end), which corresponds to the central value β_{zc} according to

$$\beta_{z0} = \beta_{zc} + \frac{L^2}{4\beta_{zc}}, \tag{2}$$

where L is the undulator length. Central β_z should not be too small in the center of the MU straight section. Otherwise, $\beta_z(s)$ will grow very fast and reach an unacceptable high value at the undulator end.

Another reason why we have to avoid too small β_{z0} is that is closely relates to the averaged $< \beta_z >$: the lower β_{z0} in the straight section, the higher $< \beta_z >$ around the ring. Computer simulation has shown that to get the large enough lifetime we need to keep β_{z0} in the range of 0.5÷0.8 m as it is demonstrated in **Fig.2a**.

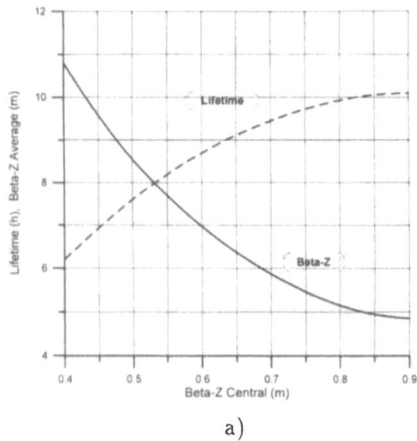
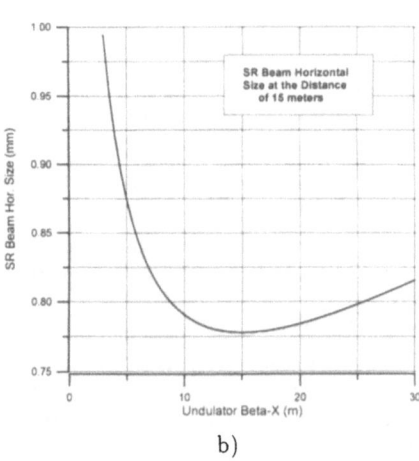

a)   b)

Fig.2 a) Elastic scattering lifetime and $< \beta_z >$. Here E=2.2 GeV, P=1 nTorr, undulator gap is 2 mm, undulator length is 0.7 m.; b) Horizontal radiation spot size at L=15 m vs. horizontal beta function in MU.

The value of β_x in the MU can be estimated by minimizing the radiation spot size at a sample. The transverse beam half-size at the distance L from the source point can be estimated as

$$d_x^2 = \sigma_x^2 + L^2(\sigma_x'^2 + \sigma_r'^2). \tag{3}$$

Here we assumed that for 10-keV X-rays the radiation beam size σ_r is negligible compared with the beam size σ_x, but the beam spread σ_x' and central cone radiation opening angle σ_r' have the same order of magnitude. Fig.2b shows the radiation spot size at L =15 m from the MU as a function of β_x value at the center of the straight section. The dependence has a flat minimum for $\beta_x = 16 \div 22$ m but grows up for small β_x.

High field wiggler can drastically affect the electron beam and proper choice of the lattice function values in the wiggler straight section is very important. To avoid undesirable increasing of beam emittance, a horizontal dispersion function in wiggler has to be matched to zero. To diminish the effect on the lattice the wiggler should be located in a small β_z region. The experience shows that it is convenient to choose the value of the vertical beta-function in a wiggler $\beta_z < 5$ m.

To increase the spatial resolution in angiography experiments using a superconducting wiggler, it is highly desirable to have the beam source of a small enough size $\sigma_x \simeq 0.2 \div 0.3$ mm. In our case it means that in a superconducting wiggler β_x has to be less than 11 m.

3 Machine configuration

The TB(NA) cell has the reflective symmetry and includes three bending magnets and two quadrupole lenses which provide proper lattice functions in the bending magnets to produce rather low horizontal emittance. Eight cells form the ring; eight straight sections 2 meters long are available to accommodate the MU and accelerator equipment.

To site the superconducting wigglers four 3 m straight sections are arranged. In the center of these sections $\beta_x = 10$ m and $\beta_z = 4$ m that is convenient enough for a strong field wiggler location. The circumference of the ring is $C = 120$ m. The schematic layout of the facility and the lattice functions for one-forth of the ring are depicted in Fig.3.

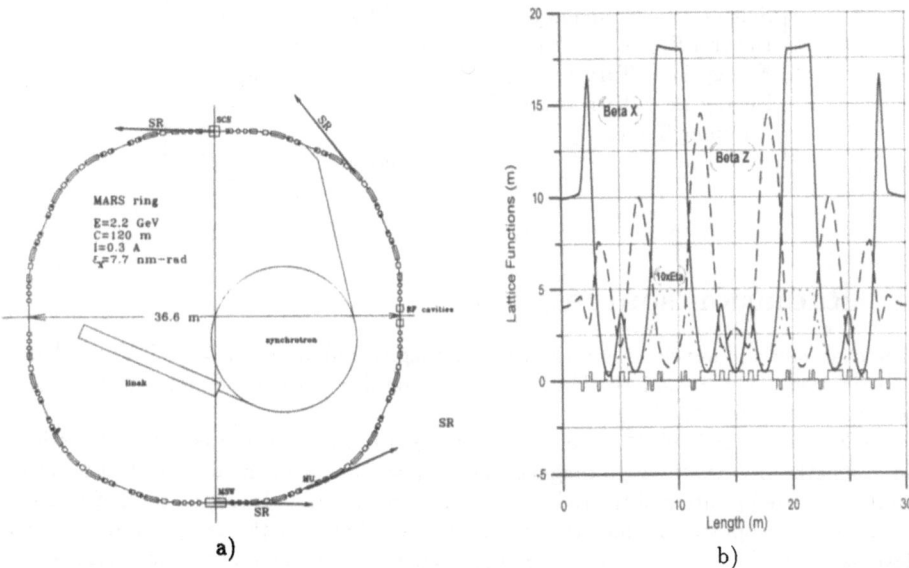

Fig. 3 a) The schematic layout of the medical storage ring. b) The lattice functions for the ring quarter.

The closed orbit is formed by 28 parallel face bending magnets. 20 magnets are regular type with the magnetic length of $l_m = 1.4$ m; the rest 8 are dispersion zeroing half-length magnets. Both types have the same crossection and field amplitude which is equal to $B_0 = 1.3726$ T at $E = 2.2$ GeV. To limit the vertical beta and to decrease the vertical chromaticity the magnets have the field index $k = -0.59$ m^{-2}.

To focus the beam there are 72 quadrupole lenses combined in 7 families. Quadrupole singlet provides adjustment of the lattice functions inside the bending magnets and dispersion zeroing. Quadrupole doublet and triplet match the lattice functions in the straight sections.

Eight 2 m dispersive straight sections accommodate focusing sextupoles to compensate natural chromaticity and a 1.6 m section is available for mini-undulators (β_z is easily tuned here in the range of 0.3÷0.7 m).

The main parameters of the storage ring are listed in Table 1.

Table 1: Main parameters of the storage ring.

Nominal Electron Energy	E (GeV)	2.2
Nominal Beam Current	I (mA)	300
Circumference	C (m)	120
Revolution Frequency	f_0 (MHz)	2.498
Harmonic Number	h	200
RF Frequency	f_{rf} (MHz)	499.6
RF Voltage at 2.2 GeV	U_{rf} (MV)	1.8
Natural Emittance at 2.2 GeV	ε (nm-rad)	7.7
Betatron Tunes	ν_x, ν_z	11.2, 6.15
Natural Chromaticity	ξ_x, ξ_z	-26.3,-14.3
Momentum Compaction	α	0.004
Energy Spread at 2.2 GeV	σ_E/E	0.00093
Synchrotron Tune	ν_s	0.01
Synchrotron Frequency	f_s (kHz)	25
Natural Bunch Length	σ_s (cm)	2.3
Energy Loss/Turn (mag.)	ΔU_m (keV)	387.7
Energy Loss/Turn (mag.+IDs)	ΔU_m (keV)	490.1
Damping Times	$\tau_{x,z,s}$ (ms)	3.0,4.5,3.1
Life time	τ (hours)	>10

4   Radiation sources

The characteristic wavelength of the bending magnet radiation is $\lambda_c = 2.8$ Å and characteristic energy is $\varepsilon_c = 4.4$ keV. The spectral photon flux of the bending magnet radiation is shown in Fig.4.

A 3-pole shifter is planned to be inserted into the dispersion-free straight section 3 m in length. Besides the high magnetic field $B_0 = 7.5 \div 8$ T, the distinct feature of the shifter is a fixed position of the radiation point from central pole for any level of magnetic field. This advantage provides the stable radiation beam at the sample while the field level is changed. A pair of warm steering magnets are located at the both sides of the straight section and provide the electron trajectory deviation as shown in Fig.5.

The main shifter parameters are presented in Table 2

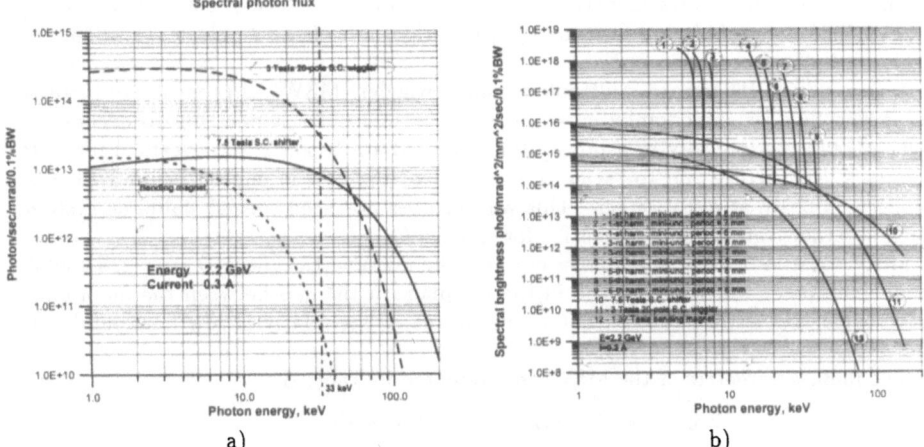

Fig.4 a) Spectral photon flux integrated over vert. angle per mrad of hor. angle, 0.1% BW
($E = 2.2$ GeV, $I = 0.3$ A). b) Spectral brightness.

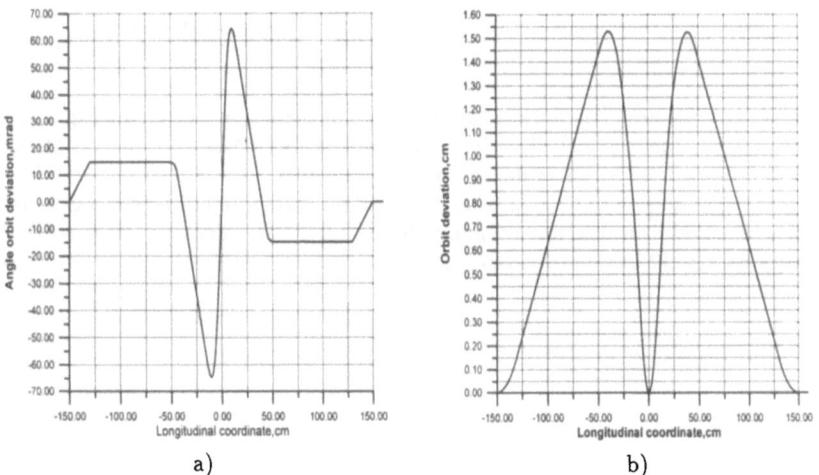

Fig.5 Beam trajectory inside the shifter: a) angle, b) x-coordinate.

Table 2: Main parameters of the strong field shifter

Maximum field on beam axis (T):	
– central pole	7.5 (8.0)
– side pole	1.75
– steering magnets	0.5
Pole gap (mm)	48 (40)
Vertical aperture of vacuum chamber (mm)	28 (20)
Horizontal aperture (mm)	≈ 100

The critical radiation wavelength from the 7.5 T shifter at 2.2 GeV is $\lambda_c = 0.51$ $\mathring{A}$ $(\varepsilon_c = 24$ keV). The spectral photon flux and spectral brightness of the 3-pole superconducting wiggler radiation are shown in Fig.4.

A new kind of ID, named multipole scanning wiggler (MSW), is proposed to increase the photon flux for angiography experiments. The main idea is not only to decline the electron beam periodically in a horizontal plane but to deflect it in a vertical plane to produce a 2-D picture and to "scan" the exposure area by the photon beam as it does the electron beam at a TV screen. This wiggler does not need special wobbling system, which is rather complex and expensive for 2.2 GeV.

MSW consists of 21+2 main poles creating the main vertical field B_z and 22+2 additional small poles which are spaced in the midplane in the gap between the main poles and provide the vertical beam scanning by means of the relatively low horizontal field B_x.

The main parameters of the MSW are presented in Table 3

Table 3: Main parameters of the MSW

Vert./hor. field amplitude (T):	3.0/0.13
Pole gap (mm)	30
Vert./hor. vacuum chamber aperture (mm)	$20/\approx 60$
Period (cm)	14
Main/scanning poles number	(21+2)/(22+2)

The beam trajectory for horizontal and vertical planes is plotted in Fig.6. A single scanning step in the vertical direction is optimized in such way that a 2-D radiation picture is obtained with the required spatial uniformity inside the horizontal angle of $\pm$ 5 mrad (Fig.7) and no additional smearing system is required. The central vertical line in Fig.7 is emitted from the low magnetic field (0.6 T) and does not disturb the image uniformity for the 30 keV photon energy.

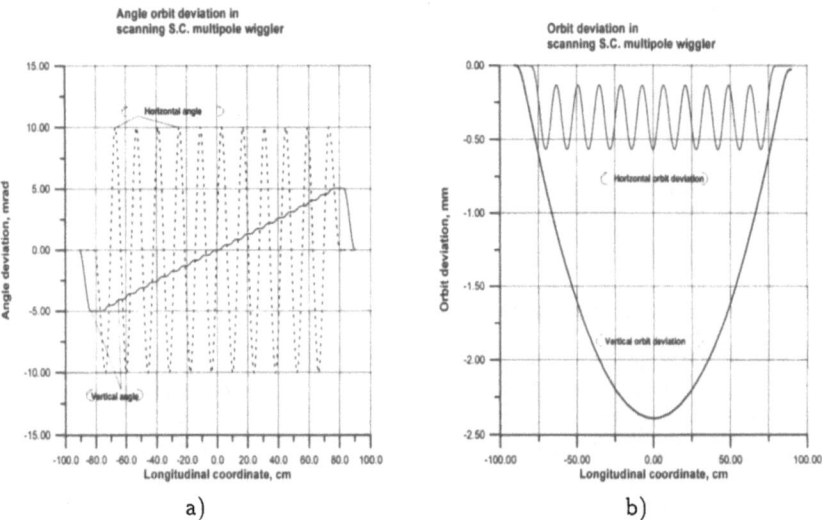

a)   b)

Fig.6 Beam trajectory in the MSW: a) angle, b) x-coordinate.

The critical radiation wavelength from the 3.0 T MSW at 2.2 GeV in forward direction is $\lambda_c = 1.3$ Å that corresponds to the critical photon energy $\varepsilon_c = 9.7$ keV. The spectral photon flux and spectral brightness of the MSW radiation are shown in Fig.4.

The mini-undulator is produced using the Ne-Fe-B hybrid magnet technology. The undulator with the gap variable down to 2 mm is placed inside the vacuum chamber.

The 1.6 m straight sections accommodate mini- undulators. Parameters of the mini-undulators with the different period lengths are presented in Table 4. In Fig.7 the central cone spectral photon flux from the mini-undulators for different periods is shown.

The main radiation characteristics of light beams from different radiation sources at 2.2 GeV are summarized in Table 5.

Here BM is the bending magnet, SCS is the superconducting shifter, MSW is the multipole scanning wiggler, and MU-n is the mini-undulator radiating at n-th harmonic; λ_c is the characteristic wavelength of radiation (n-th harmonic wavelength for the undulator); ε_c is the characteristic photon energy (n-th harmonic photon energy for the undulator). $\mathcal{F}$, B and P are the spectral flux, spectral brightness and radiated power respectively. For the bending magnet the radiated power is presented for 1 mrad horizontal opening angle. For the undulator total radiated power is shown in the line MU-1 of the Table.

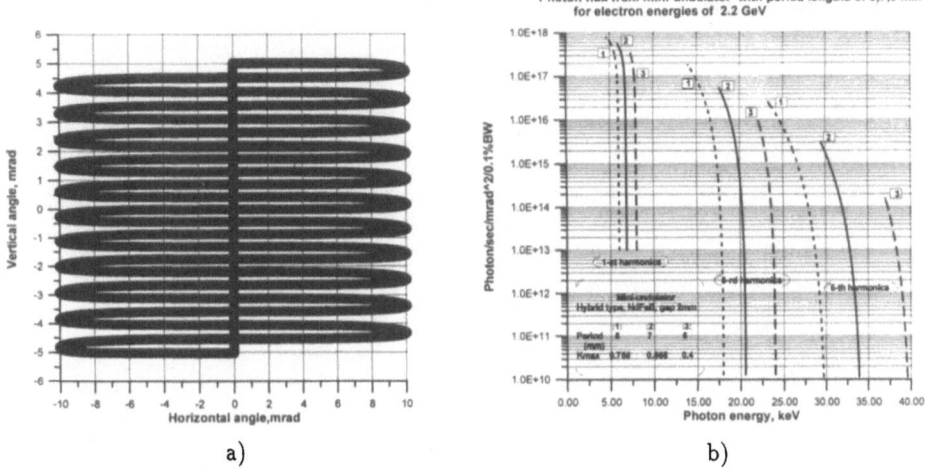

Fig.7 a) Scanning photon beam view in angle axes; b)Spectral photon flux from mini-undulators with the periods of 6,7 and 8 mm at an electron energy of 2.2 GeV.

Table 4: Mini-undulator parameters

Period length, mm	6	7	8
Maximum field, T	0.70	0.87	1.0
Maximum K	0.40	0.57	0.75
Period number	100	100	100
Length, m	0.6	0.7	0.8

Table 5: Radiation characteristics

S	λ_c (Å)	ε_c (keV)	$\mathcal{F}_c(Ph/s$ /mr/0.1%BW)	$\mathcal{B}_c$ (Ph/s/mm^2 /mr^2/0.1%BW	P_c kW
BM	2.8	4.4	1.3×10^{13}	8.5×10^{14}	0.0185(per 1 mrad)
SCS	0.5	24	1.1×10^{13}	1.2×10^{14}	14
MSW	1.3	9.7	2.1×10^{14}	1.9×10^{15}	14.6
MU-1	1.9	6.5	5.2×10^{17}	1.1×10^{18}	0.16
MU-3	0.65	19	1.8×10^{16}	5.0×10^{17}	-
MU-5	0.4	31	1.0×10^{15}	4.2×10^{16}	-

References

[1] Y.Oku et al.,"Conceptual design of a Compact Electron Storage Ring System Dedicated to Coronary Angiography", Proceedings of the 1993 Particle Accelerator Conference.

[2] P.M.Stefan et al., "Operation of a small-gap undulator on the NSLS X-ray ring", BNL-61053, 1995.

Proposal of very low cost 5-6GeV synchrotron radiation ring for medical use using permanent magnets and aluminum beam pipe without flanges and bellows

Hajime Ishimaru
KEK High Energy Accelerator Research Organization
1-1 Oho, Tsukuba, Ibaraki 305 Japan <ishimaru@mail.kek.jp>
and
G.William Foster
Fermi National Accelerator Laboratory,
P.O.Box 500 Batavia, Illinois 60510 USA <gwf@fnald.fnal.gov>

1. INTRODUCTION

We are designing a synchrotron radiation ring of medical application such an angiography for practical uses. Iodine is clinically used as a contrast agent, which has K-edge at an energy of about 33 keV.

In the very complicated design and escalated cost were justified terminating problem. In traditional accelerator technology, electro-magnets for dipole, quadrupole and some correction are used for synchrotron ring. And the vacuum beam pipes which are bakable are connected by flanges and bellows.

This paper describes the permanent magnet system including dipole and quadrupole, and a flange-less and bellow-less extruded aluminum alloy beam pipe, joined by automatic welding. The idea of this paper consists of use of permanent magnets of Fermilab 8 GeV anti-proton Recycler Ring [1] and a simple aluminum beam pipe of Fermilab Pipetron project [2]. This approach greatly simplifies the system design with the following benefits and features:

1) Drastic simplification and lower cost.
2) Extremely high reliability.

In Fermilab 8 GeV anti-proton storage ring with very low cost has been constructing using permanent magnets including dipole and quadrupole magnets along the entire ring. Circumference is 3,300 m long. Total construction cost of accelerator system without tunnel is only M$11. Aperture of the dipole magnet is 5 cm. Radius of the quadrupole is 2.5 cm. Dipole magnetic field is about 0.15-0.4 T. Field gradient of the quadrupole is 2.5 T/m maximum. Temperature stability is approximately 0.01% per 1∞C for ±15∞C . Permanent magnet consists of strontium ferrite magnet and Fe-Ni compensator alloy with an opposing temperature coefficient. This situation is very good hint to realize low cost synchrotron radiation ring.

Next generation synchrotron radiation light source has been considering using small aperture permanent magnets in Lawrence Berkeley Laboratory [3].

2. RING DESIGN

A. Lattice design

Lattice design was made for 5 GeV and 6 GeV rings with ordinary emittance machine using ordinary beam optics of FODO ($90^0/90^0$). Emittance is 3.2 x 10^{-7} mrad. Cell length is 8.12 m long. The arc consists of 28 cells. Normal cell is shown in Fig.1.

Circumference of the arc section is 227 m long. Ring has four long straight section for RF cavity, injection system, and undulators. Length of straight sections is 150 m long. Total circumference is 377 m long as same as KEK-AR. Design parameter for proposed 5 GeV or 6 GeV, and 6 GeV KEK-AR as reference is shown in Table 1.

B. Synchrotron radiation

Synchrotron radiation is extracted from the every dipole magnets. Critical energy of the synchrotron radiation for 5 GeV and 6 GeV are 17 keV and 24 keV. Energy loss per turn for 5 GeV and 6 GeV are 3.17 MeV and 5.73 MeV. Linear power density for 5 GeV and for 6 GeV with 200 mA operations, are 0.92 kW/m and 1.45 kW/m. Photon flux vs. photon energy is shown in Fig. 2. To increase brightness of synchrotron radiation, short photon beam lines will be installed.

C. Wiggler for hard X-ray

Proposed ring has four straight sections. Wiggler magnets will be inserted in two straight sections. Hard X-rays more than 33 keV will be extracted from the wiggler magnet.

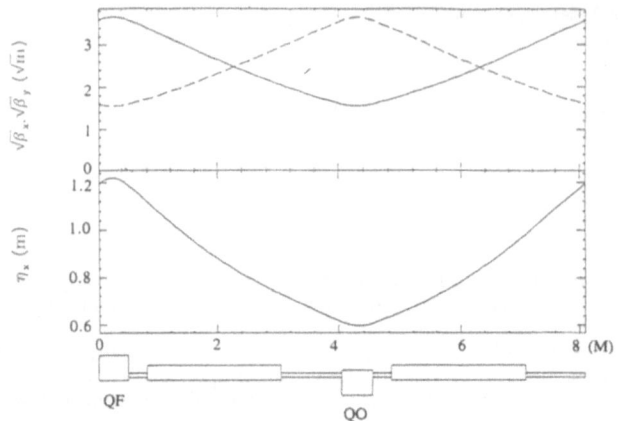

Fig. 1 Cell structure of arc section.

Table 1. Parameters of the synchrotron rings for 5 GeV or 6 GeV proposed ring, and 6 GeV KEK-AR as reference.

		Proposed	Ring	KEK-AR
Energy	:GeV	5	6	6
Dipole field	:T	0.95	1	0.87
Critical energy	:keV	17	24	21
Emittance	:10^{-7}mrad	2.57	3.26	2.55
Cell length	:m	8.12	8.12	8.2
Bending radius	:m	17.46	21.01	23
Length of dipole magnet	:m	1.97	2.26	2.6
Quadrupole field gradient	:T/m	12.13	14.56	7.7
Length of quad. magnet	:m	0.5	0.5	0.5
Circumference of arc	:m	109.7	125.7	144.5
Energy loss per turn	:MeV	3.17	5.73	4.98

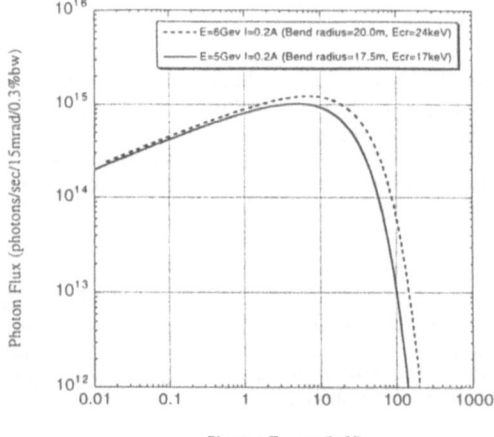

Fig. 2 Photon flux of synchrotron radiation vs. photon energy.

3. MAGNET SYSTEM

A. Hybrid permanent magnet design

The suggested design for a storage ring quality permanent magnet is a "hybrid" design pioneered by K. Halbach and used on a large-scale basis in the 8 GeV transfer line [4] and Recycler Ring projects at Fermilab. In this design [Fig. 3] the field is shaped by precision-machined steel pole tips. The field is driven by permanent magnet material which is located behind the pole tips and inside an iron flux return shell. The main advantage of this design is that the field quality is insensitive to the geometry and magnetization of the individual pieces of permanent magnet
material, due to the flux averaging of the iron pole tip. The field quality is determined mainly by the mechanical accuracy of the pole tip. A second advantage is that the permanent magnet material is away from the magnet gap and the potentially demagnetizing fields and radiation. A third advantage of this type of design is that the geometry of the pole tip can be adjusted to extract the maximum "BH energy product" from the permanent magnet material over a range of magnet gap fields and shapes.

The pole tip is the critical element in the field quality of the magnet. Low carbon steel should be used to minimize hysteritic effects. Both laminated and machined solid iron poles have been used successfully. Solid iron poles have the advantage of better flux transport along the length of the magnet, and therefore a strength which is more uniform along the length of the magnet.

B. Choice of magnet material

The important parameters for choosing the permanent magnet material are the magnetic strength required (in this case ~1 T) and the residual magnetization Br and the coercive force Hc. Other important factors include cost stability over time and temperature. Although it is possible to construct magnets which are much weaker or much stronger than the Br of the magnetic material, the hybrid configuration works best when the dipole strength is between 50% - 100% of Br.

The material with the lowest cost (per BH energy product) is Strontium Ferrite (Br ~0.4 T). This material was a good choice for the 0.2-0.3 T magnets needed for the Recycler Ring and 8 GeV Line projects at Fermilab. Neodymium-Iron-Boron [5] (Nd-Fe-B, Br ~ 1.1 T) is considerably more expensive, but some of this cost is recovered because the magnet is more compact and the iron parts are smaller. It is a good choice for the 1 T permanent magnet dipole.

C. Dipole example design

An example dipole design is shown in Fig. 3, and the resulting
magnetic field map (generated by POISSON/PANDIRA) is shown in Fig. 4. The flux return thickness was chosen to be 4 cm on the sides and 3 cm on top so that its maximum flux density was less than 1T. NdFeB "bricks" with 3 cm thickness surround the pole tips. Their orientation is such that flux is forced into the top pole tips, and flux is pulled out of the bottom pole tips. The magnet strength was adjusted to ~1 T by varying the height of the pole tips. The thickness of the bricks was chosen so that the flux density inside the bricks was ~0.7 T, which is adequately far from the demagnetizing point of the Nd-Fe-B.

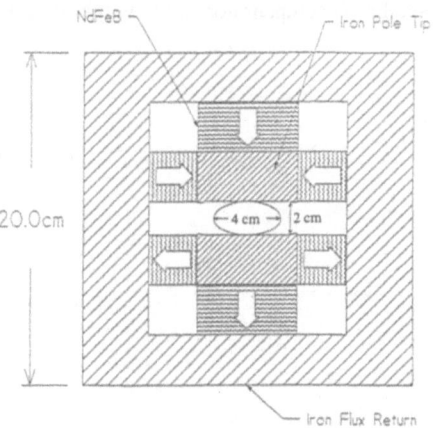

Fig. 3 Design for dipole magnet with aperture of 4 cm in horizontal and 2 cm in vertical.

The pole tip shape was generated with an optimizer which started with a flat pole tip, then added shape terms proportional to X^2, X^4 and X^6 as well as cosine like "bumps" at the ends of the pole tips. The coefficients of these terms were adjusted to minimize the RMS field defect over the design good-field aperture (+/- 1.5 cm horizontal, +/-1cm vertical in this case). The maximum defect predicted in this region by the program is less than 0.01%. Experience with the Recycler Ring prototype magnets indicates that this field quality can be achieved provided the pole tip machining tolerances are adequate.

It is important to accurately position the pole tips, particularly with respect to each other. This can be accomplished with an aluminum spacer between the pole tips (not shown), or by stainless steel or aluminum support plates at the ends of the magnet.

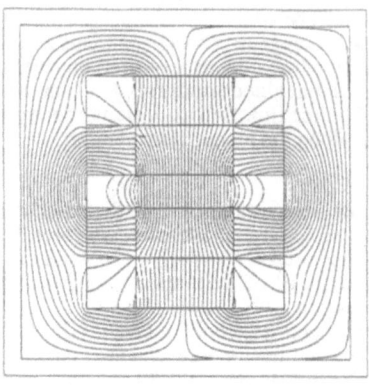

Fig. 4 Magnetic flux distribution using NdFeB with optimized pole tip.

D. Quadrupole example design

The quadrupole mechanical design (Fig. 5) and magnetic design (Fig.6) are similar. The 10 cm x 10 cm magnet is designed to fit around a 3 cm beam pipe. The field strength varies by roughly +/-1 T over an aperture of +/-2 cm, yielding a gradient of ~50 T/m. The quadrupole design also illustrates the option of "corner bricks" of permanent magnet material with a 45-degree orientation. These corner bricks (which are also an option for the dipole design) increase the strength of the magnet by ~25% but are less efficient
magnetically than the side bricks. More efficient (and complicated)
configurations of the side and top bricks are also possible. Required field strength is approximately 15 T/m. To reduce cost strontium ferrite magnet and Fe-Ni compensatory alloy will be change.

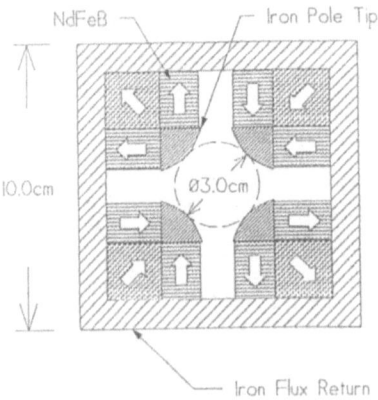

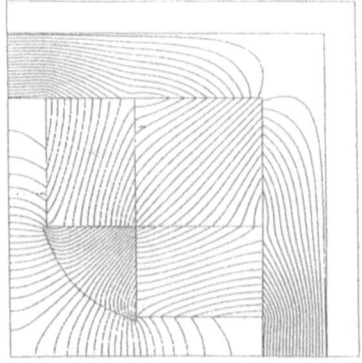

Fig. 5 Design for quadrupole magnet.   Fig. 6 Magnetic flux distribution with corner brick cycle.

E. Temperature compensation issues

Permanent magnet materials have a temperature coefficient in the range of -0.2%/∞C (Strontium Ferrite) to -0.1%/∞C (Nd-Fe-B). Typical accelerator and storage ring applications require a temperature coefficient in the range of 0.01%/∞C. Several possibilities exist: 1) a small correction windings can be placed on each magnet. 2) The temperature of the magnets can be regulated, electrically or with a water system. 3) The temperature coefficient of the permanent magnet material can be canceled by the addition
of "temperature compensation alloy" [6] (29% nickel steel) into the magnetic circuit. This is the approach taken for the Recycler Ring and 8 GeV transfer line magnets. It has been found to be effective at reducing the temperature coefficient to the level of 0.01%/∞C or below. This approach has recently been extended to Nd-Fe-B magnets [7]. It has the advantage of being entirely passive once the temperature compensation of each magnet has been adjusted. It has the disadvantage of reducing the strength of the magnet by roughly 20%, which must be made up by increasing the length of the magnet or the amount of magnetic material in it.

4. VACUUM SYSTEM

A. Beam pipe

The storage ring vacuum requirement is 10^{-9} Torr range with beam. Beam pipe with small aperture will be used extruded aluminum alloy with cooling and pump channel as ante-chamber structure in lengths of about 8.2 m of one cell.. Main pump is new type NEG strip [8] Ti-Zr-Hf housed in pump channel of ante-chamber. Activation temperature is 200-250 ∞C The beam pipe for dipole and quadrupole magnets is same cross section which has 18 mm vertical and 38 mm horizontal elliptical aperture. The beam pipe will be joined automatic welding between beam chamber and unit chamber without flanges and bellows. Inner beam pipe surface along the ring is very smooth without any gap and any step.

B. No-bellows [2]

Thermal expansion can be accommodated with an acceptable inner compression stress. Traditionally, the bellows in a electron storage ring is the most important component in the vacuum system. History has shown that the bellows for the beam chamber in synchrotron radiation rings have had many failures, such as sparking from slide contacts of the RF shield and melt-down.

The aluminum alloy beam chamber of the TRISTAN electron-positron collider was joined using automatic welding without flanges, and virtually eliminated leaks. In Japan, the super-express train, "Shinkansen" uses rails which are all welded, without gaps between rail sections. The rail has been designed to accommodate inner expansion and compression stress during temperature excursions. This situation closely represents the condition of this proposed ring.

C. Unit chamber

Beam position monitor, ion pump, vacuum gauge, roughing pumping port, and gate valve are housed in the unit chamber.

D. Beam impedance

If the wall is not smooth, beam impedance discontinuity occurs as a wake field loss. Inner beam pipe will be very smooth without any gap and any step.

E. Anchoring for beam pipe to the magnets

The beam chambers are anchored at periodic intervals to the permanent magnets and fixed at both ends of the magnets to control thermal effects. A chemical process [9] which removes water adsorption at 70∞C will be used instead of a traditional baking during NEG activation process.

5. INJECTOR, TUNNEL AND INSTALLATION

A. KEK-AR tunnel option

Tunnel and injector costs are expensive, then new proposed synchrotron radiation ring will be installed in TRISTAN accumulation ring KEK-AR. Permanent magnets system is very compact size, new proposed ring will be installed upside of the AR. Beam transfer line from injector to synchrotron ring will be used permanent magnets system as similar to 8 GeV transfer line in Fermilab.

B. Small diameter tunnel option

In ordinary accelerator, tunnel is large size, then cost for tunnel construction is high percentage. We propose small tunnel of 1.2 m in diameter using concrete pipe as similar to sewer pipe. It has two set of rail for transportation and mounting for magnets. All set of magnets and vacuum beam pipes of 8.2 m long unit cell will be transfer from ground level to the tunnel using slope tunnel on the rail. After alignment of the magnets and vacuum pipes, the beam pipes will be welded with automatic welding equipment in the tunnel.

In this case, injector is necessary. Injector cost is very expensive, then this low cost synchrotron radiation ring will be construct in Spring8 site utilizing booster synchrotron as injector.

6. SUMMARY

The proposed design using permanent magnets, aluminum beam pipe without flanges and bellows, and small tunnel using concrete pipe will satisfy the requirements for very low cost, very high reliability, high performance with a simplified design. Simple beam pipe will satisfy for reduction of components, fewer weld seams, and no flanges and no-bellows, minimum impedance, and reduced risk against leakage.

ACKNOWLEDGMENTS
The authors wish to thank to Prof. M. Ando for his encouragement, and Prof. K. Endo, Prof. S.Kamada, and Assoc. Prof. H. Fukuma for his valuable technical suggestions. Finally the authors would like to appreciate Dr. S. Matsumoto for his lattice design support.

References

[1] Recycler Ring Technical Design Handbook, FNAL-TM-1991.

[2] H.Ishimaru: Low cost warm bore vacuum chamber options, Mini-Symposium, APS Annual Meeting, Indianapolis, May 3, (1996)

[3] A.Jackson et al.: A candidate for a next generation synchrotron light source, Lawrence Berkeley Laboratory, 1997 Particle Accelerator Conference, 12-16 May 1997, Vancouver, Canada

[4] Main Injector Technical Design Handbook, FNAL.

[5] NdFeB in various grades is available from a number of vendors including Hitachi Heavy Metals. The grade chosen should take into consideration the maximum temperature during bakeout and the maximum demagnetizing force on the material (which depends on the magnetic design).

[6] "Compensator Alloy 36" from Carpenter Technologies Inc. (CarTech), Eagle Alloy (US), Telcon Inc. (UK), and other vendors.

[7] "Temperature Compensation of NdFeB Permanent Magnets", S.H. Kim and C. Doose, Argonne National Laboratory, 1997 Particle Accelerator Conf.,Vancouver BC, session 2P1.

[8] C. Benvenuti et al: Non evapolable getter films for uhv applications, Internal Note CERN-EST-SM 97-01 Aug. (1997)

[9] K.Tatenuma, K.Uchida, T.Itoh, T.Momose, and H.Ishimaru: Acquisition of clean ultrahigh vacuum using chemical treatment, to be published J. Vac. Sci. Technology (1997)

Q: What is the critical energy?

A: The critical energy is hopefully 16-17 KeV or so, for ordinary bending magnet, not wiggler.

A: We hope to make a 10 kG bending magnet using a permanent magnet with a small aperture, nearly the same as an undulator system.

Q: You have an underground tunnel, so, how do you prevent from high costs.

A: Yes I agree, but underground is not so deep, maybe two or three meters. I hope to make a slightly cheap underground. Underground is not necessary for X-ray shield, ordinary concrete pipe thickness like this is fine. Underground is no problem for X-ray radiation environment.

Q: For medical use especially in Europe, we need an economical and small storage ring, so the maximum diameter could not be more than 50 meters. Do you think it is possible to construct ?

A: Yes. I understand this in two ways. Using superconducting magnets or a small ring. Our system has magnetic field of about 10 kG, not so high. The corresponding ring is slightly larger. The total cost of a small ring using superconducting magnets is high, while a large ring using a small magnet system is very low cost which is much preferred for medical use. Our proposal doesn't use the most advanced technology such as superconducting or wiggler, and its machine operation should be easy, almost no maintenance needed, and highly reliable.

Q: Just for me to understand is, I'm not physicist, so it wouldn't decrease cost if you just have a small ring. It would not decrease this cost of 11million dollars you have said. For a small ring you need superconductor ?

A: Yes.

Q: What is the emittance of your ring?

A: Professor Ando suggested me that the emittance is not needed so small, then our lattice optics is ordinary FODO.

Q: Is it possible to build a permanent magnet sextapole ?

A: Yes

Q: Could you build a high brightness ring with permanent magnets ?

A: Dr. Bill Foster told me that he can design correction magnets, and small trim coils as well.

C: I am thinking that it might be an interesting in a small high brightness facility in a sort of 2.5GeV range injector, and would not be so expensive.

C: I think this is the important point. The concept is not limited to a high emittance machine. It could be adopted for low emittance. It's a question of tolerances and field quality, and maybe small trim coils, as you say, you can reach tolerance level adequate for a very low emittance machine. So I think it's a very interesting idea for all machines in the future not just high emittance machines.

Fluorescent X-ray Source for Diagnostic Imaging Studies

Fukai Toyofuku[1], Kenji Tokumori[2], Shigenobu Kanda[2], Katsuyuki Nishimura[3], Kazuyuki Hyodo[4], Masami Ando[4], and Chikao Uyama[5]

[1] Department of Radiological Technology, Kyushu University School of Health Sciences, 3-1-1 Maidashi, Higashi-ku, Fukuoka, 812-82 Japan
[2] Department of Oral and Maxillofacial Radiology, Kyushu University, 3-1-1 Maidashi, Higashi-ku, Fukuoka, 812-82 Japan
[3] Department of Radiological Sciences, Ibaraki Prefectural University of Health Sciences, Ami 4669-2, Ami-machi, Inashiki-gun, Ibaraki, 300-3 Japan
[4] Institute of Material Structure Science, High Energy Accelerator Research Organization, 1-1, Oho, Tsukuba-shi, Ibaraki, 305 Japan
[5] Department of Radiology, National Cardiovascular Center, Fujishirodai-5, Suita-shi, Osaka, 565 Japan

SUMMARY. In diagnostic imaging studies, the energy response of x-ray image sensors, such as newly developed screen/film systems, scintillators, storage phosphors, and CCD sensors is one of the most important characteristics. A monochromatic x-ray source with a wide energy range is necessary to determine the output of the sensor systems as a function of x-ray energy.
A fluorescent x-ray source for diagnostic imaging studies has been developed using a 6.5 GeV synchrotron radiation storage ring at Tsukuba (Japan). Fluorescent x-rays, which range from about 20 keV to 75 keV are generated by irradiating several target materials. The purity of the fluorescent x-rays can be improved to better than 95% by using Kβ attenuation filters. From the measurements using an imaging plate (IP), spatial uniformity is better than 90%. This source is also useful as a source for medical imaging such as K-edge subtraction and monochromatic x-ray CT.

KEY WORDS: Fluorescent x-ray, Synchrotron radiation, Energy subtraction, Monochromatic x-ray CT, Energy response

INTRODUCTION

Fluorescent x-ray sources using conventional x-ray tubes have been developed for diagnostic radiology studies by several researchers [1-3]. However, because of limited intensities of the sources, they have been used almost entirely for measuring the energy responses of screen/film systems. The advent of synchrotron radiation made it possible to use the fluorescent x-rays as a standard radiation field for measuring the energy responses of imaging sensors and dosimeters in the diagnostic energy region.

Fluorescent x-rays produced through K-shell ionization of high-Z target (Z>40) have energies which lie in the range used in medical diagnostic imaging. Fig.1 shows the atomic number dependencies of: Kα x-ray energy (EKα); ratio of K-shell ionization to total photoelectric effect (k), and; K fluorescence yield (ωk).
The angular distribution of fluorescent x-rays is spherically symmetric. The total number of produced K fluorescent x-ray photons per incident photon, which is the product of k and

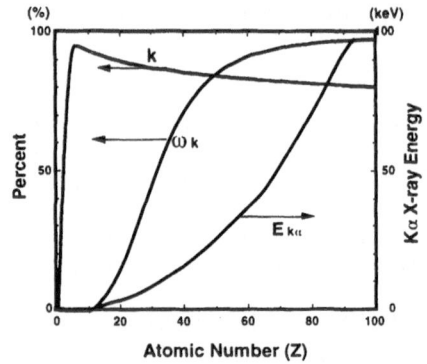

Fig. 1. Atomic number dependencies of ωk, k, and energy of Kα x-ray.

ωk, is about 0.6-0.7 in the energy range of 20 to 80 keV. Taking into account the self absorption within a target angle of 45 degrees, about a quarter of photons are emitted from the target surface when the energy of the incident photon is just above the K absorption edge of the target element. In case of the conventional x-ray tube, more than 99 percent of the incident electron kinetic energy is converted to heat, which limits the intensity of the x-rays. Therefore, considering output to input energies, the efficiency of producing the x-rays using synchrotron radiation is more than ten times higher compared with a conventional x-ray tube.

Features of fluorescent x-ray

The advantages of the fluorescent x-ray source for x-ray diagnostic imaging studies are as follows.
1. Wide beam size
Large area (more than 50cm) monochromatic beam is easily obtained, which is indispensable to cover the large detectors which are used for whole body CT and chest imaging equipments.
2. Wide energy range and rapid energy switching
From 20 to about 80keV monochromatic x-rays are obtained discretely. Energies can be quickly changed by switching the targets using a rotating target system [4,5].
3. No higher order harmonics
Higher order harmonics are not present, which is inevitable in case of Bragg diffraction monochromatization.

METHODS AND RESULTS

A fluorescent x-ray source for diagnostic imaging studies has been developed using Accumulation Ring (1.5 GeV, 30mA) at Tsukuba. Fluorescent x-rays, which range from about 20 keV to 75 keV are generated by irradiating several target materials. The incident photon beam from the bending magnet irradiates the target, the surface of which is angled at 30 - 45 degrees to the beam, to extract the fluorescent x-rays perpendicularly. The incident white x-ray is collimated by using the parallel hole collimator. Filters composed of elements having their K absorption edges between Kα and Kβ energies of the various target are used to attenuate the Kβ components preferentially . The energy spectra for Yb and Ho targets measured by using a HPGe detector are shown in Fig. 2. It is

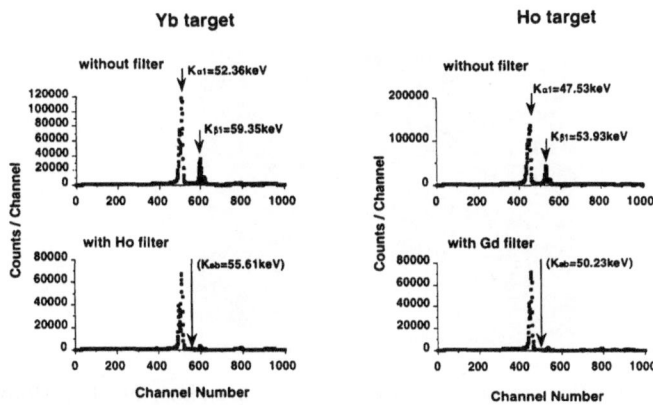

Fig. 2. Examples of fluorescent x-ray energy spectra generated by synchrotron radiation. Filters having their K absorption edges between Kα and Kβ energies are used to attenuate the Kβ components preferentially. The typical ratio of Kα to total intensity is about 95% to 98%.

136

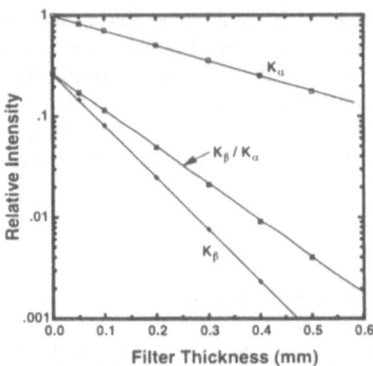

Fig. 3. Attenuation curves of Yb Kα and Kβ x-rays. The ratio of Kβ to Kα is also shown. The Kβ component is attenuated preferentially by using the Ho filter which has the K absorption edge energy between the energies of Kα and Kβ.

seen from the spectra that the Compton components are almost negligible.

Attenuation curves of Yb Kα and Kβ x-rays are shown in Fig. 3. The ratio of Kβ to Kα x-rays calculated from these curves is also shown as a function of Ho filter thickness. The Kβ component is attenuated preferentially by using the Ho filter which has the K absorption edge energy between the energies of Kα and Kβ. It is seen from Fig.3 that the intensity of Kα is reduced to about one-third if the Kβ component is reduced to one percent of the total photons.

Uniformity of the fluorescent x-ray measured by using an imaging plate is shown in Fig. 4. The diameter of the field is 20 cm at 50 cm from the focal spot. Horizontal density distribution across the center is shown under the image. The intensity of the Kα x-ray at the edge of the radiation field is estimated to be about 90% of the intensity at the center of the field.

The exposures of the fluorescent x-rays from different target materials are measured by using a shallow type ionization chamber. Photon fluence rates at 50 cm from the focal spot are calculated from the measured exposures. Typical intensities of the fluorescent x-rays which are used for K-edge subtraction of iodine, barium, and gadolinium contrast media are shown in Table 1.

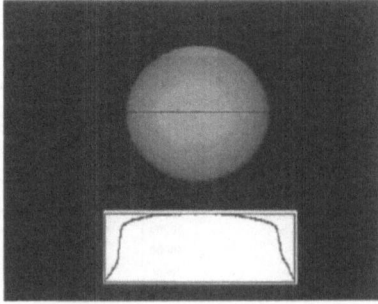

Fig. 4. Uniformity of the fluorescent x-ray measured by using an imaging plate. Horizontal density distribution across the center is shown under the image. The diameter of the field is 20 cm at 50 cm from the focal spot.

Table 1. Fluence rates of fluorescent x-rays per 30 mA ring current at 50cm from the focal spot. The diameter of the incident beam is 3mm. Specific filter is used for each target material to reduce the intensity of Kβ component preferentially.

Fluorescent X-ray	Fluence Rate (photons / sec mm² 30mA)	Kα/(Kα+Kβ) (%)
Ba (32.2keV)	6.7 x 10⁶	97
Ce (34.7keV)	8.1 x 10⁶	97
Sm (40.1keV)	7.4 x 10⁶	97.5
Ho (47.5keV)	5.5 x 10⁶	95.5
Yb (52.4keV)	4.2 x 10⁶	95
Au (68.8keV)	2.3 x 10⁶	97

DISCUSSION

There are several methods to produce monochromatic x-rays. The most popular one is crystal diffraction, which has been widely used due to the fact that the energy spread is very narrow and the energy can be changed continuously. In this method, however, it is difficult to obtain large area beams which are useful in many applications. Crystal diffraction and fluorescent x-ray methods serve as complementary one to the other in the diagnostic imaging studies. The fluorescent x-ray source is also useful as a source of medical imaging such as K-edge energy subtraction, monochromatic x-ray CT, super-magnification imaging and so forth [5,6].

REFERENCES

1. Hoffman EJ, Phelps ME (1974) Production of monoenergetic x-rays from 8 to 87 keV. Phy. Med. Biol. 19: 19-35
2. Vyborny CJ, Doi K, Metz CE, Haus AG (1977) A simple source of fluorescent x-rays for the study of radiographic imaging systems. Medical Physics 4: 482-485
3. Konishi K, Toyofuku F, Kanda S (1985) Polychromatic photon absorptiometry and its application to quantitative imaging. Proc. 16th Int. Conf. Medical & Biological Eng., Medical and Biomedical Engineering & Computing 23, suppl. Part 2, 1531-1532
4. Toyofuku F (1993) Fluorescent x-ray source using synchrotron radiation and its applications. Japanese J . Med. Phys. 13 (2): 273-280 (in Japanese)
5. Toyofuku F, Tokumori K, Nishimura K, Saito T, Takeda T, Itai Y, Hyoudo K, Ando M, Endo M, Naito H, Uyama C (1995) Development of fluorescent x-ray source for medical imaging. Rev. Sci. Inst. 66 (2): 1981-1983
6. Saito T, Kudo H, Takeda T, Itai Y, Tokumori K, Toyofuku F, Hyodo K, Ando M, Nishimura K, Uyama C (1995) Three-Dimensional Monochromatic x-ray CT. Proc. SPIE - Int. Soc. Opt. Eng. Vol. 2564: 548-57

138

Q: Where do you have a plan to install this system ?

A: At Spring-8. We started this research about 5 or 6 years ago when the Spring-8 project just started its construction. The foremost motivation to develop a fluorescent X-ray source was how we could make a large field monochromatic X-ray suitable for medical imaging using a very narrow beam from an undulator or a multipole wiggler. There are several applications, for example, K-edge subtraction imaging, magnification imaging, energy response measurement of newly developed imaging systems like digital X-ray radiography system and for future equipment.

Q: If you apply the method to a very narrow focussed beam, is it possible to perform the high resolution angiography of the magnified view in the future ?

A: At a medical station of Spring-8 which is about 250 m from the light source, the size of the undulator beam will be about 20 mm by 1.2 mm. If the take-off angle from the target is 3.4 degrees, the effective focal spot size is 1.2mm x 1.2 mm. Under this condition the photon yield will be almost the same order as the conventional x-ray CT. In order to proceed the high resolution angiography and supermagnification imaging for CT, one will need a beam focused smaller than 100 micrometers. This focussing technique looks feasible. However, since the estimated fluorescent photon intensity at 1 m from the focal spot is about 100 times lower than the maximum photon yield obtained from the Bragg reflected monochromatic X-rays using multipole wiggler X-rays this system will be of great use to CT while not much to 2D angiography.

Q: If you perform K-edge subtraction, will the existence of the K_b fluorescence bring any difficulty ?

A: The K_b fluorescence from the metal target may excite the attenuation filter so that secondary K_b and Ka X-ray is produced, but the ratio of the secondary to primary Ka X-ray is less than 10^{-2}, by that means it may cause no practical difficulty in imaging.

Q: Have you tested value of concentration of iodine or gadolinium ? What were your concentrations ?

A: We have used commercially available gadolinium whose concentration was 370 mg/ml.

Q: Did you estimate the fraction of Compton scatter of photons in your spectral ?

A: We measured the energy spectra of fluorescent x-rays by using a HPGe detector to reach a conclusion that Compton components were almost negligibly small. We haven't done Monte Carlo simulation by using, for instance, EGS4.

Remarks on the Role of Multilayer Optics and Short Period Insertion Devices for Medical Imaging Sources and Applications

Roman Tatchyn[1], Ted Cremer[1], Paul Csonka[2], David Boyers[3], and Melvin Piestrup[3]

[1]Stanford Synchrotron Radiation Laboratory, Stanford Linear Accelerator Center, Stanford, CA 94304, USA
[2]Institute of Theoretical Physics, University of Oregon, Eugene, OR 97403-5203, USA
[3]Adelphi Technology, Inc., 2181 Park Blvd., Palo Alto, CA 94306, USA

SUMMARY. Over approximately the last ten years, research and development has been conducted at the Stanford Synchrotron Radiation Laboratory (SSRL) in two areas critical to the status of Dual-energy Digital Subtraction Angiography (DDSA) and related medical imaging techniques: 1) multilayer optics, and 2) short-period insertion device technology. In this paper selected results of these experimental and theoretical studies have been reviewed, emphasizing their relevance to future DDSA systems design. A basic perspective predicated on our work is that continued development and implementation of these two technologies can favorably impact the performance and economy of existing or planned medical imaging facilities.

KEY WORDS: Dual-energy Digital Subtraction Angiography, Medical imaging, Multilayer optics, Micropole undulator, Harmonic suppression

INTRODUCTION

The purpose of this paper is to present a brief review of some of the developmental studies performed on multilayer optics and short-period insertion devices for medical imaging sources and applications at the Stanford Synchrotron Radiation Laboratory (SSRL). The basic themes unifying this work are: 1) the improvement of the clinical quality of angiograms or other (hard) x-ray diagnostic images, and 2) the improvement of the economy, performance, and scale of medical imaging installations. In the pre-1992 era the basic limitations on angiogram quality stemmed from poor signal-to-noise (S/N) performance. The principal contributing factors were: 1) high quantal noise stemming from the low number N of recorded photons/pixel ($\propto 1/\sqrt{N}$); 2) non-optimal detector performance; 3) resolution blurring from higher harmonics (66 keV, 99 keV, etc.) transmitted from the typically broadband wiggler sources employed at synchrotron radiation (SR) installations, and 4) resolution blurring stemming from mechanical rastering of the living heart through the x-ray beam over times on the order of a second.

In view of the successful optimization of detector performance by groups working at SSRL, DESY [1,2], and elsewhere [3], the approaches taken to mitigating or resolving the remaining problems at SSRL by the application of multilayer and insertion device technology were: 1) to increase the per/pixel flux without introducing artifact images at a problematical level; 2) to suppress or eliminate the transmission of higher harmonics, and 3) to develop sources that could, in principle, substantially reduce or eliminate the rastering interval. The results of our studies, including an assessment of their potential impact on the performance, economy, and scale of medical imaging facilities, are summarized below.

MULTILAYER OPTICS

In contrast to design proposals recommending more powerful wigglers [4,5], our basic multilayer-based approach to increasing per-pixel flux was to increase the bandwidth of the monochromator above- and below-edge lines from the ~0.0005-0.001 typical of Si crystals to values in the range of ~0.005-0.02 [6]. We note that the angiography group at BNL has also pursued a bandwidth-broadening strategy by bending (natural) monochromator crystals [7], but their technique is in all likelihood limited to a maximal bandwidth of ~0.005. The actual optimum bandwidth that can be utilized with our multilayer techniques [8] has not yet been conclusively established, but there are reasons to believe that with the development of advanced imaging [9,10] or computer-aided diagnostics techniques to normalize artifact images out of the angiogram, the optimal value of this parameter may be found to lie in the 0.005-0.02. range. In the research program conducted by Adelphi Technology and SSRL [8], multilayers of various bandshapes, bandwidths (extending out to 10%), and reflection efficiencies were designed, fabricated by Osmics, Inc., and tested at SSRL. A list of selected multilayer structural and performance parameters is given in Table 1.

Table 1. Absolute reflectivities and bandwidths (BWs) of selected W/Si and W/B4C uniform-period multilayers characterized at 33 keV on SPEAR. t_W=tungsten thickness; t_{Si}=silicon thickness; t_{B_4C}=boron carbide thickness.

Sample Number	t_W[Å]	t_{Si} [Å]	# of Layer Pairs	Absolute Reflectivity [%]	BW [%]
2-4	6	12	200	51	1.70
3-4	9	14	200	94	1.30
4-4	9	9	200	62	0.88
	t_W[Å]	t_{B4C}[Å]			
5-2	6	12	250	79	0.90
7-2	9	9	250	32	0.67
8-2	9	14	200	75	1.80

Reprinted with permission from [11]. ©1996 American Institute of Physics.

Based in part on the high multilayer reflectivities achieved by our program, we have recently proposed and analyzed a scheme for the suppression or elimination of higher harmonics from broadband sources [11]. As schematized in Fig. 1, the basic approach is to use two tandem reflectors

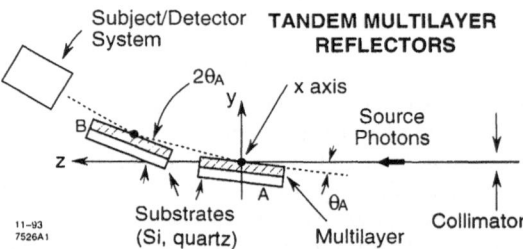

Fig. 1. Geometry of tandem multilayer reflection. Angle of incidence on B designated by θ_B.
Reprinted with permission from [11]. ©1996 American Institute of Physics.

(per monochromator element), design one multilayer with a 1:1 high-Z:low-Z material thickness ratio (suppression of even harmonics), the second with a 1:3 ratio (suppression of harmonics divisible by

3), and then optimize the materials of both to induce strong *refractive* shifting *and* suppression of the integral orders. As summarized in Tables 2 and 3 the first multilayer refractively shifts the 66 keV and 99 keV resonance angles ($\theta_n \rightarrow \theta'_n$), strongly suppressing their reflection. Since the source is a wiggler, however, the multilayer will still strongly reflect frequencies that are slightly displaced from the true harmonic values of 66 keV, 99 keV, etc. Now, if the second multilayer is designed with a different refractive shift than the first one, the harmonic frequencies reflected off the first multilayer will no longer fulfill the resonance requirement of the second, and will consequently be strongly suppressed. A graphic illustration of this process is shown in Fig. 2.

Table 2. Refractive angular order shifts at fixed harmonic energies in a W/B4C multilayer. t_W=12 Å; t_{B4C}=8 Å; N=200.

harmonic #, order	n=1	n=2	n=3
E_n [KeV]	33	66	99
θ_n [°]	0.538	0.538	0.538
θ'_n [°]	0.549	0.541	0.539
$(\theta'_n - \theta_n)/\theta_n$ [%]	2	0.48	0.15

Reprinted with permission from [11]. ©1996 American Institute of Physics.

Table 3. Refractive energy shifts at fixed incidence angle θ'_1 in W/B4C multilayer. t_W=12 Å; t_{B4C}=8 Å; N=200.

harmonic #, order	n=1	n=2	n=3
θ'_1 [°]	0.549	0.549	0.549
E'_n[keV]	33	65	97.2
E'_n/E_n	1	0.985	0.982

Reprinted with permission from [11]. ©1996 American Institute of Physics.

Refractive Fundamental and Harmonic Order Locations

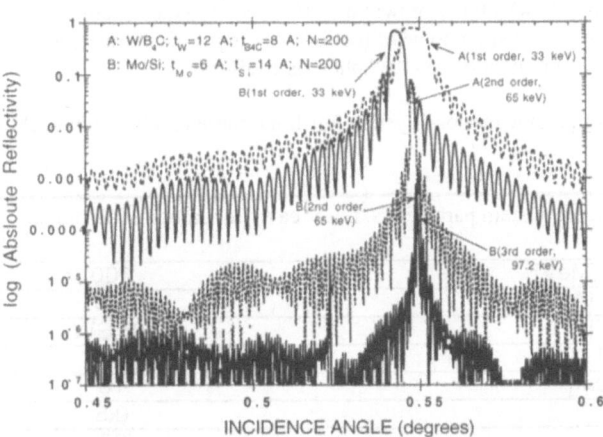

Fig. 2. Refraction-shifted spectral orders of a W/B4C and Mo/Si multilayer. The W/B4C spectral orders are all reflected out at approximately the same angle, 0.549°, while the Mo/Si multilayer demonstrates a substantial displacement between its 33 keV and higher harmonic reflection angles. Reprinted with permission from [11]. ©1996 American Institute of Physics.

We remark that this technique allows the re-optimization of wiggler parameters for conventional angiography sources and beam lines, since the basic strategy presently used for reducing harmonic contamination is to design the wiggler with a critical energy well below the K-edge of the contrast agent in question (for angiography, Iodine). With use of multilayer harmonic suppression, such wigglers can now, in principle, be designed for a maximum-flux energy of 33 keV.

SHORT-PERIOD INSERTION DEVICES

As discussed in a prior publication, short-period undulators offer a number of potential advantages over wigglers for medical imaging source applications [12]. These include: 1) an in-band flux a factor of ~2-3 higher than from a comparable wiggler; 2) for K parameters <1, substantially smaller harmonic intensities; 3) a smaller total power output with a much narrower spectral width; and 4) optimal performance on much lower energy storage rings that those utilized for conventional wigglers [13]. A major difference is the much larger angular width of a wiggler's beam, which spreads out rapidly to the typical ~10 cm width of human heart, and thus readily provides a horizontally-wide, vertically-narrow beam suitable for vertical raster-scanning. This difference, which is conventionally asserted to be a definitive advantage of the wiggler, can in fact be viewed as an advantage for the short-period insertion undulator in a source optimized for "single-shot" data acquisition [13]. This follows from the fact that the undulator beam is roughly circular, making it possible, following appropriate expansion, to "photograph" the full heart as a single image.

First, as shown elsewhere [14], the in-band power radiated by an undulator (per unit length, per unit beam current) varies inversely with E^2, where E is the electron beam energy, provided the K parameter remains fixed. To attain 33 keV with a micropole undulator (MPU), viz., an undulator with a period <1 mm, on a sub-GeV storage ring, a scheme based on a laser undulator (which can attain the necessary fields of several tens of Teslas) can be considered. The performance requirements can be determined from the following basic considerations: 1) a 10 cm x 10 cm Position Sensitive Detector (PSD) with a 100μ x 100μ pixel spacing (viz., 10^6 pixels); 2) 10^4 photons per pixel, per image; 3) an attenuation factor of 10^{-4} for 33 keV photons by the human body; 3) monochromator and detector efficiencies of ~1; 4) a line bandwidth of 1%; and 5) a data acquisition interval of 2 ms, short enough to be relatively insensitive to heart motion. Folding these numbers together indicates an angiography source flux requirement of ~5×10^{16} photons/s, 1%BW.

A nominal set of operating parameters for a system fulfilling these requirements is shown in Table 4.

Table 4. Angiography source system parameters. Laser cavity operation is assumed.

Storage Ring Energy [MeV]	600
Storage Ring Current [A]	1.5
Peak Laser Power [W]	12 GW
Laser Wavelength [μ]	100
Laser Pulse Length [cm]	10
Laser Waist [mm]	0.5
Peak Laser Field [T]	20
Laser K Parameter	0.19
X-ray Output @ 33 keV [ph/s,1%BW]	7.8×10^{16}

A possible implementation of the system, including multilayer optics optimized for this purpose, is schematized in Fig. 3. The two MPUs, one for the below-K-edge and the other for the above-K-edge line of Iodine, have slightly different extraction locations (and axes) for delivery to the appropriate multilayer. Alternatively, one location employing a fast beam kicker could be used. The divergence angles, σ_x' and σ_y', are set by the beam emittance and the focusing beta at the location of the MPUs.

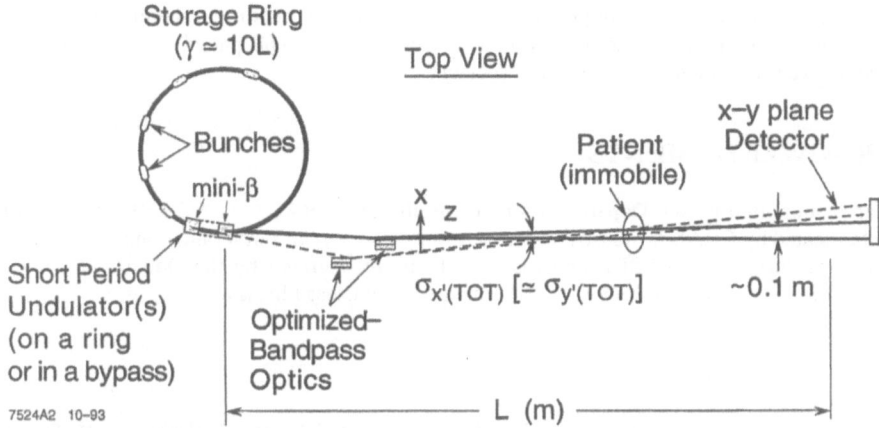

Fig. 3. Schematic of a "single-shot" angiography scheme based on short-period undulator and variable-band multilayer technologies.

For the assumed 600 MeV ring energy, a conservative assumption of $\sigma_x'=\sigma_y'\sim 1$ mr results in the attainment of a 10 cm beam waist at 50 m from the MPU. With directed design, this length could be substantially reduced. If we presume operation on a storage ring with a diameter in the 20-40 m range, it is evident that the requirements on the laser undulator, particularly in terms of required repetition rate, are very stringent, implying the necessity of substantial innovative r&d for both cavity and source development [15].

On higher energy rings, more conventional short-period, small-gap undulator technology could be employed. Here the relatively lower emission efficiency would need to be compensated with a substantially greater insertion device length than for the case of Table 4. Conventionally, this poses a problem for small-gap devices, which are limited in length to the order of the local beta function. However, special techniques for mitigating such limitations have been proposed [16], and are currently being investigated at SSRL.

DISCUSSION

We have summarized a number of results relevant to the development of medical imaging systems in the hard x-ray range based on studies at SSRL in the areas of multilayer and short-period undulator technologies. The application of multilayers to DDSA angiography monochromators appears to offer the possibility of substantial improvement in the performance of conventional systems, or even the re-optimization of wiggler-based sources for angiography applications. A key research direction related to the ultimate utility of multilayers is the development of techniques for unfolding (perhaps automatically) the images of bone and cartilage (which are, from the point of view of information theory, highly non-random classes of objects) from angiograms. The development of multilayers for improving or optimizing other aspects of medical imaging systems also appears to be a promising direction for further research. In the area of x-ray sources, the development of a single-shot imaging system through the use of short-period insertion devices appears to be a worthwhile goal to pursue. A relevant paradigm is the modern dental x-ray machine, which is relatively affordable and also works in a relatively unintrusive "single-shot" mode. Attainment of similar levels of comfort and performance in angiography could, through reduction of cost and patient trauma, make DDSA accessible to a substantially larger sector of society.

A CKNOWLEDGMENTS

Research supported by the Department of Energy through CRADA SLAC-9302. The multilayers were fabricated by CRADA Industrial Partner, Osmic, Inc. Synchrotron radiation measurements and simulations performed at SSRL and SLAC, which are operated by the Department of Energy, Offices of Basic Energy Sciences and High Energy and Nuclear Physics.

REFERENCES

1. Rubenstein E, Giacomini JC, Gordon H, Thompson AC, Brown G, Hofstadter R, Thomlinson W, Zeman HD (1990) Synchrotron radiation coronary angiography with a dual-beam, dual-detector imaging system. Nucl Instrum Meth A291: 80-85

2. Besch HJ, Bode EJ, Menk RH, Schenk HW, Tafelmeier U, Walenta AH, Xu HZ (1991) A high precision, high speed X-ray detector for the non-invasive coronary angiography with synchrotron radiation. Nucl Instrum Meth A310: 446-448

3. Thomlinson W, Gmur N, Chapman D, Garrett R, Lazarz N, Moulin H, Thompson AC, Zeman HD, Brown GS, Morrison J, Reiser P, Padmanabahn V, Ong L, Green S, Giacomini JC, Gordon H, Rubenstein E (1992) First operation of the medical research facility at the NSLS for coronary angiography Rev Sci Instrum 63(1), part 11a: 625-628

4. Burattini E, Rindi A (eds) (1988) Synchrotron Radiation Applications to Digital Subtraction Angiography (SYRDA), Italian Physical Society Conference Proceedings No. 10. Editrice Compositore, Bologna

5. Thompson AC, Zeman H, Thomlinson W, Rubenstein E, Kernoff RS, Hofstadter R, Giacomini JC, Gordon HJ, Brown GS (1988) Imaging of coronary arteries using synchrotron radiation. Nucl Instrum Meth B40-41, pt. 1: 407-412

6. Tatchyn R (1991) Preliminary Design Study for a Scanning Multilayer Mirror/Monochromator System for Diagnostic Angiography at the Iodine Ka Edge. SLAC-PUB-6412.

7. Suortti P, Thomlinson W, Chapman D, Gmur N, Siddons DP, Schulze C (1993) A single crystal bent Laue monochromator for coronary angiography. Nucl Instrum Meth A336: 304-309

8. Boyers D, Ho A, Li Q, Piestrup M, Rice M, Tatchyn R (1994) Tests of variable-band multilayers designed for investigating optimal signal-to-noise versus artifact signal ratios in dual-energy digital subtraction angiography (DDSA) imaging systems. Nucl Instrum Meth A346: 565-570

9. Zeman HD, Moulin HR (1992) Removal of harmonic artifacts from synchrotron radiation coronary angiograms. IEEET rans Nucl Sci 39(5): 1431-1437

145

10. Kulipanov GN, Mezentsev NA, Pindurin VF, Skrinsky AN, Sheromov MA, Ogirenko AP, Omigov VM (1983) Application of synchrotron radiation to the study of man's circulatory system. Nucl Instrum Meth 208: 677-683
11. Tatchyn R, Cremer T, Boyers D, Li Q, Piestrup M (1996) Multilayer optics for harmonic control of angiography beamline sources: Rev Sci Instrum. 67(9): on CD
12. Csonka PL, Tatchyn R (1992) Short Period Undulators for Human Angiography. In: Cornacchia M, Winick H (eds) Proceedings of the Workshop on Fourth Generation Light Sources. SSRL report No. 92/02, pp 555-564
13. Akisada A, Ando M, Hyodo K, Hasegawa S, Konishi K, Nishimura K, Maruhashi A, Toyofuku F, Suwa A, Kohra K (1986) An attempt at coronary angiography with a large size monochromatic SR beam. Nucl Instrum Meth A246: 713-718
14. Tatchyn R, Csonka PL, Toor A (1989) Perspectives on micropole undulators in synchrotron radiation technology. Rev Sci Instrum 60(7): 1796-1804
15. Sprangle P, Ting A, Esarey E, Fisher A (1992) Tunable, short pulse hard x-rays from a compact laser synchrotron source. J. Appl. Phys. 72(11): 5032-5038.
16. Tatchyn R (1997) A field-cancellation algorithm for constructing economical planar permanent magnet (PM) multipoles with large high-quality field apertures. Presented at: 1997 Particle Accelerator Conference 1997, Vancouver, B.C., May 12-16 1997: MS-9P121

DISCUSSION ON COMPACT SOURCES

C: We've heard a lot of interesting talks in this session. I think we have answered some of the questions and comments that I made earlier today. I think it would be nice if we have any general comments from the assembled group or general questions. It would be nice to open up general discussion among speakers, or among attendees in terms of just an open forum at this point in time. That's what this time, at least by my understanding was set aside for. I issued some challenges this morning, and earlier today. So, are there any comments from people regarding my comments related to the compact source technology which was just addressed by the last speaker. How do people here feel, for example, about the necessity of compact sources. That is certainly a key issue in some of our laboratories, and are there comments here ?

C: It occurs to me that it is definitely a trade-off about how unique the capability is that you have. So, in angiography where the image quality may end up the same as the hospital system, I can see the point, but if you look at therapy there is no problem at all with shipping patients across the country to dedicated centers. If mammography turned out to be a very unique capability at Synchrotron sources, then maybe you have to change that condition.

C: No, not according to the mammography community. You could presumably get the odd case that a physician would be willing to send their patients to a centralized location, but in general mammography colleagues say the same thing that our angiography colleagues have been saying, that if it is not in-house, then, patients are almost certainly not going to travel. That is significantly different, however, from something like a therapy once you have a diagnosis, for example , inoperable brain tumor, just as an example, which Per Spanne addressed this morning related to the macro radiation therapy program. That is a whole different situation. You can imagine having a number of centers, take just for an example the proton therapy. There are only a few centers around the world, and yet people fly there from all over the country, all over the world. Because if it is the only hope for cure of a fatal illness, then people will go and travel. But in terms of the diagnosis side of the problem, our physicians, even the mammographers, are saying no, it had better be local. And I am just wondering how wide-spread that is ? What is the feeling in Japan ? Is that also an issue here ? How about some of the medical people who are present here ? Can you answer that ? Are you willing to send your patients routinely on an eight hour journey to go and get imaged in a screening process ? This is a very serious question, because it stopped our program at Brookhaven.

C: Of course we don't routinely send our patients long way either.

C: If you think about the compact sources, I think more feasible when it comes to the mammography area where the energies needed are much lower. So, when you want to have higher energies, you end up with a machine which is no longer compact. This is what was presented a moment ago. If it works, it's a compact source, but building with such high energy is not cheap any more. So, it may turn out that compact sources will have a relatively limited use or be used where relatively small energies are needed. We don't need the highest flux for some CT applications, and this might become feasible, but hardly for angiography because it needs every photon you can get.

Ch: I should also make a comment that there are other types of compact sources that have been studied. We've been involved in a collaboration with a firm in Boston Science Research Laboratory to design a very high power, effectively rotating anode type technology machine, which, should it work in terms of delivering the photons, we would get equivalent fluxes in the

10^{11}/mm^2/sec range. The problem with that, and we have made some progress solving it, is one of optics. One should not necessarily think that it is only a compact storage ring that will produce the types of fluxes necessary. It's clear you can build a storage ring to do it, it's not yet obvious that the high power electro-static type machine will in fact perform. Unfortunately we have not received the funding to build the prototype so we cannot answer the question yet, but I would like someone to build such a device and then we could see.

C: I think it is clear that a compact source can be made if the DESY result warrants a dedicated source that should fit in the basement of a hospital, the order of 15 meters across. Such a source can clearly be made and it will produce the spectrum, identical to what you are using at hospital right now. It could be a 2GeV ring with a 6 T wiggler magnet. Two such stations could be included into such a compact ring with 40 to 50 meter circumference. If you just put the basic equations in, you come up with such a ring. You get much bigger rings when you ask for much lower emittance for other applications, for therapy, for micro beams, for undulator beams. But if you just want to do a kind of imaging you are doing at DESY, a compact ring can clearly be built. It does not push the frontier of technology, It's straight forward.

C: We'd like to give you numbers for such rings. We'll finish our study next year. If it's decided that it's worth it to continue and it is accepted by the cardiologists, then we need a compact source. We will get the following form; the photon energy is 33KeV. If you use the monochromator of Bill Thomlinson and P. Suortti, you lose a factor of two. Then, you need it if you use a line scan system in 50 cm wide line. If you use a 2D, you need it in 15 cm x 15 cm. So now we started with numbers from Dr.Dix. What can we get from one investigation ? One investigation for selective coronary angiography in Germany is 1,600 mark. All this is in Deutsche mark. They want to cut it down. That means you can't get more than 800 German marks per investigation. Then it's cheaper than selective, otherwise they never would do it. We assumed a ring has two beamlines, we think we can do 15 investigation per beamline a day, and we can work 250 days per year. It means at that ring we have 7,500 patients per year. And we get 6 million German marks.

Q: Excuse me. How many patients are there to be investigated in Germany ? In other words, how many compact synchrotron do you need from that point of view ?

A: That's difficult to say, we have 400,000 coronary angiographies per year, and 150,000 interventional therapies. We have to reach the rate of 30 percent among these patients of 150,000 interventional patients therapies per year. We have 50,000 patients per year who need a new coronary angiography, and probably a new interventional therapy, so we have at least these 50,000 patients which could be candidates for this type of angiography.

C: So, from this 6 million German marks you need 0.75 million for material, contrast material, whatever you need for investigation, then we talked to Volker Saile from Louisiana, and he said we need about 10 people from the technical side and Dr.Dill thought we should have 8 from the medical side. 1.8 million German marks for manpower. The cost for maintenance and power is 1.5 million German marks. If you assume 15 years amortization, then you can't spend more than 23 million German marks for a ring. This means 1,500 million yen or 14 million US dollars. That's the price we must meet.

C: That's actually not too far away from the price of synchrotrons which are commercially available. Oxford Instruments, for example, offers a synchrotron which is about the size of this room for about 25 million dollars. It is 25 million dollars nowadays, but probably 20 million dollars before. They didn't build many systems, but one is at IBM, and they have just sold one to Singapore.

C: That one is lower energy.

C: Right, so we'd have to add money for the insertion device.

C: What I want to point out is that people are working on cheaper synchrotrons for semiconductor industry, because they are going to need those in the future.

C: If they offer as for 25 million, it means you can build at half of the price, then add a little money for the insertion device. You may be able to build it 20 million or so.

BEAMLINES FOR MEDICAL APPLICATIONS ON THE SPRING-8

Medical Application User Group of SPring-8:
Chikao Uyama[1], Tohoru Takeda[2], Fukai Toyofuku[3], Kenji Tokumori[4], Masami Ando[5],
Kazuyuki Hyodo[5] Yuji Itai2, Hideaki.Shiwaku[6], Katsuyuki Nishimura[7],
and
SPring-8 Project Team:
Hiromichi Kamitsubo[8]

1 Research Institute, National Cardiovascular Center, Fujishirodai, Suita-shi, Osaka, 565 Japan
2 Institute of Clinical Medicine, University of Tsukuba, Tennodai, Tsukuba-shi, 305 Japan
3 School of Health Sciences, Kyushu University, Maiduru, Higashi-ku, Hukuoka-shi, 812 Japan
4 Department of Dentistry, School of Medicine, Kyushu University, Maiduru, Higashi-ku, Hukuoka-shi, 812 Japan
5 Photon Factory, High Energy Accelerator Research Organization, KEK, Oho, Tsukuba-shi, 305 Japan
6 Department of Synchrotron Radiation Facilities Project, Japan Atomic Energy Research Institute, SPring-8, Kamigori-cho, Ako-gun, Hyogo-ken, 678-12 Japan
7 Department of Radiological Sciences, Ibaraki Prefectural University of Health Sciences, Ami-chou, Inashiki-gun, Ibaraki-ken, 300-03 Japan
8 Japan Synchrotron Radiation Research Institute, Kanaji, Kamigori-cho, Ako-gun, Hyogo-ken, 678-12 Japan

SUMMARY. Three medical application beamlines of the SPring-8 are planned to be installed. The first beamline is a beamline from a bending magnet. The remaining two beamlines are from insertion devices. Medical application user group of SPring-8 recommends that those beamlines should be from a wiggler and undulator. Our proposal is as follows: the first goal of the beamline is to develop a coronary cineangiographic system. Single-energy X-ray exposure with energy above K-edge of iodine (contrast medium) is proposed to reduce exposure dose. X-ray with this energy produces cineangiogram with high contrast. To reduce, furthermore, exposure dose to the patient, 37 keV monochromatic X-ray has been proposed, even though its image contrast might slightly deteriorate. A multipole wiggler should be installed in the medical beamline, mainly because we use nonsymmetric monochromator to obtain wide exposure field. Another beamline should be from an undulator. The first application of this beamline is a divergent and monochromatic X-ray source which is necessary for taking diagnostic images of human subjects. The X-ray source will be generated by fluorescent X-ray. Another application of this beamline will be development of diagnostic imaging system using a expanded X-ray by multi-layer and super mirror. Diagnostic imaging systems to be developed using both beamlines will be: 1. Monochromatic coronary angiography, 2. Monochromatic X-ray CT, based on transmitted, Compton scatter, Thomson scatter, fluorescent, and energy subtraction, 3. Microangiography, 4. Tumor detection imaging, 5. Phase-contrast X-ray imaging whose sensitivity is much higher than that of the absorption-contrast imaging, and so on.

KEY WORDS: monochromatic coronary angiography, medical beamline, middle distance beamline, large exposure field by fluorescent X-ray, exposure dose

INTRODUCTION

Three beamlines for medical use are scheduled to be installed in SPring-8. According to the primary plan, these beamlines will be from a bending magnet, wiggler and undulator. A Biomedical Imaging Center with facilities set up for the development of instrumentation dedicated to clinical examination was completed this year [1].

The Biomedical Imaging Center is located at about 200 m from a supposed wiggler, so that the width of X-ray field at a target position can be expanded to 15 cm for monochromatic coronary angiography.

The first beamline supplying an X-ray beam to this center will be from the bending magnet. This beamline will be completed in two years. The remaining two beamlines are from insertion devices which are currently under discussion. Our proposal for two beamlines including insertion devices are as follows:
1. A wiggler beamline that is dedicated to a synchrotron radiation coronary angiography (monochromatic coronary angiography), and
2. An undulator beamline that is planned to obtain a large X-ray field by applying fluorescent X-ray technique.

WIGGLER BEAMLINE-monochromatic coronary cineangiography

The monochromatic coronary angiography system in Japan is a cineangiographic system. To realize the system, the following three requirements should be satisfied:
(1) Complications caused by the conventional selective angiographic procedure should be reduced by applying monochromatic coronary angiography through intravenous or intraaortic injection.
(2) The exposure dose should be less than that of current coronary angiography.
(3) The image quality obtained by monochromatic coronary angiography should be equal to or better than that by conventional angiography [2].

To meet item (1), we will inject contrast medium through vein or through the ascending aorta, not by catheter insertion into the coronary arterial orifice.

Takeda et. al. reported a coronary angiographic image with good quality in a dog using aortographic injection [2]. This image will be superior to images obtained by venous injection of contrast medium, because none of the coronary arteries are overshadowed by the left ventricle image. To realize monochromatic coronary angiography, the following alternative systems were proposed.

Monochromatic coronary angiography using 33 keV X-ray

The photon density fulfilling item (3) at an energy of 33 keV should be 6×10^{10}/mm^2/sec at 15×15 cm^2 field. Kitamura [3] proposed wigglers under the following prerequisites.
1. Photon density is simultaneously maximized at 33 keV and minimized at 99 keV (third harmonics).
2. Homogeneity of photon density over 15×15 cm^2 area at 225 m from the insertion device should
   be satisfied.
Wiggler I in Fig. 1 shows the spectrum optimal to the prerequisites described above. Photon density at 33 keV is 3.7×10^{10}/sec/mm^2 in 1% b.w./100 mA at 225 m. Wiggler I almost meets the photon density necessary for monochromatic coronary angiography. The exposure dose is estimated to be almost the same as that by the conventional one.

Table 1 [3] summarizes photon flux and parameters of wigglers optimal to contrast agent elements taking account the prerequisites. Wiggler M in Fig. 1 generates maximum photon density at 33 keV, the third harmonics of which are not, however, restricted to be minimum.

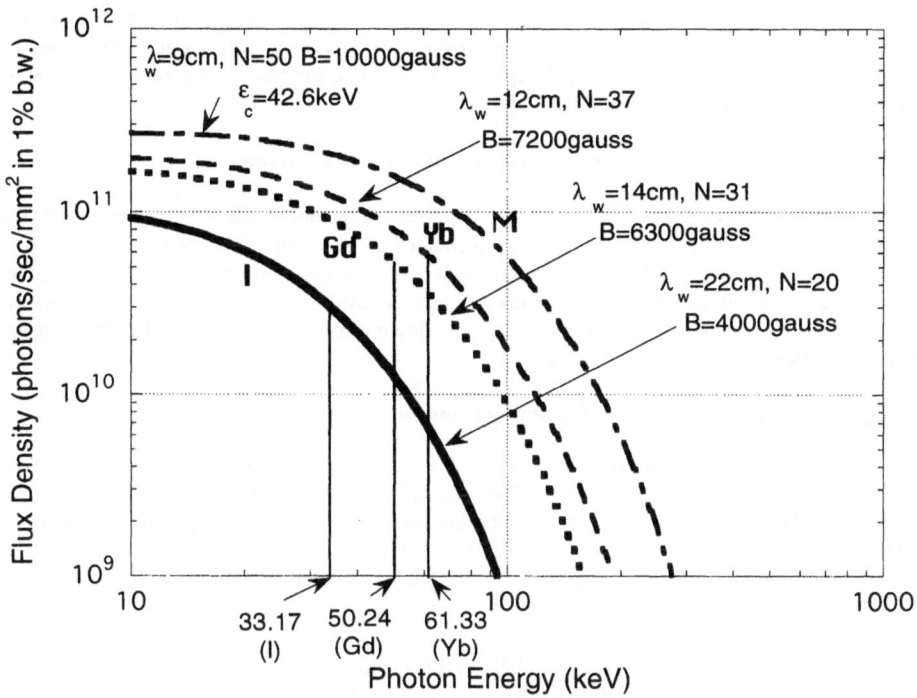

Fig. 1. Flux density of wigglers [3]
An X-ray beam is supposed to be expanded to 15 × 15 cm² at 225 m from the light source.
(Copyright 1997, Japan Society of Medical Electronics and Biological Engineering, Tokyo, reproduced
with permission)

Table 1. Wigglers optimal to elements of contrast agent and their average flux density [3]

element of contrast agent	K-absorption energy (keV)	ε_c keV	period cm	period number	magnetic field	photon flux at Kab / sec in 1% b.w.	average flux density /sec/mm² in 1% b.w.
I	33.17	17	22	20	4000	8.4×10^{14}	3.7×10^{10}
Gd	50.24	26	14	32	6200	1.2×10^{15}	5.3×10^{10}
Yb	61.33	31	12	37	7300	1.3×10^{15}	5.7×10^{10}

beam energy: 8 GeV, beam current: 100 mA, exposure field: 15×15cm². (Copyright 1997, Japan
Society of Medical Electronics and Biological Engineering, Tokyo, reproduced with permission)

Monochromatic coronary angiography using 37 keV X-ray

Since the photon density at 33 keV obtained by the wiggler I is slightly lower than that we expect,

152

exposure of X-rays at 37 keV was proposed because of the reduced attenuations in transmitting through a body, one half of the level at 33 keV. Even though image contrast at 37 keV may be slightly inferior to that at 33 keV, 37 keV exposure is practical because of the reduced exposure dose and more transmitted photons through a body.

Monochromatic coronary angiography using an undulator light source

An alternative technique to obtain 33 keV X-ray involves using undulator X-ray whose total flux curve is shown in Fig. 2. The photon density over a field of 15 × 15 cm² is estimated to be 1.3 × 10^{11}/sec/mm² in 1% b.w., assuming that beam current in the storage ring is 100 mA and that two mirrors, multilayer or supermirror [4,5], are used to expand an X-ray beam. The supermirrors are multilayers structures where the thickness of the layers down through the structure changes so that wide-band reflection occurs.

Present Opinion on Insertion Device for monochromatic coronary angiography

X-ray field expansion using a multilayer or supermirror for 33 keV or higher energy has not yet been established[5]. However, the present technique utilizing a wiggler light source and nonsym-metric reflection monochromator was applied to 4 subjects last year and confirmed to be practical [6]. Since the monochromatic coronary angiography is considered to be the first clinical application of synchrotron radiation, the wiggler insertion device should be installed for the medical beamline.

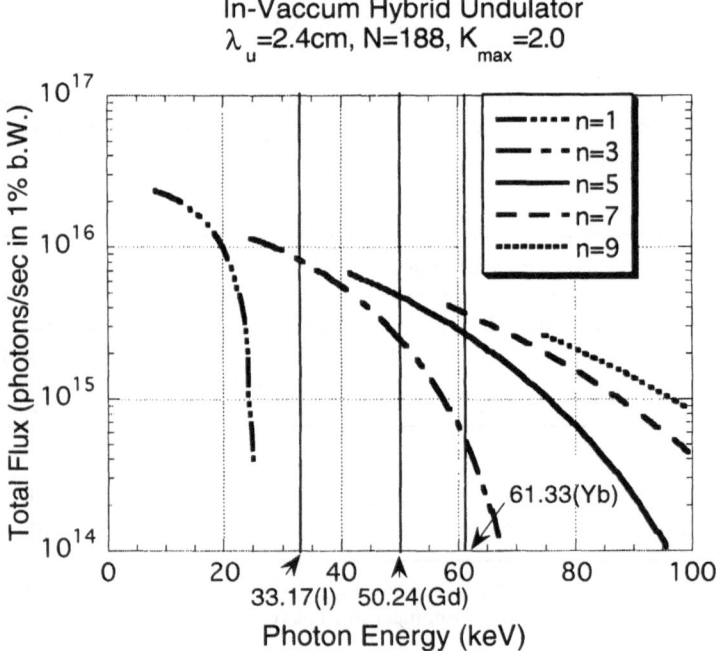

Fig. 2. Total flux of undulator U024V [3].
U024V shown in this figure is an in-vacuum hybrid undulator with parameters, λ_u=2.4 cm, N=188, K_{max}=2.0. "n" indicates a harmonic number. (Copyright 1997, Japan Society of Medical Electronics and Biological Engineering, Tokyo, reproduced with permission)

UNDULATOR BEAMLINE - large exposure field [7]

Some of medical applications using an SR light source require an exposure field larger than 30 cm wide. One possible solution to realize this is to place a long distance between the light source and an object, when using the wiggler. An alternative technique is an application of fluorescent X-ray whose light source is an undulator.

Figure 3 shows a schematic diagram of fluorescent X-ray source. Figure 4 demonstrates that a ytterbium target irradiated by an SR beam emits K_α and K_β X-ray. To attenuate K_β X-ray, a holmium filter with a K-absorption energy between K_α and K_β of ytterbium was inserted. The resulting spectrum is shown in the right side of Fig. 4. Monochromaticity greater than 99% can easily be achieved by this method.

The fluorescent photon density was estimated assuming that the undulator U024V shown in Fig. 2 was used. The total flux of the undulator when K=1.0 is shown in Fig. 5 [8]. The photon flux through the aperture of $10\,\mu$ rad$\times 10\,\mu$ rad is shown in Fig. 6. Assuming the photon flux shown in Fig. 6, the fluorescent photon density using the target elements shown in Table 2 was calculated. The beam size at 200 m (the position of Biomedical Imaging Center) from the undulator with an

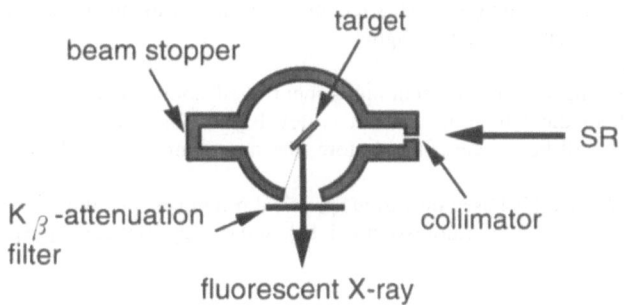

Fig. 3. Schematic diagram of fluorescent X-ray source.

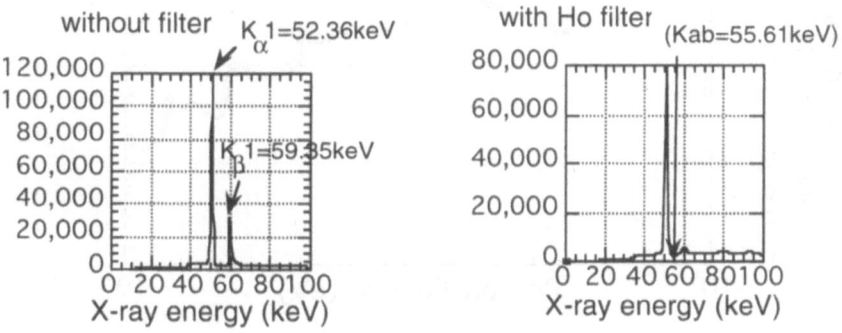

Fig. 4. Fluorescent X-ray spectrum of ytterbium target irradiated by SR beam.

left: spectrum without filter   right: spectrum with Ho filter

aperture of 10μ rad$\times 10\mu$ rad is 2×2 mm^2. Although the photon yield in Table 2 was not fully utilized because of the filter attenuation (see Fig. 4), the photon density using the fluorescent X-ray is practical for medical use.

PROPOSED DIAGNOSTIC IMAGING SYSTEM

We proposed in this paper two different monochromatic light sources, sheet-shaped and cone-shaped X-ray. The X-ray monochromatized by a single or double crystal monochromator can be selected at any energy by changing crystal angle or by replacing a crystal, in the range necessary for diagnostic imaging between 30 keV and 80 keV. The wiggler gains an advantage on this point over the undulator.

The cone-shaped (divergent) and monochromatic light source obtained by fluorescent X-ray emits at discrete energy inherent in elements. However, various elements cover practically whole energy range for diagnostic imaging. The important thing is that cone-shaped monochromatic X-ray exposes over a whole body, not at small size object by the present technique.

In the near future, multilayers and supermirrors will probably provide expanding tools of X-ray in the energy range of medical imaging. This technique promises us much more photon number at necessary X-ray energy for diagnostic imaging.

Those light sources and expansion techniques mentioned above will enable us to use various approach by which medical imaging system is developed. The imaging system closest to the clinical applications will be, as described before, the monochromatic coronary angiography [9]. Another proposals are:
1. Monochromatic X-ray CT's based on various physical principles, i.e., transmitted [10], Compton scattering, Thomson scattering, fluorescent [11,12], and energy subtracted [13],

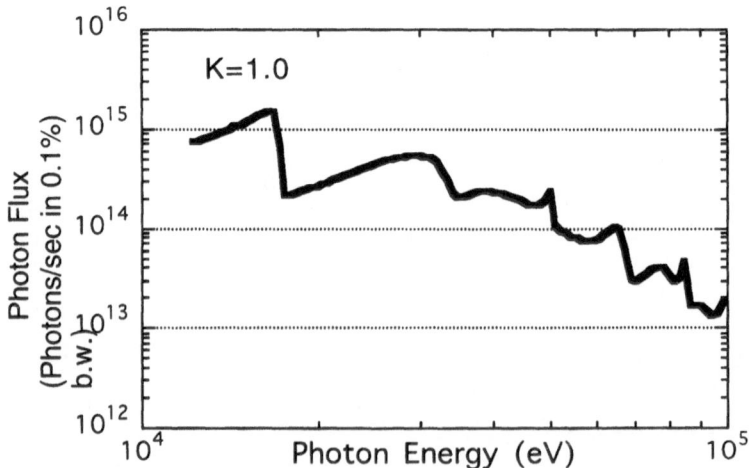

Fig. 5 Photon flux of undulator U204V (K=1.0) [7]. (Copyright 1996, Hideo Kitamura in Japan

Synchrotron Radiation Research Institute, Hyogo, reproduced with permission)

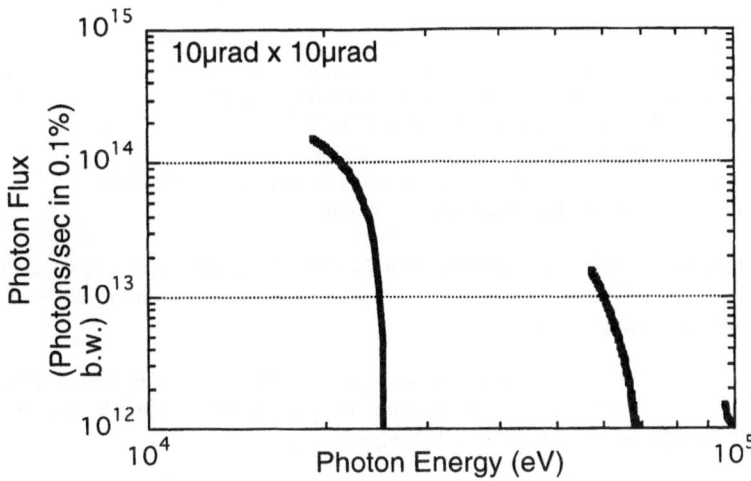

Fig. 6 Photon flux of undulator U024V with aperture of $10\,\mu\,\mathrm{rad} \times 10\,\mu\,\mathrm{rad}$

Table 2. Monochromatic X-ray source using fluorescent X-ray

target element	Ba	Ce	Sm	Ho	Yb	Au
monochromatic X-ray energy (keV)	32.2	34.7	40.1	47.5	52.4	68.8
total fluorescent X-ray (photons/sec)	1.81×10^{16}	1.57×10^{16}	1.03×10^{16}	5.35×10^{15}	4.75×10^{15}	1.40×10^{15}
fluorescent photon density at 1 m from the target (photons/s/mm^2)	2.89×10^{9}	2.50×10^{9}	1.64×10^{9}	8.52×10^{8}	7.56×10^{8}	2.22×10^{8}

SR light source: undulator U024V, aperture: $10\,\mu\,\mathrm{rad} \times 10\,\mu\,\mathrm{rad}$
Current X-ray tube: 120 kVp, 4 mm Al filter, 20 degree W target, mean photon energy = 56.5 keV, photon flux at 75 cm = 6.46×10^{6} photons/mA/s/mm^2, usual current in operating X-ray CT = 200 ~800 mA.

2. Microangiography [14,15,16],
3. Tumor detection imaging,
4. Phase-contrast X-ray imaging [17,18,19],
and so on.

Unsolved issues in the monochromatic coronary angiography are:
1. Injection site of contrast agent, venous [6,21] or aortic injection [2].
2. Energy of exposed X-ray to a subject, 33 keV or 37 keV.
3. Development of technique and procedure to reduce exposure dose.
4. Development of new contrast agents synthesized of gadolinium and ytterbium.
Those issues should be resolved through clinical applications.

The microangiography is also a new technique on the points that arteries in a heart and brain with diameter of less than 100 μm may be observed in situ and that a high definition TV camera improved angiographic image quantity.

Monochromatic X-ray CT's are expected to create new diagnostic images to detect pathological difference of tumors [22]and to assist radiation treatment planning for particle therapy informing electron density distribution in a brain and other organs.

CONCLUSION

Two insertion devices should be installed in the beamlines for the Biomedical Imaging Center.
1. One insertion device is a wiggler. X-ray with energy higher than 30 keV should be introduced to the Biomedical Imaging Center without monochromatizing to realize monochromatic coronary angiography.
2. The other insertion device is an undulator whose beam should be conveyed to the Biomedical Imaging Center to generate fluorescent X-ray by the nonmonochromatized beam with energy higher than the K-absorption energy of the target element.

REFERENCE
1. Planning Section in SPring-8 Project Team (1996) Construction of Biomedical Imaging Center in SPring-8 (Japanese), SPring-8 Information . 1(2), 12-17
2. Takeda T, Umetani K, Doi T, Echigo J, Ueki H, Ueda K, Itai Y (1997) Two-dimensional Aortographic Coronary Arteriography with Above-k-Edge Monochromatic Synchrotron Radiation. Acad Radiol 4: 438-445
3. Kitamura H (1997) Insertion Device for Medical application in SPring-8. Dedicated to Coronary Angiography(Japanese). Jpn J Med Electr & Biol Eng 11(7):4- 9
4. Joensen KD, Hoghoj P, Christensen FE, Gorenstein P, Susini J, Ziegler E, Freund AK, Wood JL (1994) Multilayered supermirror structures for hard x-ray synchrotron and astrophysics instrumentation. Proc SPIE 2011: 360-372
5. Kohmura Y, Uruga T, Kimura H, Ishikawa T (1996) Hard X-ray focusing by high-reflectivity non-planar supermirrors. In: Yokomizo H, Date S, Kashihara Y, Nishino Y, Suzuki M, Taniuchi T, Toyokawa H, Okamoto Y, Sakaue M, Tanaka G(eds) SPring-8 Annual Report 1996, Japan Synchrotron Radiation Research Institute, Hyogo, 220-221.
6. Ohtsuka S, Sugishita Y, Takeda T, Itai Y, Hyodo K, Ando M (1998) Dynamic intravenous coronary angiography using synchrotron radiation and its clinical application (Japanese). Med Imag Technol 16 in press.
7. Toyofuku F, Nishimura K, Saito T, Takeda T, Itai Y, Hyodo K, Ando M, Endo M, Naito H,

Uyama C (1995) Development of a fluorescent X-ray source for medical imaging. Rev Sci Instrum 66:1981-1983

8. Kitamura H (1996) In-vacuum hybrid undulator U024V (Japanese) In: Insertion Device Handbook '96. Japan Synchrotron Radiation Research Institute, Kamigori-cho Hyogo-ken, 206-227

9. Akisada M, hyodo K, Hasegawea S, Konishi K, Nishimura K, Maruhashi A, Toyofuku F, Suwa A, Kohra K (1986) An attempt at coronary angiography with a large size monochromatic SR beam. Nucl Instrum Meth. A246: 713-718

10. Takeda T, Itai Y, Hayashi K, Nagata Y, Yamaji H, Hyodo K (1994) High spatial resolution CT with a synchrotron radiation system. JCAT 18:98-101

11. Takeda T, Maeda T, Yuasa T, Wu J, Ito T, Kishi K, Hyodo K, Dilmanian FA, Akatsuka T, Itai Y (1997) Fluorescent scanning tomographic image with monochromatic synchrotron X-ray. Med Imag Technol 14: 183-194

12. Takeda T, Akiba M, Yuasa T, Kazama M, Hishino A, Watanabe Y, Ito T, Hyodo K, Dilmanian FA, Akatsuka T, Itai Y (1996) The fluorescent X-ray computed tomography with parallel collimator. Med Imag Technol 14: 385-386

13. Kazama M, Takeda T, Akiba M, Yuasa T, Hyodo Kazuyuki, Ando Masami, Akatsuka T, Itai Yuji (1997) Performance study of monochromatic synchrotron X-ray computed tomography using a linear array detector. Med Imag Technol 15: 615-624

14. Mori H, Hyodo K, Tobita K, Chujo M, Shiozaki Y, Sugishita Y, Ando M (1994) Visualization of penetrating transmural arteries in situ by monochromatic synchrotron radiation. Circulation 89: 863-871

15. Mori H, Hyodo K, Tanaka E, Uddin-Mohammed M, Yamakawa A, Shinozaki Y, Nakazawa H, Tanaka Y, Sekka T, Iwata Y, Handa S, Umetani K, Ueki H, Yokoyama T, Tanioka K, Kubota M, Hosaka H, Ishikawa N, Ando M (1996) Small vessel radiography in situ with monochromatic synchrotron radiation. Radiology 201:173-177

16. Takeshita S, Isshiki T, Mori H, Tanaka E, Eto K, Miyazawa Y, Tanaka A, Shinozaki Y, Hyodo K, Ando M, Kubota M, Tanioka K, Umetani K, Ochiai M, Sato T, Miyashita H (1997) Use of synchrotron radiation microangiography to assess development of small collateral arteries in a rat model of hinelimb ischemia. Circulation 95: 805-808

17. Momose A, Fukuda J (1995) Phase-contrast radiographs of nonstained rat cerebellar specimen. Med Phys 22:375-380

18. Momose A (1995) Demonstration of phase-contrast X-ray computed tomography using an X-ray interferomater. Nucl Instrum Meth A352: 622-628

20. Momose A, Takeda T, Itai Y, Hirano K (1996) Phase contrast X-ray computed tomography for observing biological soft tissues. Nature Medicine 2: 473-475

21. Ohtsuka S, Sugishita Y, Takeda T, Itai Y, Hyodo K, Ando M (1997) Dynamic intravenous coronary angiography by using synchrotron radiation and its application to measuring coronary blood flow. Jpn Circ J 61:432-440

22. Phelps ME, Hoffman EJ, Ter-pogossian MM (1975) Attenuation coefficients of various body tissues, fluids, and lesions at photon energies of 18 to 136 keV. Radiology 117: 573-583

Q: What is the field of the wiggler?

A: 0.4 Tesla for iodine, while 0.63 Tesla for gadolinium.

Q: What is the optical size of the other source, because that determines your ultimate resolution for imaging. I understand your undulator beam hits the target, which is then viewed at some angle. How much can you assess that, and how small can you make the spot?

A: The current size is 2 times 2 millimeters. If we are close to the undulator, then we can get a much smaller size.

Proposal of a New Beamline, AR-NW2, Dedicated to Medical Applications at the AR

Kazuyuki HYODO, Shigeru YAMAMOTO, and Masami ANDO

Institute of Material Structure Sciences, High Energy Accelerator Research Organization (KEK)
1-1 Oho, Tsukuba, Ibaraki 305 JAPAN

SUMMARY We propose a dedicated dual multi-pole wiggler beamline, AR-NW2, at KEK for medical applications, including clinical applications. The design goal is to built a versatile beamline, where we can choose either a single SR beam for angiography, micro-angiography or monochromatic CT etc. , or a dual SR beam for stereo-angiography and energy subtraction for lung cancer etc., as well as clinical stations, thus meeting the needs of several medical imaging techniques. We have developed a method to optimize the parameters of a MPW, and have determined the optimal parameters of a dual-MPW at AR-NW2. The method used to optimize the parameters of a MPW, the beamline layout and its performance are described in this paper.

KEY WORDS: Coronary angiography, Multi-pole wiggler, Asymmetrical reflection, Monochromatic x-ray, Dual synchrotron radiation beam

1. INTRODUCTION

We have been developing a two-dimensional imaging system for intravenous coronary angiography using synchrotron radiation (SR) [1,2]. An advantage of our system is that two-dimensional dynamic imaging of the cardiovascular system can be achieved by using the asymmetrical reflection of a crystal and a two-dimensional imaging system. The practical applicability of the system has been confirmed in animal experiments at AR-NE5A by using SR produced by a bending magnet at the accumulation ring (AR). The first human examinations of intravenous coronary angiography using the two-dimensional imaging system were performed at the AR-NE1, a multi-pole wiggler (MPW) beamline, on May 23rd and 29th in 1996 under collaboration between The University of Tsukuba and KEK [3,4]. The advantage of the two-dimensional imaging system for coronary angiography was confirmed by the examinations. It was easy to distinguish between coronary arteries and pulmonary arteries in dynamically moving images.

We needed to use SR produced by the MPW for human examinations in order to obtain a sufficient intensity of 33 keV x-ray photons, though the horizontal beam size was limited to 80 mm at the patient's position due to the vertical aperture of the beamline, NE1, which was originally designed for a magnetic Compton-scattering experiment. It was difficult to construct a large clinical station for human examinations due to the limited space of the AR experimental hall. Clinical doctors from The University of Tsukuba have strongly requested us to construct a beamline and clinical stations dedicated to human examinations[5], where they can obtain an intense monochromatic x-ray beam. There exists a 5 m-straight section at the north-west part of the AR, which is the last straight section of the AR, where we can construct a new insertion device beamline without having prepare to a new experimental hall and a large space for constructing clinical stations, where primarily the electron-positron collision experiment for the high energy physics project was planned.

We propose to construct a dual-MPW which can produce a single or dual SR beam, as well as a beamline dedicated to medical applications using the straight section. The possibility of using a dual SR beam produced by an ellipsoid MPW[6] has already been confirmed by phantom experiments [7,8]. In order to utilize several merits of two-dimensional imaging methods, source properties (geometrical and spectral) of the SR need be optimized. Although the monochromaticity and high brightness obtained by undulators may introduce new features into the two-dimensional angiography system, some other research and development (e.g. the development of a beam-expansion system comprising special mirrors or a beam-kicker system for the two-dimensional scan) are required. Here, we try to find a way to use wiggler radiation and optimize its source parameters, since a flat-shaped beam cross-section can be easily converted to a square-shaped one by a usual asymmetrically cut diffraction crystal.

2. BEAM CHARACTERISTICS REQUIRED FOR MEDICAL APPLICATIONS

The beam characteristics required in each imaging method at AR-NW2 are shown in Table 1. A large monochromatic x-ray field is needed for angiography and monochromatic x-ray imaging; on the other hand, an intense sheet beam is needed for monochromatic CT. A monochromator will be placed 15 m apart from the center of a MPW, and a clinical station for angiography, stereo-angiography and energy subtraction will be constructed at about 35 m apart from the center of the MPW, as shown in section 4.

Table 1. Beam characteristics required in each imaging system

Beam divergence (horizontal)	larger than 3.4 mrad	larger than 120 mm at 35 m apart from the center of the MPW for angiography
Beam divergence (vertical)	larger than 0.2 mrad	larger than 3 mm at 15 m apart from the center of the MPW for angiography and monochromatic CT
Intensity	larger than 2×10^{10} photons/mm^2/s at 33 keV	
Beam divergence between the dual beam	larger than 0.5 mrad	larger than 7.5 mm at 15 m apart from the center of the MPW for stereo-angiography and energy subtraction
The degree of contamination of higher harmonics from a single Si crystal	less than 1 % for 33 keV photons	

3. INSERTION DEVICE

3.1. Geometrical constraints

Since the beam shape from the wiggler is flat, in order to use it for 2-dimensional imaging the x-ray beam must be expanded by an asymmetrically cut monochromator in the vertical direction. The vertical size, $2v$, of the area is given by

$$2v = 2\,\ell_m \sigma_{y'}\, b\,, \tag{1}$$

where ℓ_m is the length between the source point and the asymmetrically cut monochromator, $\sigma_{y'}$ is the standard deviation of the angular divergence of the electron beam passing through the MPW, and b is an asymmetry factor of the monochromator for beam expansion of the x-ray beam.
A deflection parameter of the wiggler, K, which is defined by

$$K = 0.934\, B_0(\text{T})\, \lambda_u(\text{cm})\,, \tag{2}$$

is determined by the length of the beamline, ℓ, and the required width, $2h$, of the area to be illuminated is

$$K = \gamma\, \Psi_0 = \gamma h/\ell\,. \tag{3}$$

Here, $B_0(\text{T})$ is the peak value of the magnetic field, $\lambda_u(\text{cm})$ is the period length in the MPW, γ is the Lorentz factor of electrons, and Ψ_0 is the maximum deflection angle of the electron orbit in the MPW. If a critical energy of the wiggler radiation,

$$\varepsilon_c(\text{eV}) = 1.735 \times 10^{-4}\, \gamma^2\, B_0(\text{T})\,, \tag{4}$$

is given by other conditions, such as constraints on the spectral properties of the radiation (see next section), the basic parameters of the MPW can be completely determined through the above relations when γ is given.

3.2. Spectral properties of the MPW

The angular flux density of radiation from a MPW, with a period number of N, into the (φ, ψ) directions, which are measured from the central axis of the wiggler in the horizontal and vertical planes, respectively, is given by [9]

$$\frac{d^2N(\omega, \varphi, \psi)}{d\Omega\, d\omega/\omega} = 3.46 \times 10^6 \times 2\, N\, \gamma^2\, I(A)\, (N_{//} + N_\perp) \quad \text{(photons/sec/mrad}^2\text{/0.1\%bw)}, \tag{5}$$

where

$$N_{//} = \frac{1}{2\pi\gamma^2\sigma_{x'}\sigma_{y'}} \int_{-K}^{K} d\xi \left(\frac{\omega}{\omega_c(\xi)}\right)^2 \int_{-\infty}^{\infty} d\zeta \left(1 + \zeta^2\right)^2 K_{2/3}^2(\eta) \exp\left[-\frac{(\gamma\varphi - \xi)^2}{2\gamma^2\sigma_{x'}^2} - \frac{(\gamma\psi - \zeta)^2}{2\gamma^2\sigma_{y'}^2}\right], \tag{6}$$

$$N_\perp = \frac{1}{2\pi\gamma^2\sigma_{x'}\sigma_{y'}} \int_{-K}^{K} d\xi \left(\frac{\omega}{\omega_c(\xi)}\right)^2 \int_{-\infty}^{\infty} d\zeta\, \zeta^2 \left(1 + \zeta^2\right) K_{1/3}^2(\eta) \exp\left[-\frac{(\gamma\varphi - \xi)^2}{2\gamma^2\sigma_{x'}^2} - \frac{(\gamma\psi - \zeta)^2}{2\gamma^2\sigma_{y'}^2}\right], \tag{7}$$

with

$$\eta = \frac{\omega}{2\,\omega_c(\xi)}\left(1 + \zeta^2\right)^{3/2}, \tag{8}$$

$$\omega_c(\xi) = \omega_{c,0}\sqrt{1 - \left(\frac{\xi}{K}\right)^2}. \tag{9}$$

Here, $I(A)$ is the beam current given in Ampere, and $\omega_{c,0}$ is the critical frequency of the wiggler radiation in the case of an on-axis observation. In eqs. (6) and (7), $K_{1/3}(\eta)$ and $K_{2/3}(\eta)$ are the fractional-order Bessel functions. The exponential factors indicate the probability-distribution function of the angular divergence in the electron beam; $\sigma_{x'}$ and $\sigma_{y'}$ give the standard deviation of the distribution in the horizontal and vertical directions, respectively. In order to study the basic principles of wiggler radiation, we simply estimate the on-axis properties of the spectrum. In this case, the angular flux density, $\mathcal{D}$, is given by

$$\mathcal{D}(\omega) = \frac{d^2N(\omega, 0, 0)}{d\Omega\, d\omega/\omega}. \tag{10}$$

This equation can be further approximated as follows, instead of the angular convolution in eqs.(6) and (7):

$$\mathcal{D}(\omega) = \left[\frac{d^2N(\omega, 0, 0)}{d\Omega\, d\omega/\omega}\right]_{\text{natural}} \frac{\sigma_{p'}}{\Sigma_{y'}}, \tag{11}$$

where

$$\left[\frac{d^2N(\omega, 0, 0)}{d\Omega\, d\omega/\omega}\right]_{\text{natural}} = 3.46 \times 10^6 \times 2\, N\, \gamma^2\, I(A) \left(\frac{\omega}{\omega_c}\right)^2 K_{2/3}^2\left(\frac{\omega}{2\omega_c}\right). \tag{12}$$

The effective angular divergence of the radiation from the MPW, $\Sigma_{y'}$, is given as a convolution of the angular divergence of the electron beam passing through the wiggler, $\sigma_{y'}$, and the intrinsic angular divergence of each photon, $\sigma_{p'}$ [8],

$$\Sigma_{y'} = \sqrt{\sigma_{y'}^2 + \sigma_{p'}^2}, \tag{13}$$

where

$$\sigma_{p'} = \frac{1}{\sqrt{3}\,\gamma}\sqrt{\frac{\omega_c}{\omega}}. \tag{14}$$

3.3. Constraints based on the spectral properties

Two constraints should be considered concerning the spectral properties of the MPW. One is concerned with the intensity in terms of the angular flux density of photons having an energy of $\varepsilon_1 = \hbar\omega_1$ at the radiation($\hbar$ is Planck's constant).

The other constraint is $\mathcal{D}(\omega_3)/\mathcal{D}(\omega_1)$,which describes the degree of contamination of higher harmonics of a crystal monochromator used to separate photons having frequency ω_1 . In order to prevent contamination and to reduce $\mathcal{D}(\omega_3)/\mathcal{D}(\omega_1)$, the critical energy, ε_c , (or lower critical frequency, ω_c) must be lowered. However, a lower ε_c usually gives a lower intensity of photons having the energy at which the imaging is made. Therefore, the critical energy should be optimized so as to give a lower $\mathcal{D}(\omega_3)/\mathcal{D}(\omega_1)$ and a higher $\mathcal{D}(\omega_1)$ under the given conditions of an accelerator and a beamline including experimental facilities. Under the assumption given in the last section, the ratio can be expressed as

$$\mathcal{D}(\varepsilon_3)/\mathcal{D}(\varepsilon_1) = r(\varepsilon_c/\varepsilon_1)\, \mathcal{R}(\varepsilon_c/\varepsilon_1,\, \gamma\sigma_{y'}) \,, \tag{15}$$

where

$$r(\varepsilon_c/\varepsilon_1) = \frac{\left[\dfrac{d^2 N(\omega_3, 0, 0)}{d\Omega\, d\omega/\omega}\right]_{natural}}{\left[\dfrac{d^2 N(\omega_1, 0, 0)}{d\Omega\, d\omega/\omega}\right]_{natural}} = 9\,\frac{K_{2/3}^2\left(\dfrac{3}{2}\dfrac{\varepsilon_1}{\varepsilon_c}\right)}{K_{2/3}^2\left(\dfrac{1}{2}\dfrac{\varepsilon_1}{\varepsilon_c}\right)} \,, \tag{16}$$

$$\mathcal{R}(\varepsilon_c/\varepsilon_1,\, \gamma\sigma_{y'}) = \frac{\sigma_p(\varepsilon_3)}{\Sigma_y(\varepsilon_3)} \Bigg/ \frac{\sigma_p(\varepsilon_1)}{\Sigma_y(\varepsilon_1)} = \frac{1}{\sqrt{3}}\,\sqrt{\frac{3\,\gamma^2\,\sigma_{y'}^2 + \varepsilon_c/\varepsilon_1}{3\,\gamma^2\,\sigma_{y'}^2 + \varepsilon_c/3\,\varepsilon_1}} \,. \tag{17}$$

Both factors r and $\mathcal{R}$ are shown in Fig.1: $\mathcal{R}$ is a function of the accelerator parameter as well as the critical energy, whereas r gives $\mathcal{D}(\omega_3)/\mathcal{D}(\omega_1)$ in the case $\gamma\sigma_{y'}=0$.

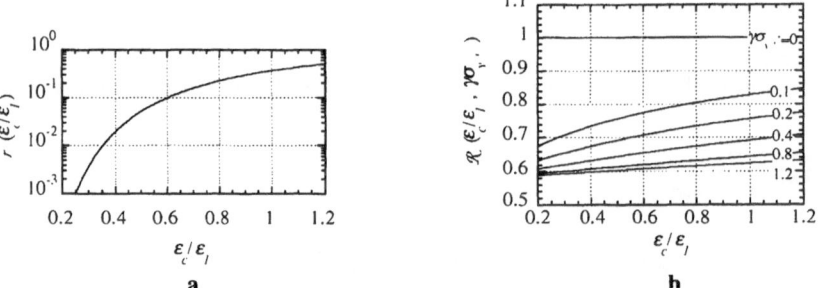

Fig.1. **a** and **b** show the relationship between $\varepsilon_c/\varepsilon_1$ and factors r and $\mathcal{R}$, respectively. The ratio $\varepsilon_c/\varepsilon_1$ should be optimized so as to give a lower $\mathcal{D}(\omega_3)/\mathcal{D}(\omega_1)$ and a higher $\mathcal{D}(\omega_1)$ under the given conditions of the accelerator and beamline.

From equation (12), the angular flux density can be rewritten as

$$\mathcal{D}(\varepsilon_c/\varepsilon_1) = \mathcal{A}(\varepsilon_c/\varepsilon_1)\, \mathcal{G}(\varepsilon_c/\varepsilon_1,\, \gamma\sigma_{y'})\, \gamma^2\,\frac{2L}{\lambda_u} \,, \tag{18}$$

where

$$\mathcal{A}(\varepsilon_c/\varepsilon_1) = 3.46 \times 10^6 \times I(\mathrm{A})\left(\frac{\varepsilon_1}{\varepsilon_c}\right)^2 K_{2/3}^2\left(\frac{\varepsilon_1}{2\,\varepsilon_c}\right) \,, \tag{19}$$

$$\mathcal{G}(\varepsilon_c/\varepsilon_1,\, \gamma\sigma_{y'}) = \frac{\sqrt{\varepsilon_c/\varepsilon_1}}{\sqrt{3\,\gamma^2\,\sigma_{y'}^2 + \varepsilon_c/\varepsilon_1}} \,. \tag{20}$$

When $\varepsilon_c/\varepsilon_1$ or ε_c is determined based on the constraint on $\mathcal{D}(\omega_3)/\mathcal{D}(\omega_1)$ we can determine the two basic parameters of the MPWs, K and λ_u by solving eqs.(2) and (4). However, we further need to think about the absolute intensity of the flux density. This causes an over-constrained condition in the determination of the wiggler parameters, which usually becomes unsolvable. If we can set the beam energy, γ, as another variable parameter, however, a new set of three parameters can be obtained through three independent constraints. The ratio of the required angular flux density, $\mathcal{D}^*\left(\varepsilon_c/\varepsilon_1\right)$, for clinical applications at $\varepsilon_c/\varepsilon_1$ to $\mathcal{g}\left(\varepsilon_c/\varepsilon_1\right)$ gives a new relation between γ and λ_u at a given length L of the MPW,

$$\frac{\mathcal{D}^*\left(\varepsilon_c/\varepsilon_1\right)}{\mathcal{g}\left(\varepsilon_c/\varepsilon_1\right)} = \gamma^2 \frac{\sqrt{\varepsilon_c/\varepsilon_1}}{\sqrt{3\,\gamma^2\,\sigma_{y'}^2 + \varepsilon_c/\varepsilon_1}} \frac{2L}{\lambda_u}, \tag{21}$$

which is useful for finding the optimal wiggler parameters when combined with eqs.(2) and (4). The function $\mathcal{g}\left(\varepsilon_c/\varepsilon_1\right)$ is shown in Fig.2. The relation between $\mathcal{D}^*\left(\varepsilon_c/\varepsilon_1\right)$ and the required areal flux density at the patient position, $\mathcal{D}_{patient}$, is written as

$$\mathcal{D}^*\left(\varepsilon_c/\varepsilon_1\right) = \ell\,\ell_m\,b\,\mathcal{D}_{patient}. \tag{22}$$

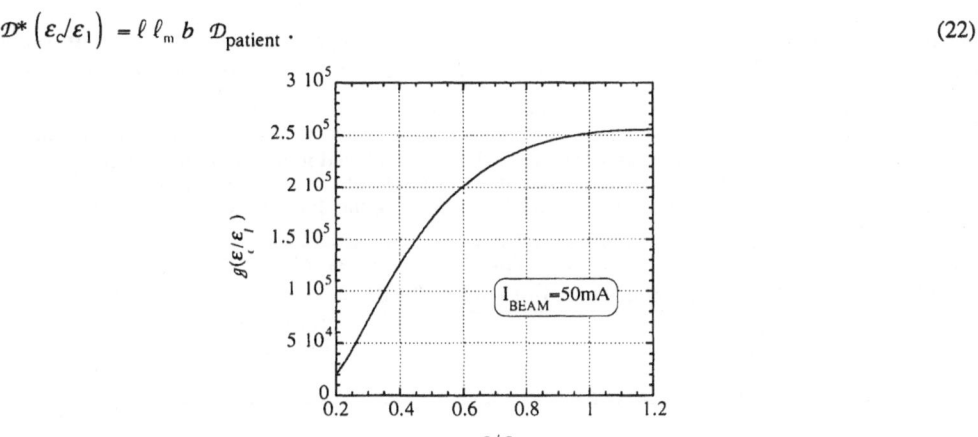

Fig.2. Relationship between $\varepsilon_c/\varepsilon_1$ and $\mathcal{g}\left(\varepsilon_c/\varepsilon_1\right)$. The function $\mathcal{g}\left(\varepsilon_c/\varepsilon_1\right)$ is useful for finding the optimal wiggler parameters when combined with eqs.(2) and (4).

3.4. Practical case in the AR

Consider the case using the AR which can be operated at 5 to 6.5 GeV for SR experiments with a 50 mA beam current. We show below a selection of the parameters of the dual MPW, which should be designed for the use of two-dimensional angiography. Since the length of beamline AR-NW2, which has been newly constructed, is 35 m, the deflection angle is given as $\Psi_0 = h/\ell = 2.1$ mrad. Similarly, the vertical beam divergence, $\sigma_{y'}$, should be 100 μrad, since the asymmetric monochromator is located the 15 m-point from the center of the MPW, and the required vertical size, $2v$, is 120 mm in this case; the asymmetry factor, b, is 40.

As shown in Fig.1, the degree of contamination of higher harmonics from a crystal monochromator, $\mathcal{D}(\omega_3)/\mathcal{D}(\omega_1)$ is well suppressed to less than 0.01 if $\varepsilon_c/\varepsilon_1$ is selected to be 0.388 with the effect of $\gamma\sigma_y$, (Fig.1b). This means that $\varepsilon_c = 12.87$ keV when iodine is used as a contrast material, where the K-edge absorption energy is 33.17 keV. The value of $\mathcal{g}\left(\varepsilon_c/\varepsilon_1\right)$ can be determined as 1.196×10^5 by using Fig.2. We can then determine the optimal values of $\lambda_u(\text{cm})$, $B_0(\text{T})$ and γ using the following three equations derived from eqs. (2), (4) and (21)' (under the assumption that $\gamma^2 \sigma_y'^2 \gg \varepsilon_c/\varepsilon_1$):

$$B_0(\text{T})\,\lambda_u(\text{cm})\Big/\gamma = \Psi\%_{0.934} = A(\text{T cm}) , \qquad (2')$$

$$\gamma^2 B_0(\text{T}) = \frac{\varepsilon_c(\text{eV})}{1.725 \times 10^{-4}} = B(\text{T}) \qquad (4')$$

and

$$\frac{\gamma}{\lambda_u(\text{cm})} = \frac{\mathcal{D}^*}{g}\frac{\sqrt{3}\,\sigma_y}{\sqrt{\varepsilon_c/\varepsilon_1}}\frac{1}{2L(\text{cm})} = C(\text{cm}^{-1}). \qquad (21')$$

$\lambda_u(\text{cm})$, $B_0(\text{T})$ and γ can be determined by using the parameters A, B and C, as shown in the following equations:

$$\lambda_u(\text{cm}) = \sqrt{\frac{B}{AC^3}} , \qquad (23)$$

$$B_0(\text{T}) = AC \qquad (24)$$

and

$$\gamma = \sqrt{\frac{B}{AC}} . \qquad (25)$$

Preliminary results are given in Table 2 for the case $\varepsilon_c = 12.87$ keV, $L = 200$ cm. If we set $\mathcal{D}^* = 8.4 \times 10^{13}$ photons/s/mrad²/0.1% bw, $\mathcal{D}_{\text{patient}}$ can be calculated as 2×10^{10} photons/s/mm² /0.5% bw using the parameters $\ell = 35$ m, $\ell_m = 15$ m and $b = 40$, and equation (22). This value agrees with the required flux density at the patient position, which is shown in Table 1. We can choose either a single SR beam or a dual SR beam if the same type two MPWs are placed in the straight section of the AR along with vertical stearing magnets to change the exit angle of the SR beam from each MPW, as shown in Fig. 3. The spectrum available at the AR-NW2 using the dual-MPW is shown in Fig. 4.

Table 2. Example of parameters of a MPW for AR-NW2 in the case of $\varepsilon_c = 12.87$ keV, $L = 200$ cm, $\mathcal{D}^* = 8.4 \times 10^{13}$ photons/s/mrad²/0.1% bw, $\ell = 35$ m, $\ell_m = 15$ m and $b = 40$.

γ	8219 (4.2 GeV)
$\lambda_u(\text{cm})$	16.8 cm
$B_0(\text{T})$	1.10 T

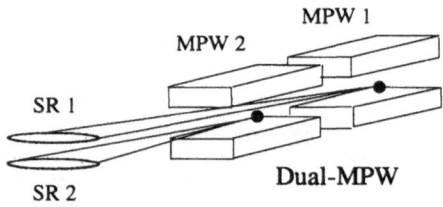

Fig. 3. Schematic diagram of a dual-MPW to produce a single or dual SR beam

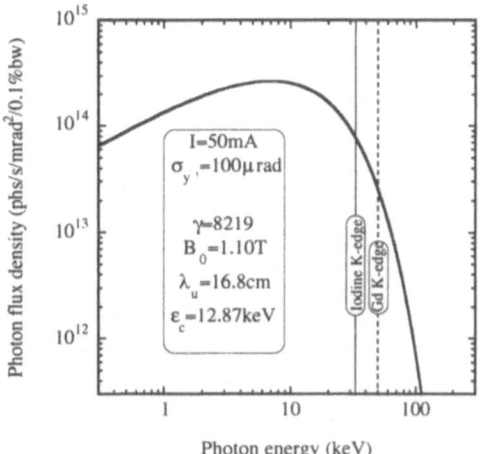

Fig. 4. Spectrum produced by a dual-MPW at the AR-NW2

4. BEAMLINE LAYOUT AND OPTICAL COMPONENTS

The arrangement of the optical components and clinical stations are shown in Figs. 5 and 6. The beamline provides a monochromatic beam and can be operated in the two modes: (1) **the A1 mode**, using station A1, which will be located on the surface level in the north experimental area in the AR 35 m apart from the center of the MPW, and (2) **the A2 mode**, using station A2, which will be located in the north experimental hall for the high-energy physics project 28 m apart from the center of the MPW. The characteristics of the monochromators and detectors for each mode are summarized in Table 3.

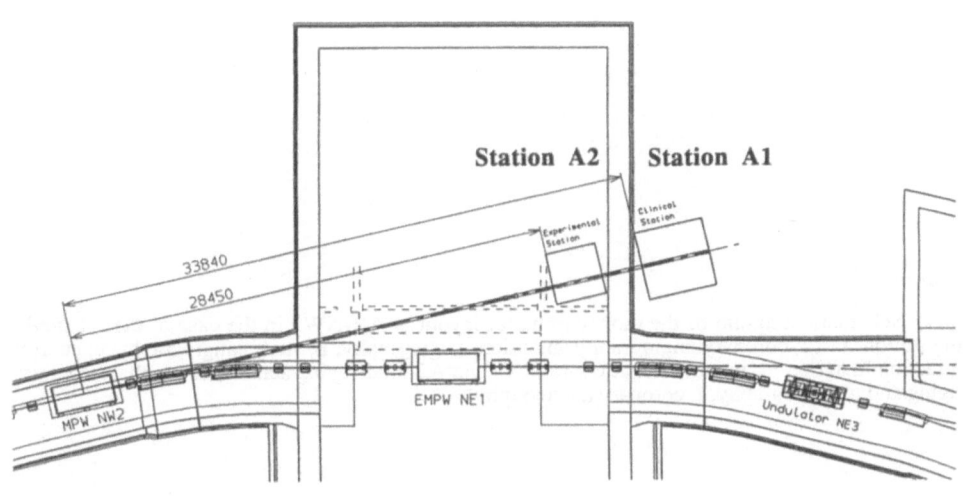

a top view

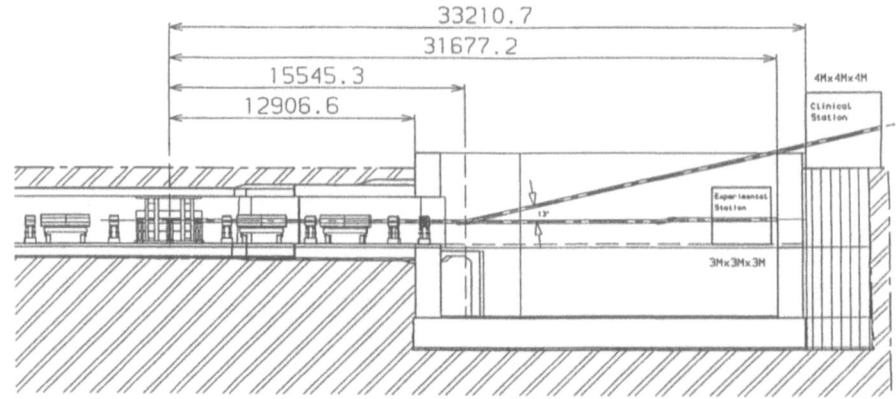

b side view

Fig. 5. Schematic diagram of beamline AR-NW2 designed by a CAD system.
a: top view, **b**: side view

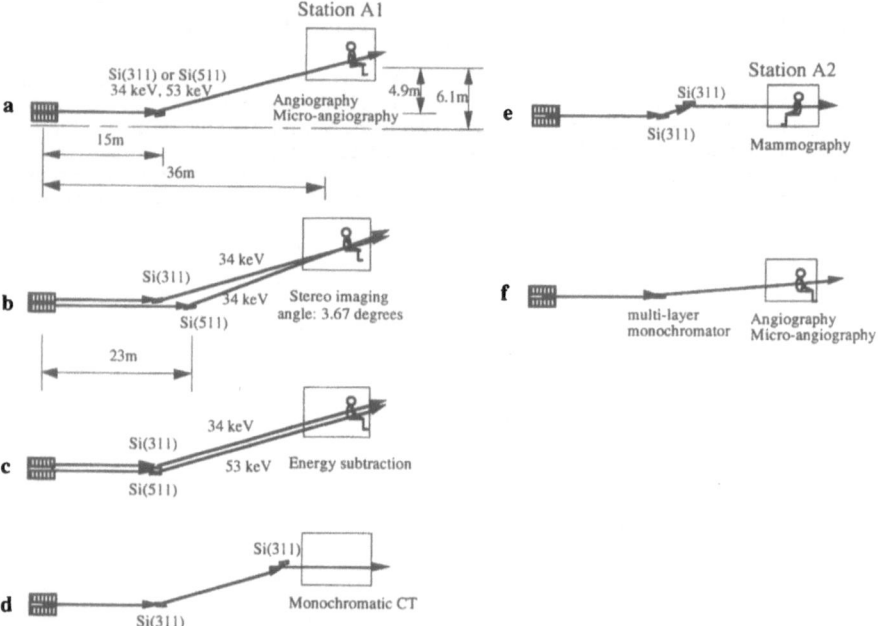

Fig.6. Schematic diagram of the monochromator layout at AR-NW2 in the case of the A1 mode using station A1 (**a**; coronary angiography and micro-angiography; **b**; stereo-angiography, **c**; energy subtraction imaging; **d**; monochromatic x-ray CT) and A2 mode using station A2 (**e**; phase contrast imaging and mammography; **f**; coronary angiography)

Table 3. Characteristics of the monochromators and detectors for medical imaging system

clinical station	imaging method	SR beam	optics	x-ray energy	detector	spatial resolution
A1	angiography	single	single crystal	33 - 55 keV	II - (CCD, HARP)TV	0.2 mm
	stereo-angiography	dual	dual crystal	33 - 40 keV	II - (CCD, HARP)TV	0.2 mm
	micro-angiography	single	single crystal	33 - 55 keV	screen - HARP TV	0.03 - 0.05 mm 0.2
	energy subtraction	dual	dual crystal	33 - 55 keV	II - (CCD, HARP)TV	mm
	monochromatic CT	single	double-crystal	25 - 60 keV	CCD, CdTe	0.5 - 1 mm
A2	fluorescent CT	single	double-crystal	25 - 60 keV	CCD, CdTe, Ge	0.5 - 1 mm
	high resolution CT	single	double-crystal	25 - 60 keV	CCD	0.001 - 0.005 mm
	phase contrast imaging	single	double-crystal	30 -100 keV	screen - HARP TV	0.03 - 0.05 mm
					II - (CCD, HARP)TV	0.2 mm
	mammography	single	double-crystal	18 - 33 keV	screen - HARP TV	0.03 - 0.05 mm
	angiography	single	multi-layer monochromator	33 - 37 keV	II - (CCD, HARP)TV	0.2 mm

II : Image Intensifier, HARP : High-gain Avalanche Rushing amorphous Photo conductor

(1) A1 mode

Two-dimensional intravenous angiography uses an asymmetrically cut single Si crystal with (311) reflecting planes for 34 keV photons above the K-edge energy of iodine or (511) reflecting planes for 52 keV photons above the K-edge energy of gadolinium, to expand the vertical SR beam size to larger than 120 mm at the patient position, as shown in Fig. 6 (a). All images will be taken above the K-edge energy of the contrast materials. These crystals will be placed 15 m apart from the center of the MPW, where the vertical beam size is 3 mm. A contrast material using gadolinium is considered to be useful for angiography examinations in order to decrease the radiation dose onto patients and also to increase the signal-to-noise ratio in an image. Since the Bragg angle for both crystals is the same, 6.5 degrees, it will be easy to change the energy of photons by exchanging the crystal without changing any other situations of the beamline. An image-intensifier (II)-TV system can be used as a two-dimensional imaging detector. We can choose a HARP (High-gain Avalanche Rushing amorphous Photo conductor)-TV camera, which is a photo-tube camera manufactured by NHK having a dynamic range of greater than 10,000, as a TV camera for an II-TV system instead of a conventional CCD-TV camera, which has a dynamic range of 500. Micro-angiography, where the spatial resolution is 30 - 50 micrometer, can be performed using a screen - HARP TV system instead of a conventional II-TV system [10,11]. Stereo-angiography uses two crystals in which the upper and lower crystals are placed so as to reflect 34 keV and 40 keV photons using the upper and lower SR beams produced by the dual-MPW, respectively, as shown in Fig. 6 (b). It will be useful to distinguishing between coronary arteries and the left ventricle or aorta in the case of intravenous coronary angiography. Energy subtraction, which uses, for example, 34 keV and 53 keV photons, will be useful for detecting small lung cancers. In this case, two crystals are used to obtain two monochromatic energy photons in the same reflecting angle, as shown in Fig. 6 (c) . The reflected beam from the lower crystal, 53 keV photons, penetrates through the upper crystal having a thickness of 1 mm, with a transmission rate of 76 %. The monochromator for monochromatic x-ray CT will be a double-Si(311) crystal, as shown in Fig. 6 (d) [12,13].

(2) A2 mode

An asymmetrically cut crystal with a large view area will be used for phase-contrast imaging and mammography, as shown in Fig. 6 (e). Because the needed photon flux density is much less than that required for angiography of a human heart, we can use a double-crystal monochromator to obtain an outgoing monochromatic x-ray beam parallel to the ground level. Fluorescent CT and high-resolution CT also require a double-crystal monochromator with as symmetrically cut crystal [14]. It will be possible to use a multi-layer monochromator for angiography in this mode using station A2, as shown in Fig. 6 (f). We have been developing a multi-layer monochromator to obtain a larger integral intensity than that of a Si crystal with a lapped surface, whose energy resolution, $\Delta E/E$, is 4.5×10^{-3}. In the case of intravenous coronary angiography using one monochromatic energy above the K-edge of the contrast material, it is not necessary to use a Si crystal to obtain monochromatic x-ray photons. The available photon flux is easily increased without increasing the ring current if a monochromator is used which can reflect photons over the range of 1 keV at 33 keV. It will be useful not only for coronary angiography, but also for many other imaging methods.

5. CONCLUSIONS

We have proposed constructing a new beamline for medical applications at the AR, especially for clinical examinations. We have demonstrated a method to optimize the parameters of a MPW; also, suitable parameters of the dual-MPW for medical applications at AR-NW2 have been determined. The beamline provides a single SR beam or a dual SR beam produced by the dual-MPW for many purposes of medical imaging.

ACKNOWLEDGMENTS

The authors would like to express their thanks to many colleagues and collaborators, such as H. Fukuma, Y. Itai, Y. Sugishita, S. Ohtsuka, T. Takeda and S. Wu, with whom they have discussed the new beamline.

REFERENCES

1. Akisada M, Ando M, Hyodo K, Hasegawa S, Konishi K, Nishimura K, Maruhashi A, Toyofuku F, Suwa A, Kohra K (1986) Nuclear Instruments and Methods. A246: 713-718
2. Hyodo K, Nishimura K, Ando M (1991) Coronary angiography project at the Photon Factory using a large monochromatic beam. In: Ebashi S, Koch M, Rubenstein E (eds) Handbook on synchrotron radiation, Vol 4. Elsevier Science Publishers B. V., Amsterdam, pp 55 - 94
3. Hyodo K, Ando M, Oku Y, Yamamoto S, Ohtsuka S, Sugishita Y, Takeda T, Itai Y, Tada J : in press in Journal of SR
4. Ohtsuka S, Sugishita Y, Takeda T, Itai Y, Tada J, Hyodo K, Ando M (1997) Intravenous coronary angiography using synchrotron radiation. Heart View 1-11:1326-1330 (in Japanese)
5. private communications with Y. Sugishita, S. Ohtsuka, Y. Itai and T. Takeda
6. Yamamoto S, Kawata H, Kitamura H, Ando M, Sakai N, Shiotani N (1989) First production of intense circularly polarized hard x rays from a novel multi-pole wiggler in an accumulation ring. Phys. Rev. Lett. 62(23): 2672-2674
7. Hyodo K, Shiwaku H, Yamamoto S, Kitamura H, Ando M (1992) A new proposal on use of the dual beam produced by an elliptic-MPW (EMPW) for angiography. Rev. Sci. Instrum. 63: 601
8. Hyodo K, Shiwaku H, Yamamoto S, Kitamura H, Ando M (1994) K-edge subtraction coronary angiography system using the dual linearly polarized synchrotron radiation beams from an elliptic multipole wiggler. In: Chance B, Deisenhofer J, Ebashi S (eds) Synchrotron radiation in the biosciences. Oxford Univ. Press, London, pp 557 - 565
9. See *e.g.* Hoffman A (1986) Theory of synchrotron radiation. SSRL ACD-note #38 , and Kim K-J (1989) Characteristics of synchrotron radiation. Proceedings of the A.I.P. conference #184: 565-632
10. Mori H, Hyodo K, Tobita K, Yamakawa A, Shinozaki Y, Tanioka K, Kubota M, Ando M (1994) Visualization of penetrating transmural arteries in situ by monochromatic synchrotron radiation. Circulation 89: 863-871
11. Mori H, Hyodo K, Tanaka E, Uddin-Mohammed M, Yamakawa A, Shinozaki Y, Nakazawa H, Tanaka Y, Sekka T, Iwata Y, Handa S, Umetani K, Ueki H, Yokoyama T, Tanioka K, Kubota M, Hosaka H, Ishiwaka N, Ando M (1996) Small-vessel radiography in situ with monochromatic synchrotron radiation. Radiology 201: 173-177
12. Nagata Y, Yamaji H, Hayasi K, Kawashima K, Hyodo K, Kawata H, Ando M (1992) High energy, high resolution monochromatic x-ray computed tomography system. Research on Nondestructive Evaluation 4: 55-78
13. Takeda T, Akatsuka T, Hyodo K, Hiranaka Y, Zeniya T, Yuasa T, Satoh M, Wu J, Ishiwaka N, Itai Y (1992) Synchrotron radiation x-ray computed tomography to detect tracer material. Medical Imaging Technology 10(3): 299-300
14. Takeda T, Ito T, Kishi K, Maeda T, Yuasa T, Wu J, Kazama M, Hyodo K, Akatsuka T, Itai Y (1994) Preliminary experiment of the fluorescent x-ray computed tomography with synchrotron radiation. Medical Imaging Technology 12(4): 537-538

C: That was comprehensive plans for medical work on the accumulator ring and I hope it can proceed. It would be nice to finally make use of the large experiment halls that were put into Accumulator Ring, but I believe never used for high energy physics. I think this is a good suggestion.

Q: Can you keep enough space within the experimental station just for emergency medical treatment or something else?

A: There is a large space near the experimental station. We hope we can construct many medical facilities around the clinical stations.

Scanning Slit Radiography System with Synchrotron Radiation

Katsuyuki Nishimura[1], Tatsuya Fujisaki[1], Kenji Tokumori[2], Fukai Toyofuku[2], Tohoru Takeda[3], Kazuyuki Hyodo[4], Masami Ando[4] and Chikao Uyama[5]

[1] Ibaraki Prefectural University of Health Sciences (IPU), Ami-cho, Inashiki-gun, Ibaraki 300-03, Japan
[2] Kyushu University, Higashi-ku, Fukuoka-shi, Fukuoka 812, Japan
[3] The University of Tsukuba, Tsukuba, Ibaraki 305,Japan
[4] High Energy Accelerator Research Organization (KEK), Tsukuba, Ibaraki 305, Japan
[5] National Cardiovascular Center Research Institute, Suita, Osaka 565, Japan

SUMMARY. From the study of performance of scanning slit X-ray radiography, the following results were obtained. (1) It is confirmed that, by choosing proper width of electronic slit on 2-dimensional detector, effect of scattered radiation can be almost removed. (2) With the narrower incident beam and the narrower electronic slit width, the more the contrast increases. (3)Stripe like artifact appearing on the case of narrow slit width can be removed by interpolation processing. (4) From the PSF (point spread function) calculated by Monte Carlo simulation, scatter rejection performance parameters were calculated.

KEY WORDS: Synchrotron radiation, Scanning slit, Scatter rejection performance parameters

INTRODUCTION

Scanning slit X-ray radiography, in which 1-dimensional synchrotron radiation field is scanned together with the electronic slit scan on 2-dimensional detector area, can make use of all photons in primary beam for image formation and provide high S / N images, compared with other X-ray imaging modalities, because of the capability of rejecting scatter rays. In this paper, the performance of scanning slit X-ray radiography combined with SR is discussed from the view points of theoretical derivation of image processing to obtain image information, and the calculation of scatter rejection performance parameters for the results of phantom experiment as well as Monte Carlo simulation.

THEORY OF IMAGE PROCESSING[1]

Let $g(x)$ be a 1-dimensional X-ray beam profile which is related to radiation dose. Then the image of an object $O(x,y)$ at each step i is expressed as

$$f_i(x,y) = O(x,y)g(x - x_i) \qquad (1)$$

If the 1-dimensional X-ray beam is scanned stepwise, the resulting image is expressed as a summation of Eq.(1) over i.

$$F(x,y) = \sum_i f_i(x,y) = O(x,y)\sum_i g(x - x_i) = O(x,y)G(x), \qquad (2)$$

where $G(x) = \sum_i g(x - x_i)$. If the step width is sufficiently smaller than the beam width, $G(x) = a$ (constant). So, the image of the object is calculated as

$$O(x, y) = \frac{F(x, y)}{a} \qquad (3)$$

If the step width is comparable to the beam width, it is obtained with the correction of spatial variance of input field as,

$$O(x, y) = \frac{F(x, y)}{G(x)} \qquad (4)$$

On the other hand, when the weighted summation by an electric slit function $h(x - x_i)$ is replaced for the summation in Eq.(2), the following equation is obtained.

$$F_h(x, y) = \sum_i h(x - x_i) f_i(x, y) = O(x, y) \sum_i g(x - x_i) h(x - x_i) \qquad (5)$$

Here, putting $G_h(x) = \sum_i g(x - x_i) h(x - x_i)$, the image of the object is obtained as

$$O(x, y) = \frac{F_h(x, y)}{G_h(x)}. \qquad (6)$$

Therefore, by choosing a proper width of the electric slit of 2-dimensional detector (namely a width of window function), the effect of scattered radiation can be eliminated using the above equation.

EXPERIMENTAL METHOD

Phantom Experiment

The imaging system was placed at the beamline NE5 of AR(Accumulation Ring) in KEK, where the synchrotron radiation from a bending magnet was supplied. The geometrical arrangement of the imaging system is shown in Fig.1. A single crystal monochromator was placed at the distance of 15.5 m from the radiation source. The 2-dimensional detector comprising I I (RTP9211G, Toshiba Co.) and TV camera (XC-77RR, Sony Co.) was placed at 3 m from the monochromator. In front of the detector a plate-like bone phantom containing the stripes of bone material with thickness of 0.5, 1.0, and 1.5 cm was placed.

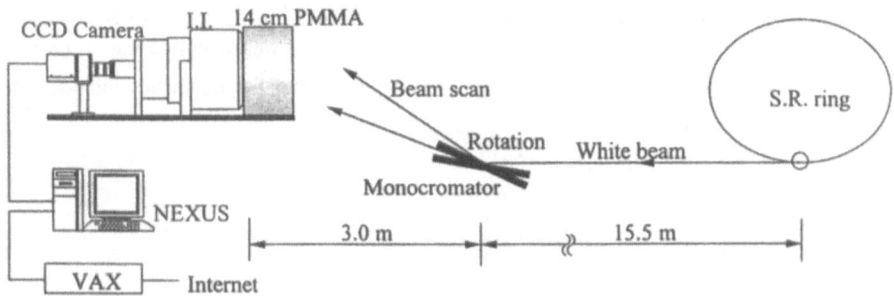

Fig.1   Geometry for the bone phantom experiment.

The scanning of SR beam is simulated by a mechanical change in angle of reflection lattice plane (311) of Si single crystal. The reflected monochromatic X-ray beam, the width of which is 8 mm, was scanned stepwise with the step width of 1.7 mm. The obtained data were transferred from a VAX computer system in KEK to an INDY computer system in IPU via Internet.   Electronic scanning slit was realized in the image processing where spatial window function was applied to the original data. The processing was done by the home-made C program as well as commercially available image processing software (DrView, Asahikasei Info. System Co.) on the INDY computer system.

Monte Carlo Simulation

Scatter rejection performance parameters were calculated by using the general purpose Monte Carlo code system, Electron Gamma Shower Code System version 4 (EGS4). Distributions of energy absorption were obtained with respect to concentric cylindrical bins, since statistic error was estimated large for the pixel-by-pixel simulation for dose distribution in fluorescent substance on 2-dimensional detector. And from these distributions, the 2-dimensional PSFs, $e_s(x, y)$ only for scattered photons and $e_t(x, y)$ for all photons including primary and scattered ones, were calculated. It was assumed that energy of primary beam was 33 keV, the object was made of polymethylmethacrylate (PMMA), and X-ray I I was open to external photons through Al window with the thickness of 0.5mm and detected these photons by fluorescent material CsI with the thickness of 141 mg/cm^2. For the EGS4 parameters, the lower limit energies of photon (PCUT) and that of electron (ECUT) were set at 10 keV and 521 keV respectively, and the step size of electron (ESTEP) was set to be 1 % of electron energy. The number of history (NCASE) was 1×10^7 history. The cross section data for the present model were calculated with the program PEGS4 (Preprocessor for EGS4).

The values of total absorption dose and scattering absorption dose are necessary for calculating scatter rejection performance parameters. These were obtained by convolving the modified beam profile function by a slit, $g(x)h(x)$, with PSF data $e_t(x, y)$ and $e_s(x, y)$. In the case of scanning slit radiography, after taking convolution between the modified beam profile and PSF, the absorption dose distributions, E_t and E_s, were obtained by scanning the convolved function. These quantities, expressing the scatter rejection performance parameters, such as scatter-to-primary ratio $(S / P)_D$, scatter transmission $(T_s)_D$, and contrast improvement factor $(K)_D$ were obtained by the following equations[3]. The suffix D means that the quantities include detector characteristics.

$$(S / P)_D = \frac{E_s(+)}{E_p(+)} \tag{7}$$

$$(T_s)_D = \frac{E_s(+)}{E_s(-)} \tag{8}$$

and

$$(K)_D = \frac{T_p}{T_t} = T_p \cdot \frac{E_t(-)}{E_t(+)}, \tag{9}$$

where s, p, t indicate scattered, primary, and total radiations, respectively. Symbols (+) and (−) mean "with" and "without" the slit. The primary transmission T_p is expressed as $E_p(-)/E_p(+)$ and the total transmission T_t as $E_t(-)/E_t(+)$.

RESULTS

Phantom Experiment

Synthesized images of bone phantom without slit and with slits for various window width are shown in Fig.2a-c. In the image (Fig.2a) which is simulating large field radiography, the contrast between the potions of bone and PMMA only is found low, leading to the necessity of eliminating scattered radiation. Although with the decreasing the window width the better improvement in sharpness was obtained, stripe artifacts appear in the image with narrow window width (Fig.2b,c). This was caused by the superposition of window function with raw data at each step along the perpendicular direction. By interpolating neighboring slit images, the artifact disappeared (Fig.2d) .

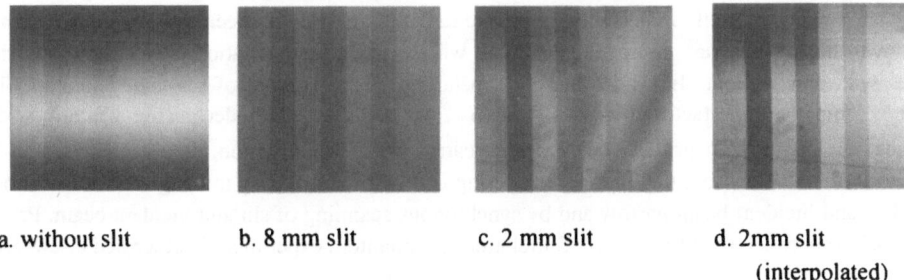

a. without slit   b. 8 mm slit   c. 2 mm slit   d. 2mm slit
(interpolated)

Fig.2   Processed images with and without window function

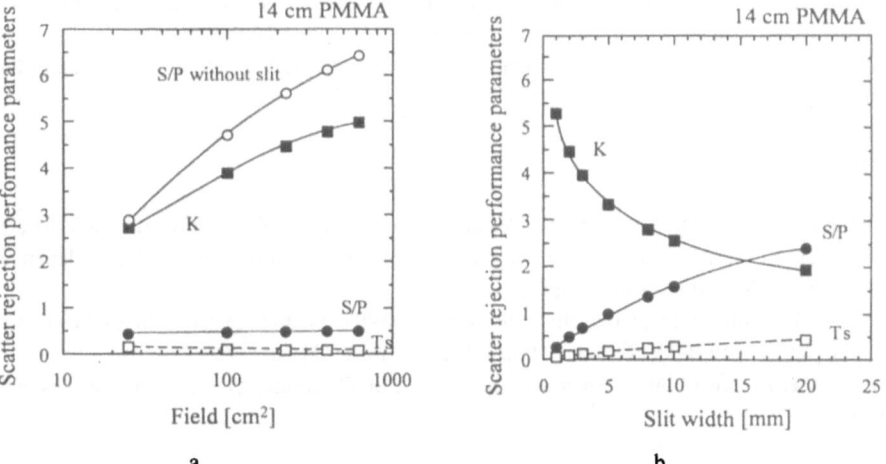

Fig.3   Scatter rejection performance parameters for the system with single slit.

Scatter rejection performance parameters

Scatter rejection performance parameters calculated for the results of Monte Carlo simulation are shown in Fig.3. Fig.3a shows them as a function of field size for the window width of 2 mm. Fig.3b shows them as a function of window width for the field of 15×15 cm^2. In Fig.3a, open circle indicates the $(S/P)_D$ in the case without window function, namely without using scatter rejection mechanism, which is suppressed in the case with window function as shown by the curve with solid circle. Contrast improvement factor becomes larger than 4 for a window width of smaller than 2 mm. This is comparable to the case of using grids with high grid-ratio. From these result it is shown that the scattered radiation can be eliminated largely with use of slit method, especially for large field.

DISCUSSION

It is confirmed from the result of the phantom experiment and the calculation of scatter rejection performance parameters that the contrast and the sharpness of the images are improved with decreasing window width and also that dynamic range increases with decreasing window width. It is shown that the contrast improvement factor, which is related to a ratio between total absorbed doses with and without slit, varies largely depending on the amount of scattered radiation. The contrast improvement factor increases and $(S/P)_D$ decreases with decreasing window width, because the contrast for primary beam, which carries image information, does not depend on the presence of slit. Therefore the effect of scattering can be minimized by making the widths of both window and incident beam narrow and by synchronous scanning of slit and incident beam. Precise comparison between the Monte Carlo Simulation and phantom experiment is described elsewhere[2].

So far the scanning slit method has been considered to be inferior to a grid method or an air-gap method because of time resolution. It will be overcome with the development of rapid SR beam scan and rapid acquisition system. In the grid method or air-gap method which has been used to remove the effect of scattering, the increase of incident photon is necessary to improve S/N, leading to the increase of radiation exposure to patients. It is expected that images with high S/N and high contrast can be obtained by scanning-slit X-ray radiography without increasing radiation exposure to patients.

REFERENCES

1. Nishimura K, Fujisaki T, Uyama C, Hyodo K, Toyofuku F, Tokumori K and Ando M (1996) SR Scanning Beam Radiography with II-TV System. Abstracts of 1st Korea-Japan Joint Meeting on Medical Physics (Seoul Korea) 23-24
2. Fujisaki T, Nishimura K, Urahashi S, and Ueda S (1997) Scatter Rejection in SR Scanning Slit Radiography with II-TV System. Jpn. J. Med. Phys. **17**[3] 161-172
3. Dinko Plenkovich (1989) Electronic Scanning-Slit Fluorography. Acta Radiol. Suppl.**373** 5-46

Accuracy of Attenuation Coefficients in Monochromatic X-ray CT

Kenji Tokumori[1], Fukai Toyofuku[2], Shigenobu Kanda[1], Katsuyuki Nishimura[3], Kazuyuki Hyodo[4], Masami Ando[4], and Chikao Uyama[5]

[1] Department of Oral and Maxillofacial Radiology, Kyushu University 3-1-1 Maidashi, Higashi-ku, Fukuoka, 812-82 Japan
[2] Department of Radiological Technology, Kyushu University School of Health Sciences, 3-1-1 Maidashi, Higashi-ku, Fukuoka, 812-82 Japan
[3] Department of Radiological Sciences, Ibaraki Prefectural University of Health Sciences, Ami 4669-2, Ami-machi, Inashiki-gun, Ibaraki, 300-3 Japan
[4] Institute of Material Structure Science, High Energy Accelerator Research Organization, 1-1, Oho, Tsukuba-shi, Ibaraki, 305 Japan
[5] Department of Radiology, National Cardiovascular Center, Fujishirodai-5, Suita-shi, Osaka, 565 Japan

SUMMARY. We have developed a monochromatic x-ray CT system which consists of a fluorescent x-ray source generated by synchrotron radiation, a CdTe array detector a rotating table and a computer system. We performed phantom experiments at NE5 station (KEK, Japan) and compared the experimentally obtained CT values with the theoretically calculated values. The measured and theoretically calculated CT values (linear attenuation coefficients) were within 6 % agreement over a wide range of iodine concentrations.

KEY WORDS: Fluorescent x-ray, Synchrotron radiation, CT, CdTe array detector

INTRODUCTION

A monochromatic x-ray CT system has several advantages [1-4].
1) There is no beam hardening effect.
2) The CT value shows a linear attenuation coefficient.
3) Subtraction images can be obtained using dual monochromatic energy x-rays.
Especially, 1) and 2) give important clinical diagnostic information in the head and neck regions. Our final purpose is a development of a monochromatic x-ray 3D CT system which can be used for the clinically diagnosis. In such clinical systems, it must have a large radiation field. Therefore, we have applied a fluorescent x-ray source.

Using fluorescent x-rays generated by synchrotron radiation, we have produced medical images of phantoms[5] . A fluorescent x-ray source can generate monochromatic x-rays which range from about 20 keV to 70 keV by irradiating several target materials with a white X-ray beam. We have developed a monochromatic x-ray CT system using this source, and investigated a useful technique for clinical diagnosis . The purpose of this study is to evaluate the accuracy of CT values of the monochromatic x-ray CT system developed here.
We performed phantom experiments and compared the experimentally obtained CT values with the theoretically calculated values.

MATERIALS AND METHODS

The system consists of a fluorescent x-ray source, a rotating table, a CdTe array detector (Matsushita Industrial Equipment Co., Japan) and a computer system (Macintosh Quadra 650, Apple Computer, Japan) (Fig. 1). Measurements were taken using synchrotron radiation at NE5 station (AR (6.5GeV), KEK, Tsukuba, Japan) (Fig. 2). Several phantoms which contain iodine contrast media of different concentrations were measured.

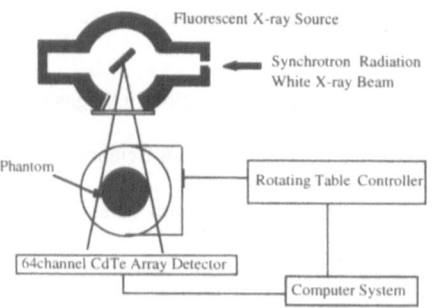

Fig. 1. Schematic diagram of the CT system

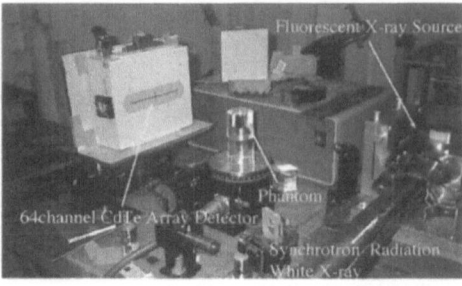

Fig. 2. Photograph of the CT system

Fluorescent x-ray source

The fluorescent x-ray generated by irradiating the target material offered a large beam size due to its divergent characteristic . It was possible to obtain a two dimensional projection image [6]. However, in this study, we used a fan beam fluorescent x-ray. In this experiment, we used the fluorescent x-rays from a gadolinium (Gd) target ($K_{\alpha 1}$=43.0keV). A Samarium (Sm) foil filter was used to attenuate the K_{β} x-ray preferentially.

CdTe array detector

The CdTe array detector has 64 detector elements. The size of each detector element is 2mm(w) x 2mm(h). Each element has two discriminators (upper discriminator and lower discriminator) and two 16-bit counters (upper counter and lower counter). Each discriminator rejects pulses smaller than the chosen energy limits. All pulses in between the upper and lower energy limits were obtained by subtracting the upper counter value from the lower counter value. By changing the energy limits, we can get an incident x-ray spectrum.

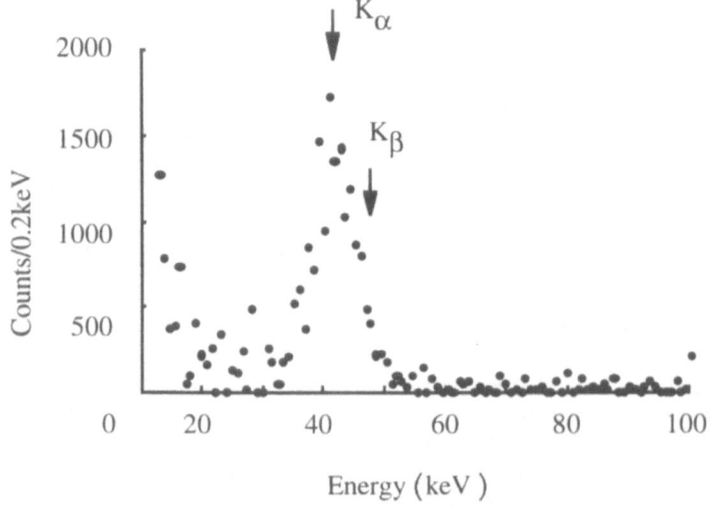

Fig. 3. Energy spectrum of the fluorescent x-rays from the Gd target ($K_{\alpha 1}$=43.0keV) with the Sm foil filter measured by using a CdTe array detector

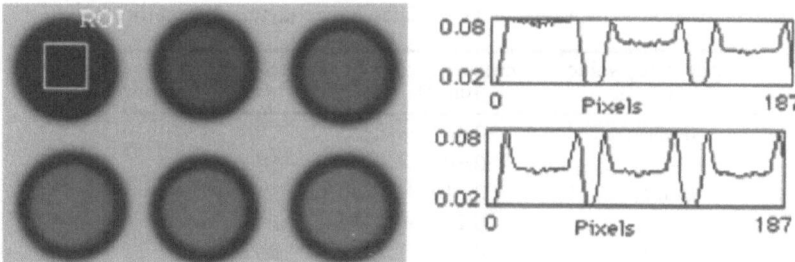

Fig. 4. CT images and profiles of the phantoms with different iodine concentrations

Computer system

The CdTe array detector and the rotating table are controlled by the computer system. Photon counting data measured by the CdTe array detector were stored in the computer system, and the rotating table was then rotated by 3 degrees and the process repeated. After 120 scans, the CT images were obtained by using the filtered-backprojection algorithm. All programs were written in C language (Symantec C++, Symantec Co., USA).

Phantoms

We used nine cylindrical phantoms with 20mm diameter. One of the phantoms was filled with water, and the others filled with iodine contrast media with different concentrations.

RESULTS

An energy spectrum of the fluorescent x-rays from the Gd target ($K_{\alpha 1}$=43.0keV) with the Sm foil filter was measured by using a CdTe array detector (Fig. 3). The energy resolution of this CdTe detector is about 12keV FWHM. Because of this poor energy resolution, it is impossible to

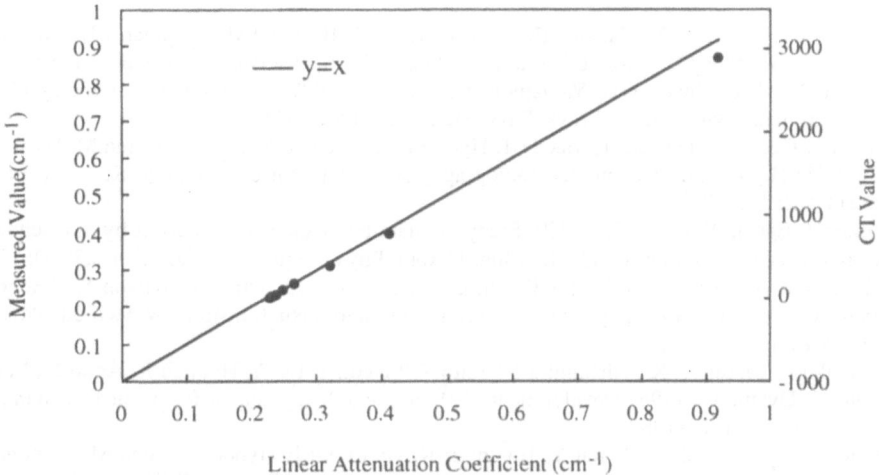

Fig. 5. Measured and calculated linear attenuation coefficients relationship

Table 1. Comparison of measured and calculated linear attenuation coefficients

calculated value (cm^{-1})	measured value (cm^{-1})	relative error (%)
0.920	0.869	5.96
0.412	0.395	4.33
0.321	0.310	3.43
0.266	0.262	1.57
0.248	0.243	1.93
0.239	0.233	2.69
0.234	0.228	2.37
0.232	0.220	2.28
0.230	0.223	3.28

separate the K_β from K_α. We also measured the same fluorescent x-rays using a HPGe detector system and found that the ratio of K_α to the total (K_α and K_β) K x-ray photons was about 98%. The lower and upper discriminator limits were 20keV and 57keV respectively.

Using this system, We obtained eight CT images of phantoms that had different iodine concentrations (Fig. 4) and one CT image of phantom that filed with water. The mean CT values were obtained by averaging over the ROI (23x23pixels), and they were compared with the theoretical values (linear attenuation coefficients) (Fig. 5, Table 1).

CONCLUSION

The measured and theoretically calculated CT values (linear attenuation coefficients) were within 6 % agreement over a wide range of iodine concentrations. All the measured CT values were smaller than the theoretically calculated values, however, that may be attributed to the effect of scattering radiations.

REFERENCES

1. Dilmanian FA, Wu XY., Parsons EC, Ren B, Kress J, Button TM, Chapman LD, Coderre JA, Giron F, Greenberg D, Krus DJ, Liang Z, Marcovici S, Petersen MJ, Roque CT, Shleifer M, Slatkin DN, Thomlinson WC, Yamamoto K, Zhong Z (1997) Single- and dual-energy CT with monochromatic synchrotron X-rays. Phys. Med. Biol. 42(2): 371-87
2. Itai Y, Takeda T, Akatsuka T, Maeda T, Hyodo K, Uchida A, Yuasa T, Kazama M, Wu J, Ando M (1995) High contrast computed tomography with synchrotron radiation. Rev. Sci. Instrum. 66(2) PT. 2: 1385-7
3. Hirano T, Eguchi S, Usami K, (1989) Study of quantitative elemental analysis by monochromatic X-ray CT using synchrotron radiation. Jpn. J. Appl. Phys. Regul. Pap. Short Notes,28(1): 135-9
4. Thompson AC, Llacer J, Campbell Finman L, Hughes EB, Otis JN, Wilson S, Zeman HD, (1984) Computed tomography using synchrotron radiation. Nucl. Instrum. & Methods Phys. Res. Sect. A,222(1-2): 319-23
5. Toyofuku F, Tokumori K, Nishimura K, Saito T, Takeda T, Itai Y, Hyoudo K, Ando M, Endo M, Naito H, Uyama C (1995) Development of fluorescent X-ray source for medical imaging, Rev. Sci. Inst. 66(2): 1981-1983
6. Saito T, Kudo H, Takeda T, Itai Y, Tokumori K, Toyofuku F, Hyodo K, Ando M, Nishimura K, Uyama C (1995) Three-dimensional monochromatic X-ray CT. Proc. SPIE - Int. Soc. Opt. Eng. 2564: 548-57

Reconstruction Algorithm for Fluorescent X-Ray CT and Its Application to the Actual Data by Synchrotron X-Ray

Tetsuya Yuasa[1], Tohoru Takeda[2], F. Avraham Dilmanian[3], Kazuyuki Hyodo[4], Takao Akatsuka[1], and Yuji Itai[2]

[1]Faculty of Engineering,Yamagata University, Yonezawa, Yamagata, 992 JAPAN
[2]Institute of Clinical Medicine, University of Tsukuba, Tsukuba, Ibaraki, 305 JAPAN
[3]Medical Department, Brookhaven National Laboratory, Upton, NY, 11973 USA
[4]Photon Factory, National Laboratory for High Energy Physics, Tsukuba, Ibaraki, 305 JAPAN

SUMMARY. We describe a new attenuation correction method for fluorescent x-ray computed tomography (FXCT) applied to image nonradioactive contrast materials *in vivo*. The principle of the FXCT imaging is that of computed tomography of the first generation. In order to detect smaller iodine concentrations, attenuation correction is needed, because we can not observe net fluorescent x-rays radiating from contrast materials without attenuation within an object. We present a correction method based on the measurement process. The derivative equation system is solved by the least squares method using the singular value decomposition. The attenuation correction method is applied to the projections obtained from the experiment using the synchrotron radiation to confirm its effectiveness.

KEY WORDS: fluorescent x-ray, computed tomography, singular value decomposition, least squares method, synchrotron radiation

INTRODUCTION

Fluorescent x-ray analysis method has been used in tracer element detection studies, with sensitivities reaching one picogram per gram of certain elements [1]. However, these measurements require a thin sample and, therefore are limited to measurements near the surface. Fluorescent x-ray tomography employing an x-ray tube has been used to study iodine in samples of several mm in diameter [2], while x-ray fluorescence microtomography employing synchrotron radiation has been used in studies of Fe and Ti in 8mm samples, and in detection of iron in a bee head [3].

We used monochromatic x-rays produced by a synchrotron radiation (SR) source. Advantages of such a source over an x-ray tube are: 1) high brilliance, 2) broad continuous spectrum and 3) small beam divergence. Another advantageous property of SR for FXCT is its linear polarization. The polarized nature of SR allows reducing the spectral background originating from Compton scattering in the plane of the storage ring by positioning the detector at 90 degrees to beam in the plane of the polarization. For these reasons, SR-FXCT has higher sensitivity compared to conventional fluorescent analysis with an x-ray tube beam. We could delineate a 4-mm-in-diameter channel filled with 500μgI/ml contrast material in an acrylic rounded phantom which size is 20mm in diameter without attenuation correction [4-6]. However, in order to analyze contrast materials quantitatively at smaller concentration inside larger objects, attenuation correction is indispensable.

The attenuation correction method in this paper is an extension of the algebraic reconstruction technique (ART) used in the early days of x-ray transmission CT. The merits of this method are as follows:
1) objects with inhomogeneous distributions of attenuation coefficients for incident and fluorescent x-rays can be treated,
2) statistical fluctuation of the measured count can be considered, and
3) error analysis of results based on the statistical method can be performed.

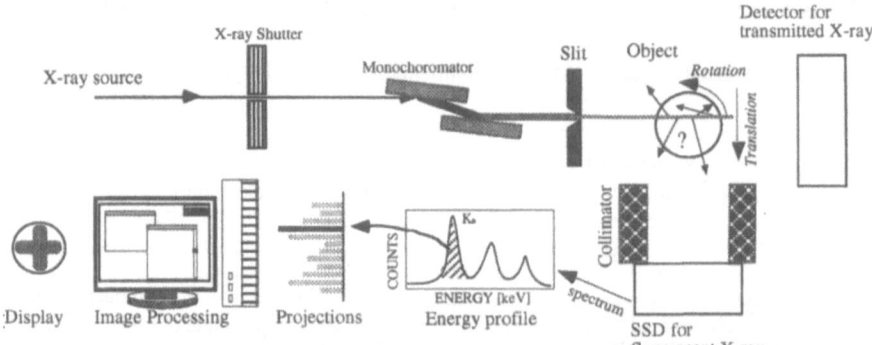

Fig. 1. Schematic diagram of SR-FXCT

EXPERIMENTAL SETUP OF SR-FXCT

The schematic diagram of a typical SR-FXCT system is shown in Fig. 1. White x-ray beam from a source is monochromatized using a monochromator. It is collimated into a pencil beam using a slit before it impinges on the object. Fluorescent x-ray is emitted isotropically by the de-exciting contrast atoms along the line of the incident beam, with an intensity proportional to the product of the iodine concentration in the incident beam and the incident x-ray flux. It is detected in a solid state detector operating in a photon-counting mode. The detector is collimated to reduce the amount of stray radiation being detected. The net counts in the characteristic x-ray fluorescent spectral lines at each projection point constitute the CT projections. The detector is positioned perpendicular to the incident beam for reducing Compton scattering background in the spectrum. The energy of the incident beam is carefully tuned so that the fluorescent spectral line does not overlap with the Compton scatter peak. Projections are acquired at constant angular steps using a translation-rotation motion of the object over 180 degrees.

ATTENUATION CORRECTION AND IMAGE RECONSTRUCTION METHOD

The object is assumed to be 2- dimensional. Three matrices, d_j, μ^I_j and μ^F_j ($j=1, 2, \cdots, N$) fixed to the object (Fig. 2) are prepared, where j ($j=1, 2, \cdots, N$) is the index identifying the pixel, and d_j, μ^I_j and μ^F_j are the tracer-element concentration to be estimated, the linear attenuation coefficient at the energy of the incident x-ray, and that of the fluorescent x-ray, respectively. Note that μ^I_j and μ^F_j are known from the transmission CT image. Also, let us number each incident x-ray S_i with the index i that runs from 1 to M. M is the number of projection data. S_i is then the set consisting of the indices identifying pixels which are intersected by the ith ray (Fig. 3). Taking note of the jth pixel being struck by beam S_i, let us follow the process as follows:
Step 1) The incident x-ray is attenuated by the shaded pixels in Fig. 4. Here, S_{ij} is defined as the set of the indices denoting these pixels, which is apparently the subset of the set S_i. Defining the length of the line

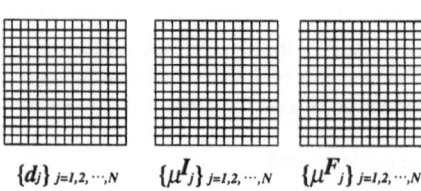

$\{d_j\}_{j=1,2,\cdots,N}$ $\{\mu^I_j\}_{j=1,2,\cdots,N}$ $\{\mu^F_j\}_{j=1,2,\cdots,N}$

Fig. 2. Three matrices prepared for FXCT reconstruction.

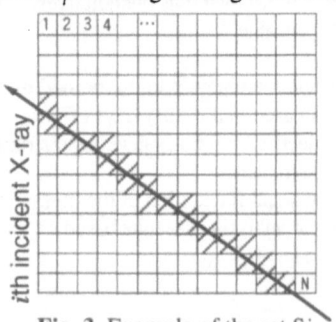

Fig. 3. Example of the set Si.

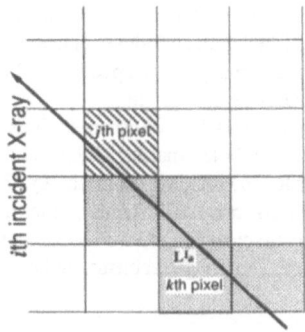

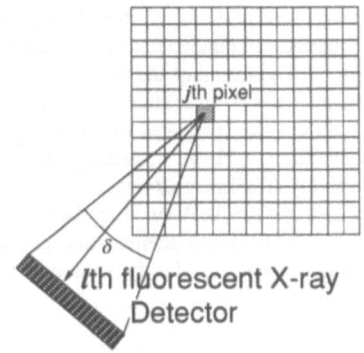

Fig. 4. Example of the set S_{ij}.　　　　　　**Fig. 5.** Definition of the angle δ.

segment such that the ith x-ray is intersected with the kth pixel ($k \in S_{ij}$) as L^I_{ik}, the incident x-ray flux in front of the ith pixel is written as $f_{ij} = I_o \exp(-\Sigma_{k \in S_{ij}} \mu^I_k L^I_{ik})$.

Step 2) The fluorescent x-ray is radiated isotropically, whose absorbed flux is in proportion to the product of the flux of the x-ray entering the jth pixel and concerning this phenomenon $\omega \mu_{ph} f_{ij} L^I_{ij}$, and the iodine concentration d_j. Let us define the angle at which the jth pixel is viewed by the detector as δ (Fig. 5). The x-ray absorbed flux is $\omega \mu_{ph} (\delta/2\pi) f_{ij} d_j L^I_{ij}$.

Step 3) We consider the attenuation process up to the detector. For a predefined integer, K, let $\Delta\delta = \delta / K$. Here, the fan-shaped fluorescent x-ray is approximated by K individual x-rays. We define the index identifying the angle of the fluorescent x-rays as l ($1 \leq l \leq K$). Considering the jth pixel ($j \in S_j$) and the lth fluorescent x-ray, we consider the attenuation of the lth ray from the jth pixel to the detector (Fig. 6). Let T_{ijl} be a set of indices consisting of the pixels which are intersected with the lth fluorescent x-ray. These pixels denoted as the shaded pixels in Fig. 6, attenuate the lth fluorescence x-ray before they reach the detector. Let L^F_{ijm} be the length of the line segment such that the lth ray is intersected

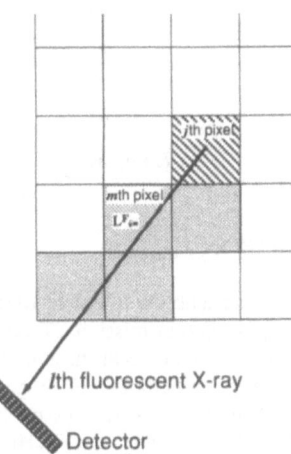

Fig. 6. Example of the set T_{ijl}.

with the mth pixel ($m \in T_{ijl}$). The lth ray is subject to the attenuation by $\exp(-\Sigma_{m \in Tijl} \mu^F_m L^F_{ijm})$. Hence, the x-ray flux reaching the detector from the jth pixel is $g_{ij} = \omega \mu_{ph} (\Delta\delta/2\pi) \Sigma^K_{l=1} \exp(-\Sigma_{m \in Tijl} \mu^F_m L^F_{ijm})$. Accordingly, the x-ray photons measured for the ith ray $I_i = \Sigma_{j \in Si} f_{ij} g_{ij} L^I_{ij} d_j = \Sigma_{j \in Si} h_{ij} d_j (i = 1, 2, ..., M)$, where $h_{ij} = f_{ij} g_{ij} L^I_{ij}$. The matrix representation is: $I = H d$, where $H = (h_{ij}) (i = 1, 2, ..., M, j = 1, 2, ..., N)$, $I = (I_i) (i = 1, 2, ..., M)$, and $d = (d_j) (j = 1, 2, ..., N)$. The algebraic equation system is solved using the least squares method with the singular value decomposition [7].

EXPERIMENTAL RESULTS

The experiment was carried out at the bending magnet beam line of BLNE-5A of the Tristan Accumulation Ring (6.5GeV, 10-30mA) in Tsukuba, Japan. The incident beam energy was tuned to 33.4keV to image iodine (K-edge of 33.17keV). The measured photon flux in front of the object was approximately 7×10^7 photons mm^{-2}s^{-1} for a storage-ring current of 30mA. The incident monochromatic x-ray beam was a fixed horizontal pencil beam, collimated to 1mm (horizontal)×2mm (vertical) size using a tantalum slit. For the detection, emitted fluorescent x-ray was collimated with a long, cylindrical, slit-like collimator of 1/4 diameter-to-length ratio (25×100mm^2). The distance between the sensor and the object was 250mm. The HPGe detector was positioned in the horizontal plane perpendicular to the beam. The acrylic rounded phantom was 20mm in diameter and included a cross-shaped axial channel filled with an iodine contrast material at 200µgI/ml (Fig. 7). The scanning and the rotation steps were 1mm and 5 degrees, respectively. Projections were generated from the K_α line, after subtracting the multiple scattering background.

Three 22×22 matrices were prepared, one for the reconstructed image, and the two others for linear attenuation coefficients. Each pixel size was 1mm×1mm. H, I and d were a 792×484 matrix, a 792×1 and a 484×1 vectors, respectively. The linear attenuation coefficients of water for the incident beam energy (33.4keV) and the fluorescent one (28.3keV) were, respecively, set to 0.0316mm^{-1} and 0.03851mm^{-1}. Since the iodine solution is diluted and the linear attenuation coefficients of acrylic are close to those of water, we regarded the object as homogeneous for the attenuation part of the program. The image reconstructed by our algorithm is shown in Fig. 8.

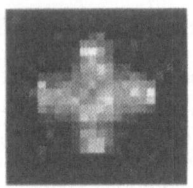

Fig. 7. Physical phantom.　　　　　**Fig. 8.** SR-FXCT image.

CONCLUSION

The method's capability to image 10 µg/ml amounts of iodine in the subject is 1-2 orders of magnitude better than that in transmission CT, and gives the method the potential of becoming usable for functional imaging of such organs as the heart or the brain at a sub-millimeter spatial resolution. The nuclear-medicine funtional imaging methods, i.e., Single Photon Emission Computed Tomography (SPECT) and Positron Emission Tomography (PET), do not have such a good resolution (typical spatial resolutions for SPECT and PET are 8 mm and 4.5 mm FWHM, respectively). Realization of FXCT could, therefore, contribute to the basic and clinical research in radiology.

REFERENCES

1. Iida A, Gohshi Y (1991) Tracer element analysis by x-ray fluorescent. In: Handbook on Synchrotron Radiation, Vol.4, Ebashi S, Koch M, Rubensein E (eds) North-Holland, Elsevier Publisher, Amsterdam, pp 307-348
2. Cesareo R, Mascarenhas S (1989) A new tomographic device based on the detection of fluorescent x-rays. Nucl. Instr. Meth., A277: 669-672
3. Boisseau P, Grodzins L (1987) Fluorescence tomography using synchrotron radiation. Hyperfine Interactions 33: 283-292
4. Takeda T, Maeda T, Yuasa T, Akatsuka T, Ito K, Kishi K, Kazama M, Hyodo K, Itai Y (1995) Fluorescent scanning x-ray tomography with synchrotron radiation. Rev. Sci. Instrum. 66(2): 1471-1473
5. Takeda T, Maeda T, Yuasa T, Wu J, Ito T, Kishi K, Hyodo K, Dilmanian FA, Akatsuka T, Itai Y (1996) Fluorescent scanning x-ray tomographic image with monochromatic synchrotron x-ray. Medical Imaging Technology 14-2:183-194
6. Takeda T, Akiba M, Yuasa T, Kazama M, Hoshino A, Watanabe Y, Hyodo K, Dilmanian FA, Akatsuka T, Itai Y (1996) Fluorescent X-Ray Computed Tomography with Synchrotron Radiation Using Fan Collimator. SPIE Vol. 2708: 685-695
7. Yuasa T, Akiba M, Takeda T, Kazama M, Hoshino A, Watanabe Y, Hyodo K, Dilmanian FA, Akatsuka T, Itai Y (1997) Reconstruction Method for Fluorescent X-Ray Computed Tomography by Least Squares Method Using Singular Value Decomposition. *IEEE Trans. on Nucl. Sci.* 44-1: 54-62

Closing Remark

Junnichi Chikawa
Centre for Advanced Science and Technology Harima Science Park City,
Kanaji, Kamigori-cho, Ako-gun, Hyogo-ken, 678-1201, JAPAN

In his talk, Dr.Yamasaki showed x-ray photographs of a patient's lung, one taken 30 years ago and one recently, which brings us to the conclusion that there has been no significant progress in x-ray imaging technology employed in hospitals. This fact may suggest that economical compact SR sources should be developed urgently for use in hospitals in order to materialize the practical use of various new methods of using synchrotron radiation, such as coronary angiography and bronchography with energy subtraction, fluorescent x-ray CT, and multiple-energy computed tomography using monochromatic beams.

Progress of these imaging methods and some small medical SR sources were reported in the conference. Another important outcome of the conference is the advent of new imaging techniques by phase contrast and refraction contrast. In fact, x-ray imaging made by absorption contrast has been used for the past one hundred years, ever since the discovery of x-ray by Roentgen in 1895. We are now facing a new pattern of x-ray imaging which is essentially different from absorption contrast.

The new methods are based on image contrast due to the differences of refractive index distributed within an object. The refractive index for x-rays deviates very slightly less than one. In principle, this is proportional to the density of materials. The phase contrast is due to the phase shift of x-rays passing through an object using a Bonse-Hart monolithic interferometer; the phase shift is converted to intensity variations by interference with the reference beam. The observed images are formed by density distribution in the object. The method is very sensitive to density variations; the sensitivities are 1000 times higher for light elements compared with absorption contrast. This high sensitivity means that the optical system must be stable, within tolerances much lower than the x-ray wavelength.

For refraction contrast imaging, two methods have been proposed. One is to detect very small angle deviations of the beam refracted by an object. The incident beam from an SR source is made parallel and monochromatized by the first double crystal arrangement. The x-ray beam passing through the object is analyzed by the second double crystal arrangement. The X-ray beam is refracted by the gradient of density in the direction perpendicular to the x-ray beam trajectory, and the angle deviation from the incident beam is proportional to the integral of the density gradient along the x-ray propagation trajectory.

The other method of imaging by refraction is to observe a narrow shadow formed along the edges of an object in between the refracted and the incident beam direction; the shadow results from the second derivative of the density in the direction transverse to the propagation trajectory, and the contrast is extremely enhanced at the edges of an object.

To observe the shadows, spherical waves from a point-shaped x-ray source are more convenient than plane waves; high resolution will be achievable by making the x-ray source small because the resolution can be nearly equal to the x-ray focal size. It has been proposed to make such a point-shaped x-ray source with a small metal target placed at the exit of a tapered glass capillary focusing an SR beam from an undulator; the focusing efficiency of the capillary is greater than 25%, and hard x-ray photons absorbed by the heavy metal target are converted into fluorescent x-rays with high efficiency, very close to 100%. For radiation therapy, one may pierce the capillary into the center of cancer tissue to irradiate locally by adjusting the appropriate photon energy of the SR beam.

The refraction contrast is due to the difference in density (refractive index) between the object and its environment. For example, a bone has a density of 1.7 ~2.0. If we assume that the environment (human body) is similar to water, having a density of 1, the contrast is formed by a difference of 0.7 ~ 1.0. For a bronchus and stomach however, air having nearly zero density is contained, and the contrast is due to the density difference of about 1. This means that bronchi and stomachs can be imaged like bones. Since no absorption agent is needed, the methods are suitable for a regular cancer check-up.

For the new methods which require high-energy photon beams, using a large SR facility such as the SPring-8 should be considered, connecting to a hospital by an "information highway" network which affords remote control from the hospital.

In many SR facilities, the main subject of medical application has been angiography. Recently, four patients were examined successfully by a joint team from the University of Tsukuba and KEK, using SR at the 5.0 GeV accumulation ring at KEK. The results have been reported, and the importance of real-time observation has been emphasized. It is now an important issue whether or not the new imaging techniques mentioned above are applicable to angiography.

For blood vessels, however, the average density of blood is 1.06, and therefore the density difference from the environment is as small as 0.06. One favourable factor is that the refraction contrast is insensitive to the volume of blood in the heart, although an outline of the heart is imaged and vessels on the heart are, in principle, imaged. The technique of injecting small bubbles of air into blood vessels, which is used primarily for sonar diagnosis, may also be useful for the imaging.

In conclusion, we are now at the crossroads of comparing the imaging methods by absorption contrast with the new methods, and may understand this workshop as being the occasion to question which direction within traditional imaging or within the new methods should be taken for medical diagnosis.

Workshop Programme

Haga, Hyogo, Japan Aug.8-11, 1997

Oral Presentation

August 8th (Fri)
14:00-15:45   Registration at Counter of SRI'97 in Himeji Citizen Hall
16:00   Leave from Himeji by bus
18:00   Arrive at Haga
18:30-20:00   Welcome Dinner

August 9th (Sat)
07:30-08:15   Breakfast

Opening Ceremony Session Chairperson: Chikao Uyama/Masami Ando
08:20-08:30   Opening Remark by Michio Kono MD President HAGA97, Kobe Univ

Session I
Chairperson: Per Spanne / Tohoru Takeda
08:30--10:30   Session I Activity Report and Perspective Views
08:30-09:30   I-I   Medical activity at DESY intravenous coronary angiography
                      by Wolf-Rainer Dix PhD and Thorsten Dill MD DESY
09:30-10:00   I-2   Perspective view of medical applications in Japan
                      by Yuji Itai MD, University of Tsukuba
10:00-10:30   I-3   Medical activities in Japan-clinical coronary cineangiography
                      by Yasuro Sugishita MD, University of Tsukuba

10:30-10:45   Coffee Break

Session II
Chairperson: Yoshisada Fujiwara / Richard Garrett
10:45--12:00   Session II Activity Report
10:45-11:00   II-I   Medical activities at NSLS by William Thomlinson PhD, BNL
11:00-11:30   II-2   First tests on substraction bronchography study at the angiography station
                      of the VEPP-III storage ring by Valery Fedorovitch Pindyurin PhD BINP
11:30-12:00   II-3   Medical activities at ESRF by Per Spanne PhD ESRF
12:00-12:15   II-4   Present status of medical applications of SR by William Thomlinson

12:15-13:20   Lunch

Session III
Chairperson: Yuji Itai / William Thomlinson
13:20--15:30   Session III Panel Discussion -- What Applications
Using Synchrotron Radiation are Expected by Medical Doctor
13:20-13:40   III-I   What Radiologists need for SR medical application
                       by Katsuhito Yamasaki MD Kobe University
13:40-14:00   III-2   Small Vessel Radiography in Situ Using Monochromatic Synchrotron
                       Radiation   by Hidezo Mori MD Tokai University
14:00-14:20   III-3   Synchron radiation coronary angiography with aortographic approach

by Tohoru Takeda MD University of Tsukuba

14:20-14:40   III-4   Beamlines for Medical Applications on the Spring-8
by Chikao Uyama PhD National Cardiovascular Center

14:40-15:00   III-5   A Plan of a Synchrotron Light Source Dedicated to Medical Applications at
NIRS   by Masami Torikoshi PhD NIRS

15:00-15:45   Discussion

15:45-16:30   Poster / Coffee Break

Session IV-A

Chairperson: Katsuyuki Nishimura / Wolf-Rainer Dix

16:30-16:50   IV-1   Perspective for Medical Applications of Phase-Contrast X-Ray Imaging
by Atsushi Momose PhD, Hitachi

16:50-17:20   IV-2   New methods of X-ray imaging based on phase contrast
by Stephen Wilkins1 PhD, Dachao Gao1, Tim Guretev2, Andrew Pogany1
and Andrew Stevenson1, (1:CSIRO, DMST, 2:CSIRO, FFP)

17:10-17:30   IV-3   Synchrotron Radiation Applications in Medical Research Diffraction
Enhanced X-ray Imaging by William Thomlinson PhD BNL

17:30-19:00   Dinner

Session IV-B

Chairperson: Takao Akatsuka / Pekka Suortti

19:20-19:40   IV-4   Contrast Analysis of Coronaries using 2D Monochromatic X-rays for
Proposal of Optimized Dedicated Synchrotron System for IVCA
by Yasunari Oku PhD student GUAS/Kawasaki Heavy Industries and
Kazuyuki Hyodo and Masami Ando PhD's KEK

19:40-20:00   IV-5   Intracellular localization of cisplatin in ovarian cancer cells by x-ray
microimagin A feasibility study
by Kuniko Kihara and Hiroshi Kihara PhD's Kansai Medical University

August 10th (Sun)
07:30-08:15   Breakfast

Session V-A

Chairperson: Herman Winick / Shigeru Yamamoto

08:30--12:00   session V Instruments, Proposals and Plans

08:30-08:50   V-1   Proposal of very low cost 5 GeV electron storage ring for medical use
using permanent magnets and aluminum beam pipe without flanges and
bellows by G.W.Foster PhD Fermi Lab and H.Ishimaru PhD KEK

08:50-09:10   V-2   Conceptual design of the MARS (Medical Application Radiation Source)
by E.Levichev, N.Mezentsev PhD's Budker Institute of Physics, and
A.Iwata,S Kamiya PhD's Kawasaki Heavy Industries

09:10-09:30   V-3   Proposal of New Beamline AR NW2 Dedicated to Medical Applications at
the AR by Kazuyuki Hyodo, Shigeru Yamamoto and Masami Ando PhD's
KEK

09:30-09:50   V-4   Scanning Slit Radiography System with Synchrotron Radiatio by
Katsuyuki Nishimura PhD Ibaraki Prefectural University of Health Science

09:50-10:05   Poster / Coffee Break

10:05-10:20   Photograph

Session V-B
Chairperson: Hiroshi Kihara / Stephen Wilikins
10:20-10:40   V-5   Fluorescent x-ray source for diagnostic imaging studies
                      by Fukai Toyofuku PhD Kyushu University
10:40-11:00   V-6   Improvement of X-ray phosphor screens resolution by microstructuring
                      screen surfaces by V.I.Kondratyev, M.V.Kuzin, G.N.Kulipanov,
                      V.V.Lyakh, N.A.Mezentsev, L.A.Mezentseva, V.P.Nazmov, and Valery
                      Fedorovitch Pindyurin PhD's Budker Institute of Nuclear Physics,
                      Novosibirsk and by Yu.T.Pavlyukhin, A.A.Sidelnikov, and B.P.Tolochko
                      PhD's Institute of Solid State Chemistry, Novosibirsk
11:00-11:20   V-7   Reconstruction Algorithm for Fluorescent X-Ray CT and Its Application to
                      the Actual Data by Synchrotron X-ray by Tetsuya Yuasa[1], Tohoru Takeda[2],
                      F.Avraham Dilmanian[3], Kazuyuki Hyodo[4], Takao Akatsuka[1] and Yuji Itai[2]
                      (1Yamagata Univ, 2University of Tsukuba, 3BNL, 4KEK)
11:20-11:40   V-8   Proposal of therapy using microbeam by Junichi Chikawa CAST
11:40-12:00   V-9   Remarks on the Role of Maltilayer Optics and Short Period Insertion Device
                      for Medical Imaging Sources and Applications
                      by R.Tatchyn, T.Crewer, P.Csonka, D.Boyers and M.Piestrup

12:00-14:00   Lunch
14:00-16:00   Sightseeing

Session VI
Chairperson: Chikao Uyama / Masami Ando
16:00-17:30   Session VI Discussion, Review and Summary
17:30-18:00   Closing Remark by Junichi Chikawa PhD Chair HAGA97
18:30-20:00   Farewell Dinner (BBQ)

August 11th (Mon)
07:30-08:15   Breakfast
08:45   Leave from Haga to Himeji or Harima by bus

Session Summary I

Chairperson: Per Spanne / Tohoru Takeda

Drs. Dix and Dill presented the resuls of system of NIKOS-IV and human coronary imaging. Image quality of IV CAG is good to diagnose the coronary artery. They tried the backheal venous injection, and reported that image quality was almost same as SVC injection. Total diagnostic ability is reported about 86%. IV CAG may be suitable to follow up the PTCA and CABG.

Q : What is the criteria of the coronary stenosis, 50, 75, 90 or 99% ?
A : Dr. Dill said severe stenosis.

Dr. Itai presented the history and current status of application of synchrotron radiation to medicine in Japan; 1. varios angiographic results performed by intravenous and aortographic approaches, 2. various types of monochromatic computed tomography such as high spatial resolution, high contrast resolution CT, Thomson scattered, fluorescent x-ray and phase-contrast CT.

Q : Dr. Dill asked about the risks with arterial injection ?
A : The motality of intravenous CAG is almost the same as aortographic CAG, whereas the morbidity of anortographic CAG is higher than that of intravenous CAG. But to think the image quality and diagnostic ability, aortographic approach is thought to be an important method of coronary artery.

Dr.Sugishita presented the resuls of animal experiment and human coronary cine angiography. The merit of this CAG technique is the visualization of coronary arteries by conventional cine angiography.
Dose of x-ray exposure may cause a problem. Total X-ray exposure in which human study was limited to less than 50 R/projection by that means that the photon flux is the order of $2x10^{10}$ p/mm2/s.

Session Summary II

Chairperson: Yoshisada Fujiwara / Richard Garrett

Dr. Thomlinson summarised the medical programs at the NSLS. They have a dedicated medical facility, SMERF (Synchrotron Medical Research Facility) where transvenous coronary angiography, bronchiography, and micro-beam therapy have been performed, and which may be used for CT in the future. Other studies, notably mammography and photon activation therapy, have been performed on other beamlines at NSLS. Currently most activity is in mammography and bronchiography.

The angiography and CT programs both have problems due to the lack of a compact source. American physicians are not interested in synchrotron radiation diagnostic techniques unless they can be installed at hospitals.

Dr. Thomlinson strongly urged that medical programs should be driven by the medical community which is the case with mammography, not by the physicists.

Dr. Pindyurin described the first bronchiography phantom images taken at the VEPP-III storage ring at BINP. The existing angiography line scan system was used, and a 0.5mm thickness of Xe could be detected. It is proposed to move this program to the VEPP-IV 6 GeV storage ring. In the discussion Dr. Thomlinson suggested that the image must be taken quickly, as Xe is absorbed into the lung in a few seconds.

Dr. Spanne described the dedicated medical facility being commissioned at the ESRF. The imaging station is 150m from the source, giving a maximum beam width of 30cm. This station will be used for coronary angiography, CT and new medical imaging modalities such as phase contrast. In addition, a second station at 36m from the source will be used for a micro-beam radiation therapy program (MRT).

Dr. Spanne presented results of preliminary animal experiments of MRT, which shows very high promise for therapy of brain tumors with little or no damage to the normal brain tissue. He also presented preliminary result of phase contrast CT.

In the final presentation, Dr. Thomlinson summarised the world-wide activity in medical applications of synchrotron radiation. He stressed the importance of dedicated medical facilities at synchotron light sources, such as those at the ESRF, Hasylab, ELETTRA and NSLS, and planned for SPring-8, and the KEK Accumulation Ring.

Session Summary III

Chairperson: Yuji Itai / William Thomlinson

Dr. Mori discussed the use of the AR for obtaining radiographs of small vessels and ducts in the heart, brain and other organs. The goal is to visualize structures down to 20-85 microns in-situ. Clinical applications would be micro-circulation disorders and evaluation of angiogenesis. This could lead to cancer diagnosis and evaluation of treatment and therapy. In-situ videos of coronary transmural arteries were shown with very high resolution using the AR source and a new HDTV avalanche detector system. Dose limitations would be controlled by decreasing the frame rate. Images have been obtained in various animal models such as dogs and goats.

In a survey of the needs of clinical radiologists, Dr. Yamasaki discussed limitations of current technologies of hospital chest x-rays and CT. New SR based systems could show advantages of higher resolution slice thickness and enhanced contrast for lesion detection.

Dr. Takeda presented the extensive work on single energy aortographic coronary angiograhy. In contrast with dual-energy subtraction venous injection angiography using SR, the system is a 2D system with the photon energy just above the k-absorption edge of iodine. The injection of the contrast agent is into the root of the aorta and was stated to be much safer than conventional selective angiography. (That point was questioned by two cardiologists who were present at the workshop.) In any event, the aortic injection produces good quality images in the dog, as shown by Dr. Takeda. The dilution factor of the contrast agent is much smaller than intravenous injection, and the use of monochromatic radiation gives 2 times the contrast over conventional sources. The dose limitations can be controlled by limiting the number of frames, and by going to higher energies.

Dr. Uyama described the status and plans of the new medical research center being constructed at SPring-8. The conventional construction of the facility is greatly advanced and is at 200 meters from the source. It will accept three beamlines: 1) a multipole wiggler line for coronary angiography, x-ray CT, phase contrast CT, etc. 2) an undulator line for creating a fluorescence source for large field whole body CT, large field imaging, etc. 3) a bending magnet line for general medical application development.

Finally, Dr. Torikoshi described the plans for a compact synchrotron dedicated to medical applications at the National Institute of Radiological Sciences. The ring would utilize superconducting bending magnets to obtain a small circumference of 50 m at an electron energy of 1.8 GeV. High field wigglers would allow coronary angiography and other clinical applications at high photon energies. The bending magnets would be used for experiments in physics and biology to support clinical applications.

191

Session Summary IV-A

Chairperson: Katsuyuki Nishimura / Wolf-Rainer Dix

In this session different methods for contrast advancement in images were presented.

In the talk by A.Momose et al. X-ray phase contrast images are compared to transmission x-ray images of soft tissue samples. It was shown that the sensitivity for structures inside soft tissue like cancer tissues is about 1000 times higher in phase contrast images. In this work the interferometry method for phase contrast imaging was applied. Up to now small samples of 5 Å~ 5mm^2 were used. A new interferometer for larger samples is under construction. A very large interferometer for mammography was proposed. For large samples and medical application an optimization of the photon energy corresponding to the sample thickness will be necessary (about 50 KeV for 10cm).

In the second presentation by S.Wilkins et al. this interferometry method based on phase contrast was compared to other phase contrast imaging methods in an overview. This included differential phase-contrast imaging with analyzer crystals and methods without crystals like inline phase contrast imaging with plane and spherical incident waves. Examples for the different methods and perspectives for medical applications are given. These perspectives are higher contrast for soft tissue images, reduced absorbed dose as well as background resolution.

Another method for remarkable back-ground reduction and, therefore, improved contrast was presented by W. Thomlinson et al. This method diffraction enhanced imaging case are analyzer crystal behind the sample in order to separate scattered radiation from absorbed radiation.

The method is well suited for thick samples and was applied to the US standard mammography phantom. The resulting images show remarkable better contrast than those from commercially available mammography units.

Session Summary IV-B

Chairperson: Takao Akatsuka / Pekka Suortti

The session consisted of two talks, where optimization on SR source for angiography and imaging cancer cells by x-ray microscopy were discussed. The talks were given by Y.Oku and K.Takemoto, respectivety.

The conclusion of the first talk was that a small storage ring with low electron energy is optimized for angiography when superconducting bending magnets and wigglers are used. That was discussed about the image quality while taking into account of scattered x-rays and third higher harmonics contamination. The second talk demonstrated the feasibility of imaging cancer cells by a phase-contrast microscope, when the tissue has been tested by cisplatin. The contrast is due to platinum against the low-Z back ground of the tissue.

Discussion

There were quite a few questions following the talk of Dr. Oku. These concerned the x-ray grid used to suppress the scattering background, blurring the contrast due to the effective source size, and 2-dimensional grid of crossed lead/wood sandwich plates was asked, and wood was chosen because of low absorption. This, however, gives rise to small angle scattering. It was noted that the effects of scattering are reduced when the distances between the source, grid, and detector are increased, but this is off-set by the penumbra of the grid. The author has written the Monte Carlo code that includes the effects of beam polarization in terms of Stokes parameters.

The questions on Dr.Takemoto's talk concerned the performances of the microscope, specimen environment, and the effect of radiation on the sample. It was explained that the theoretical limit of resolution is about 50nm, not this is not quite reached, partly due to the resolution of the CCD detector. The specimen was a wet sample in air for easy mounting and alignment. It was printed out that the energy used for phase-contrast imaging was notside the water window resulting in high absorption and potential damage to the sample. The author did not think that this was the case, and imaging by the Pt contrast reveals the cell structure even when the molecules structure of cisplatin disintegrates

193

Session Summary V-A

Chairperson: Herman Winick / Shigeru Yamamoto

Until now all medical work with synchrotron radiation has been carried out at general purpose facilities designed and operated for a wide range of non-medical basic and applied research. In a few cases (e.g., NSLS, HASYLAB) special facilities for medical work, particularly dual-energy coronary angiography, have been constructed and used on general purpose machines. The increasing medical activity at many facilities has motivated thinking about possible future facilities optimized for and dedicated to medical work, preferably of a size that can be accommodated in a hospital.

For dual-energy subtraction at the K-absorption edge of iodine (33 keV) it appears that the critical energy of the synchrotron radiation spectrum should be about 16 keV to minimize harmonic content. Such a spectrum can be produced by a high field, superconducting wiggler (~5-8 T) in a low energy ring (~1.6-1.8 GeV). The wiggler can have many poles to increase the flux. The entire facility can be very compact, with a circumference of 40-60 meters, including 2-3 wigglers with associated beam lines serving exposure stations. Such a ring could fit in a basement room of a hospital.

Several designs have been carried out for such rings. One design [1] is for a ring with an electron energy of 1.6 GeV, bending magnet field 1.5 T, with a circumference of less than 40 meters. Two angiography exposure stations are included using 5 pole, 5 T superconducting wiggler magnets as sources. Another design [2] is for a ring with an electron energy of 1.75 GeV and a circumference of 61 meters. Three angiography exposure stations are included using 3 pole, 8.3 T wiggler magnets as sources.

At Haga97 we had reports on the designs of two rings that might be used for medical applications.

H.Ishimaru described a 5 GeV ring with a circumference of about 300 meters. Since the total arc length in the 1 T bending magnets is only about 100 meters much space is available for insertion devices. The innovative features of this ring include the use of permanent magnets for the bending, quadrupole and sextupole magnets and the use of a welded vacuum chamber with no bellows or flanges. R&D has been carried out on questions such as radiation damage to and temperature stability of the permanent magnets and chemical processing of the vacuum chamber to enable high vacuum to be reached without the usual bakeout procedures. These features would result in high reliability and low cost. With a large enough stored current, each 1 T bending magnet might serve a beam line for dual-energy coronary angiography. Use would be made of the experience at Fermilab where a 3.3 km permanent magnet antiproton ring is under construction.

N.Mezentsev described the Medical Application Radiation Source (MARS), a 2-2.4 GeV ring with ~10 nm-radian emittance and ~150 meter circumference. High field (~7.5 T) superconducting wigglers would be used for dual-energy coronary angiography and there would be space for undulators and other sources for other medical applications as well as applications in non-medical areas.

While both of these proposals have very interesting features and construction of such rings might be justified for broad scientific as well as medical use, they are considered too large to fit in a hospital environment.

There was also a presentation by K.Hyodo of a proposed beam line to be built on the Accumulation Ring at KEK optimized for medical applications, particularly for two dimensional imaging for intravenous coronary angiography. His presentation was based on their scheme to find best optimized parameters for the two dimensional imaging for a system which comprises a storage ring and multipole wigglers. Based on initial results on human subjects in 1996, the two dimensional imaging approach appears promising. The proposed beam line would enable this

194

approach to be evaluated in more detail.

A presentation by K. Nishimura described the design of a scanning slit system to enhance the image quality in two dimensional imaging with synchrotron radiation, such as has been used at the AR and is planned for the new beam line described by K.Hyodo in the previous presentation. Since scattering in the subject contributes background which degrades the quality of the image when an area beam is used, this technique appears to be important and should be tried.

References:

1. H. Wiedemann, M. Baltay, R. Carr, M. Hernandez, W. Lavender, "A Compact Radiation Source for Digital Subtractive Angiography", Nucl. Instr. & Meth. A347 (1994) 515-521.

2. Y. Oku, K. Aizawa, S. Nakagawa, M. Ando, K. Hyodo, S. Kamada, H. Shiwaku, "Conceptual Design of a Compact Electron Storage Ring System Dedicated to Coronary Angiography", Proc. 1993 IEEE Particle Accelerator Conf.

Session Summary V - B

Chairperson: Hiroshi Kihara/Stephen Wilikins

There was a big discussion on beam size for diagnosis of human body. Apparently, beam generated by the third generation SR has much smaller emittance, whereas the demand for human body diagnosis is much bigger. To solve this apparent contradiction, Dr Toyofuku presented an idea to utilize low emittance beam of generating large and uniform field of view by using a fluorescent x-ray. He described ideas and some results for using an SR beam as pump for a secondary fluorescent X-ray source for a variety of X-ray imaging applications including clinical diagnosis. The idea of generating large and uniform field of view is to illuminate a target metal by beam from undulator, and to utilized emitted fluoresent x-rays. With this technique, Toyofuku could generate fluresent x-rays of 50mmÉ"in diameter and of energy from 10 to 90KeV. To get purely monochromatized x-rays he used an attenuation filter to suppress KÉ¿ x-rays. Such an approach can provide divergent beams of high uniformity with respect to angle over a large solid angle together with a high degree of monochromaticity and relative ease of changing wavelength (i.e. target). Using, say, a SPring-8 undulator as the pump for a fluorescent source of, say, $1\times 1mm2$, intensities of order 5×10^8 photons/sec/mm^2 at 1m from the secondary (i.e. fluorescent) source appear possible. Such a source can be quite useful for conventional clinical radiographic-type applications with the following advantages over parallel-beam methods:
* arbitrary large field size
* wide (monochromatic) energy range
* fast energy switching (in a few msec perhaps)
* well-suited to in-line phase-contrast imaging
* could operate with multiple experimental stations to cater for several patients being imaged simultaneously less demanding on detector performance (spatial resolution) than corresponding parallel-beam methods. The fluorescent x-ray thus generated is a very good candidate of monochromatic CT.

The suggestion of Professor Chikawa to use a tapered glass capillary (or other concentrating method) to produce a more intense secondary fluorescence source seems a very promising one. Such a source, with a size of 30 micron or less, would be very well suited to the in-line (i.e. "c rystal-less") method of phase-contrast imaging. The tapered capillary (or other focusing means) could provide an extremely intense microfocus source with many advantages over laboratory microfocus sources and parallel-beam methods using SR. In particular, higher intensities, higher chromatic coherence, better lateral spatial coherence and others. This is an exciting area proposed for development on one of the three medical beamlines presently under construction at SPring-8.

In hard x-ray region, the development of x-ray detectors is also crucially important. The key issues of the development are sensitivity in wide energy region from 10 to 90 KeV, spatial resolution, uniformity and wide dynamic range. One of the most commonly used detectors so far is the imaging plate. Dr Pindyurin described some promising new methods for using micromachining to produce pixellated image intensifyer screens and storage phosphor screens giving higher spatial resolution (better integrated MTF) than current commercial counterparts. His group is developing another type of detector based on x-ray microfabricated phosphor screen. To get high sensitivity, they fabricated the screen with high depth. To get higher spatial resolution, they used copper coating as a spatial and angular optical microfilter. Present problems relate to uniformity of response from one pixel to another and of a residual pixel mesh structure in the image. We definitely appreciate their much efforts and we look very much forward to hearing more advancement of detectors by their continuous development.

A brief outline was given by Dr Yuasa of a reconstruction algorithm for fluorescent X-ray CT obtained using SR X-ray data and this seemed an interesting and potentially attractive approach for some applications.

Organization

Organized by The Organizing Committee of HAGA'97.
Sponsored by The Japanese Society for Synchrotron Radiation Research.
Hosted by The Executive Committee of The 2nd International Conference on Industrial Applications of Synchrotron Radiation formed by Hyogo Prefecture, Harima Technopolis Foundation, Hyogo Science and Technology Association and Japan Synchrotron Radiation Research Institute.

Conference Chair
Michio KONO (Kobe Univ)

Organizing Committee
Chair: Junichi CHIKAWA (CAST)
Masami ANDO (KEK), Yuji ITAI (Univ of Tsukuba), Michio KONO (Kobe Univ)
Yasuro SUGISHITA (Univ of Tsukuba), Chikao UYAMA (NCVC)

International Advisory Board
Mitsuyuki ABE (Kyoto Hospital), Masayoshi AKISADA (Intern'l Univ of Health and Welfare)
Takao AKATSUKA (Yamagata Univ), Emillio BRATTINI (Frascati),
Dean CHAPMAN (Illinois Institute Technology), Avraham DILMANIAN (BNL)
Wolf-Rainer DIX (DESY), Yoshisada FUJIWARA (Kobe Univ)
Shunnosuke HANDA (Tokai Univ), Shin HASEGAWA (Tokyo Kogei Univ)
Yoshio HIRAKI (Okayama Univ), Yuji ITAI (Univ of Tsukuba)
Shuji KIMURA (Hyogo Adult Diseases Center), Michio KONO (Kobe Univ)
Gennady KULIPANOV (BINP), Takahiro KOZUKA (Habikino Hospital)
Edward RUBENSTEIN (Stanford Univ), Clemens SCHULZE (Paul Scherrer Institute)
Kunio SHINOHARA (Univ of Tokyo), Per SPANNE (ESRF)
Yasuro SUGISHITA (Univ of Tsukuba), Makoto TAKAMIYA (NCVC)
William THOMLINSON (BNL), Albert THOMPSON (LBL)
Hiromitsu YOKOYAMA (Kobe Univ)

Executive, Programme and Publication Committee
Chair: Masami ANDO (KEK), Chikao UYAMA (NCVC)
Secretary to Executive and Programme Committee: Katsuto YAMASAKI (Kobe Univ)
Secretary to Publication Committe: Tohoru TAKEDA (Univ of Tsukuba)
Hozuka AKITA (Kobe Univ), Kazuyuki HYODO (KEK)
Masao MATSUMOTO (Osaka Univ), Hidezo MORI (Tokai Univ)
Koichi MORI (IPU), Katsuyuki NISHIMURA (IPU)
Sadanori OHTSUKA (Univ of Tsukuba), Yasunari OKU (GUAS)
Hideaki SHIWAKU (JAERI), Junichiro TADA (SPRING-8)
Tohoru TAKEDA (Tsukuba Univ), Kenji TOKUMORI (Kyushu Univ)
Fukai TOYOFUKU (Kyushu Univ)

Acknowledgements

We would like to thank the members of the International Advisory Board and all participants from various SR facilities in the world and William Thomlinson and Wolf-Rainer Dix who made unlimited contribution not only in the ignifying stage of the Workshop but also until its publication. Special thanks should be given to the late Hajime Ishimaru who sacrificed his precious time to participate the Workshop and to present his and G.W.Foster's paper there. He was a world renowned ultra-high vacuum expert. His paper in this proceedings is, as we believe, full of his expertise and passion for invention as his other papers.

A paper reviewing process was introduced; we should express our thanks to those who have engaged in this such as Werner Brefeld, Avraham Dilmanian, Yoshisada Fujiwara, Richard Garrett, Yutaka Kihara, Nikolai Mezentsev, Atsushi Momose, Alessandro Olivo, Edward Rubenstein, Pakkari Suortti, Keiji Umetani and Stephen Wilkins. Needless to say that the above two and the Publication Committee members also involved in this task.

Mr. Taisuke Okada a Secretary to the Governor of Hyogo Prefecture who was grown up in his proud Haga town introduced its Mayor Mr. Koichiro Nakata and his staff who also kindly assisted our Workshop. It is not exaggerated that we could not hold the Workshop without a kind support from the secretaries, Miho Hirose, Noriko Murai and Mari Yasumizu at the Department of Radiology, Kobe University School of Medicine who have devoted themselves before, throughout and even after the Workshop to its success.

A financial support was very kindly arranged by several organizations; we should express our special sincere gratitude to the following: New Industry Division, Commerce and Industry, Hyogo Prefecture Department, Banyu Pharmaceutical Co., Clinical Supply Co., Daiichi Pharmaceutical Co., Daiichi Radioisotope Labs., Eisai Co., Fuji Medical System, GE Yokogawa Medical Systems, Hitachi Ltd., Hitachi Medico, Horii Pharmaceutical Ind. Ltd., Hyogo Prefecture, Kawasaki Heavy Ind. Ltd., Kodak Japan, Konica Medical Inc., Kyoto Kagaku Ltd., Nihon MediPhysics Co., Ltd., Nihon Schering Co., Philips Medical Systems, Sakai Chemical Industry Co., Sankyo Co., Ltrd., Shimadzu Co., Shionogi & Co., Ltd., Siemens-Asahi Medical Technologies Ltd., Sumitomo Metal Ind., Takeda Chemical Ind., Tanabe Pharmaceutical Co., Toshiba Medical Systems and Yamanouchi Pharmaceutical Co.

As mentioned in the preface this book has also the inclusion of a few presentations at Daigo in 1992. Let us take this opportunity to express our special thanks to Mr. Hiroshi Kuroda, the Mayor of Daigo and Mr. Sho Ishii heading the Tourist Bureau at Daigo who provided us with all kindness.

Last but not the least at all we would like to thank Kimiyo Matsuda and Reiko Otsubo for their unlimited and pleasant contribution in the successful editing process.

Publication Chair
Masami Ando and Chikao Uyama

List of Participants

ADACHI Syuji	Kobe Univ
AKATSUKA Takao	Yamagata Univ
ANDO Masami	KEK
CHIKAWA Junichi	CAST
DILL Thorsten	University Hospital Hamburg
DIX Wolf-Rainer	HASYLAB at DESY
ENDO Masahiro	National Institute of Radiological Sciences
FRANCOIS Esteve	CHU. IRM
FRANK Matthias	Lawrence Livermore Nat.Lab.
FUJIWARA Yoshisada	Kobe Univ
GARRETT Richard Frederick	Australia Nuclear Science and Technology Organization
HAGELSTEIN Michael	PEA
HONDA Osamu	Osaka Univ
HYODO Kazuyuki	KEK
IKEZOE Junpei	Ehime Univ
ISHIMARU Hajime	KEK
ITAI Yuji	Univ of Tsukuba
JOHKOH Takeshi	Osaka Univ
KAGOSHIMA Yasushi	Himeji Institute of Technology
KIHARA Hiroshi	Kansai Medical Univ
KONO Michio	Kobe Univ
KUZAY Tuncer M.	Argonne National Laboratory
MATSUMOTO Masao	Osaka Univ
MEZENTSEV Nikolai Alexandrovich	Budker Institute of Nuclear Physics
MOCHIZUKI Takayasu	Himeji Institute of Technology
MOMOSE Atsushi	Hitachi Ltd.
MORI Koichi	Ibaraki Prefectural University of Health Sciences
MORI Hidezo	Tokai Univ
MORII Yasuji	Toshiba Cooperation
MURASE Kenya	Ehime Univ
NISHIMURA Katsuyuki	Ibaraki Prefectural University of Health Sciences
NODA Asao	Kobe Univ
OKU Yasunari	Graduate University for Advanced Studies
OLIVO Alessandro	Trieste University
PINDYURIN Valery Fedorovitch	Budker Institute of Nuclear Physics

SEKKA Takafumi	Tokai Univ
SHIWAKU Hideaki	Japan Atomic Energy Research Institute
SPANNE Per	ESRF
SUGISHITA Yasuro	Univ of Tsukuba
SUORTTI Pekka	ESRF European Synchrotron Radiation Facility
TAKEDA Tohoru	Univ of Tsukuba
TAKEMOTO Kuniko	Kansai Medical Univ
TANAKA Etsuro	Tokai Univ
TANIGUCHI Mieko	Nagoya Univ
THOMLINSON William C.	NSLS
TOKUMORI Kenji	Kyusyu Univ
TORIKOSHI Masami	National Institute of Radiological Sciences
TOYOFUKU Fukai	Kyusyu Univ
TSUSAKA Yoshiyuki	Himeji Institute of Technology
UMETANI Keiji	Hitachi Ltd.
UYAMA Chikao	National Cardiovascular Center
WANG Gongli	Beijing Scientific and Radiation Facility
WILKINS Stephen William	Commonwealth Scientific and Industrial Research Organization
WINICK Herman	SSRL/SLAC
YAMAMOTO Shigeru	KEK
YAMASAKI Katsuhito	Kobe Univ
YOSHIDA Katsuya	National Institute of Radiological Sciences
YUASA Tetsuya	Yamagata Univ

Key Words List